Orthopaedic pathologies of the stifle joint

For this English edition:

Orthopaedic pathologies of the stifle joint

Plaza Antonio Beltrán Martínez nº 1, planta 8 - letra I
(Centro empresarial El Trovador)
50002 Zaragoza - Spain

First printing: March 2017

This book has been published originally in Spanish under the title:
Patologías ortopédicas de la rodilla
© 2016 Grupo Asís Biomedia, S.L.
ISBN Spanish edition: 978-84-16818-26-6

Translation:
Melissa Knudtson

Illustrator:
Jacob Gragera Artal

ISBN: 978-84-16818-60-0
D.L.: Z 403-2017

Design, layout and printing:
Servet editorial - Grupo Asís Biomedia, S.L.
www.grupoasis.com
info@grupoasis.com

GRUPO asis

Servet is the publishing house of Grupo Asís

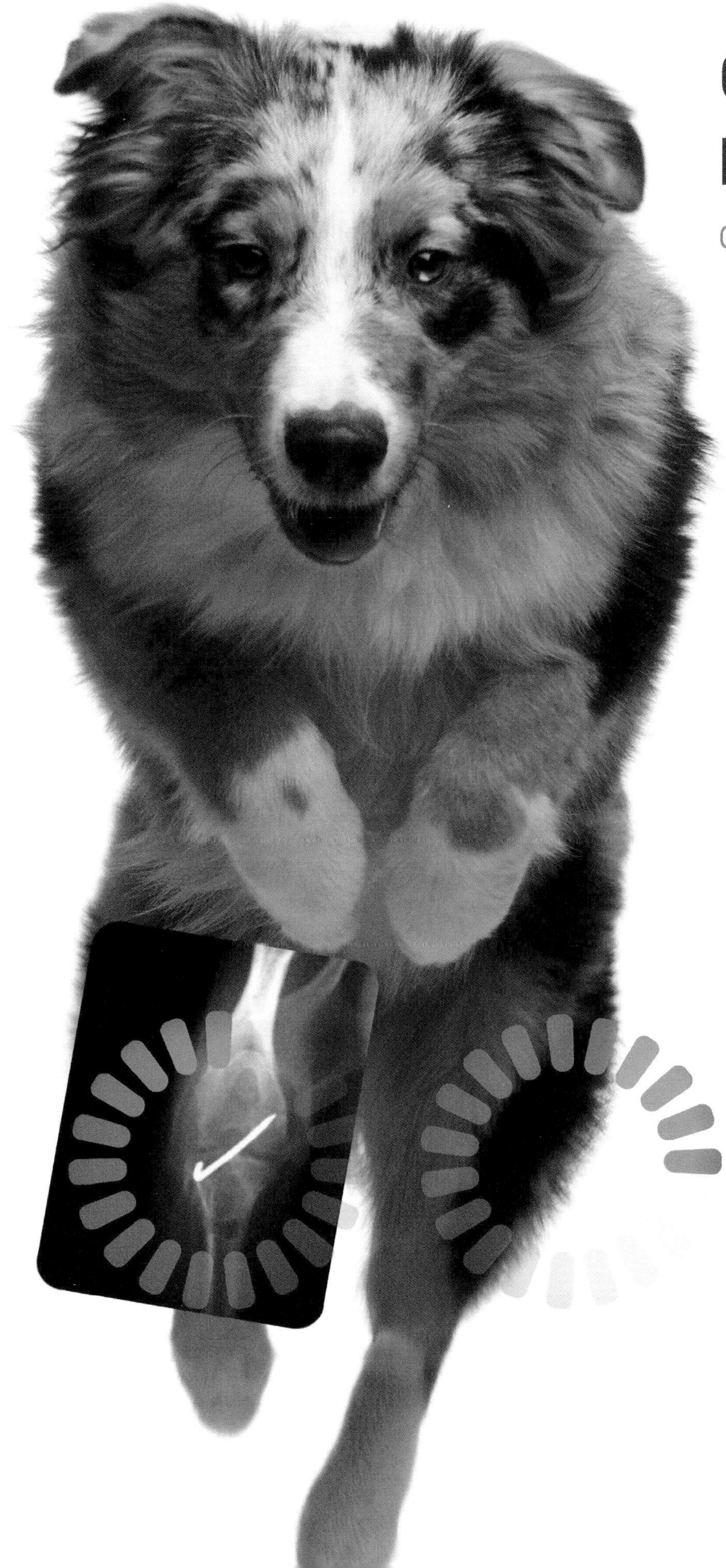

Orthopaedic pathologies of the stifle joint

José Luis Vérez-Fraguela
Roberto Köstlin
Rafael Latorre Reviriego
Salvador Climent Peris
Francisco Miguel Sánchez Margallo
Jesús Usón Gargallo

SERVET

AUTHORS

José Luis Vérez-Fraguela

Licentiate Degree in Veterinary Medicine and Doctorate Degree in Animal Medicine and Health from the Faculty of Veterinary Medicine of the University of Extremadura (UEX). Graduate in Law from the Spanish National University of Distance Education (UNED). Teacher and researcher in the Department of Surgery at the UEX. Researcher in the Experimental Surgery Unit at the University Hospital Complex of A Coruña (CHUAC). Member of the Department of Animal Medicine and Health of the UEX. Scientific adviser in veterinary orthopaedics at the Jesús Usón Minimally Invasive Surgery Centre (CCMIJU) in Cáceres (Spain). He has gained experience at universities in Europe, the United States and Japan. Spanish National Research Award in 1998. European patent in 2011. He has undertaken various subsidised research projects and is a scientific reviewer for various journals. He is also a member of the scientific committee and an organiser for different courses, conferences and monographs. He has over 70 publications, comprising books, essays and original publications, and has given countless lectures and courses. Honorary President of the Spanish Society of Veterinary Orthopaedics and Traumatology (SETOV).

Roberto Köstlin

Doctorate Degree in Veterinary Medicine from the National University of the Northeast in Corrientes (Argentina). Doctorate Degree in Veterinary Medicine and teaching qualification at Ludwig Maximilian University in Munich (Germany). Diploma from the European College of Veterinary Surgeons (ECVS). Senior Lecturer in Surgery at the University of Veterinary Medicine in Hanover (Germany). Senior Lecturer in Surgery and Ophthalmology at Ludwig Maximilian University in Munich. Member of the scientific committee and organiser for various courses and conferences. He has published several books and has over 100 scientific publications to his credit. He has given countless international lectures on every continent. Honorary Member of the Spanish Society of Veterinary Orthopaedics and Traumatology (SETOV).

Rafael Latorre Reviriego

Professor of Veterinary Anatomy. He earned his Doctorate Degree in Veterinary Medicine from the University of Murcia in 1990. He has gained experience at the University of Milan (Italy); the University of California, Davis (United States); the University of Cambridge (United Kingdom); the University of Tennessee (United States); and the University of London (United Kingdom). His work has largely focused on the clinical anatomy of the musculoskeletal system. He has made important contributions in the form of atlases and books, as well as scientific articles published in prestigious journals, mainly on diagnostic imaging of joints. Thanks to his involvement in developing and teaching anatomical plastination techniques as a working tool in clinical anatomy, he is now the President of the International Society for Plastination.

Salvador Climent Peris

Professor Emeritus at the University of Zaragoza since 2012 Graduate in Veterinary Medicine from the University of Zaragoza, 1969. Professor of Veterinary Anatomy and Embryology since 1982. He has completed terms at the Anatomy Departments of the Faculties of Medicine at the University of Zaragoza, Madrid Complutense University and the Free University of Brussels, the Faculty of Veterinary Medicine in Toulouse, and the Animal Biology Department at the University of Clermont-Ferrand (France). He has been actively involved in the set-up and development of CCMIJU in Cáceres since 1986, taking part in the design, preparation and selection of appropriate animal models for the specialisation courses in minimally invasive surgical techniques taught at the school.

Francisco Miguel Sánchez Margallo

Scientific Director of the CCMIJU in Cáceres. He earned his Licentiate Degree and Doctorate Degree in Veterinary Medicine from the UEX. Spanish Royal Academy of Doctors Award in 2001. He is a Project Manager for surgery and minimally invasive techniques related to biomaterials, medical instruments, preclinical trials, medical diagnostic imaging, endoscopy, minimally invasive surgical procedures and new surgical technologies. He is the author of multiple patents, utility models and industrial designs. He is a lecturer in various university postgraduate training programmes and director of various official master's degree programmes and university specialist courses. He is deputy director of the Singular Spanish Scientific and Technological Infrastructure (ICTS) named Nanbiosis. There, he works in close collaboration with researchers, surgeons, physicians, entrepreneurs and engineers in biomedicine as well as with various universities in Spain and elsewhere and hospitals and companies all over the world.

He is the author of over 140 articles in high-impact publications and has contributed to over 500 papers at conferences in Spain and abroad related to surgery and surgical technology. He has actively contributed to over 80 R&D projects and has led several projects in Europe and beyond. He has directed 25 doctoral dissertations and is currently directing five predoctoral students. He is the author or co-author of 16 books and over 50 book chapters related to surgery and minimally invasive surgery. At present, he is a member of the Technology Committee of the European Association for Endoscopic Surgery (EAES), the international Society for Medical Innovation and Technology (iSMIT), the Spanish Association of Surgeons (AEC), the Spanish Association of Urology (AEU), the Spanish Society of Surgical Research (SEIQ), and several Spanish and European technology platforms. He is a reviewer for many scientific publications and a member of the editorial board of several international scientific publications.

Jesús Usón Gargallo

Licentiate Degree and Doctorate Degree in Veterinary Medicine from the University of Zaragoza. He is an expert in Animal Pathology and has served for many years as a Professor in the Department of Surgical Pathology and Surgery of the Faculty of Veterinary Medicine at the University of Extremadura. In Aragon, he directed the School of Animal Surgery at the Experimental Institute of Surgery and Reproduction. With the idea of translating biomedicine to a technology project, in 1986, he moved to Cáceres. There, he established the starting point of the present-day Jesús Usón Minimally Invasive Surgery Centre (CCMIJU). He is currently the Honorary President of this centre. In addition to his teaching work, he has had a productive research career with a particular interest in minimally invasive surgery (MIS). The excellent results of his research have attracted the most renowned Spanish and foreign specialists. Today, the CCMIJU is a global landmark and a centre of reference in Spain and elsewhere for research and teaching in minimally invasive surgery.

He has directed over 40 doctoral dissertations and has contributed to 49 research projects in various fields of specialisation such as laparoscopy, endoscopy and microsurgery. He is the author of several books and many scientific articles published in high-impact journals and co-author of the “City of Health and Innovation” project, which will promote the transfer of technology between companies, technology agents and universities. He has over 20 patents and industrial designs to his credit and has directed the design of 10 mobile apps. His many awards include the Gold Medal of Merit in Work and the Gold Medal of Extremadura.

COLLABORATORS

Ayala Florenciano, M. D. DVM, PhD. Professor of Veterinary Anatomy, University of Murcia (Spain).

Bardet, J. F. DocVet, MS, Dipl ACVS. Dr. Bardet Veterinary Clinic, Neuilly-sur-Seine, Paris (France). Former president of the European Society of Veterinary Orthopaedics and Traumatology (ESVOT).

Climent Aroz, M. DVM, PhD. Professor of Veterinary Anatomy, University of Zaragoza (Spain).

Domínguez Sarceda, R. DVM. La Castellana Veterinary Clinic, Madrid (Spain). President of the Spanish Society of Veterinary Traumatology and Orthopaedics (SETOV, in its Spanish acronym).

Ferreiro Sánchez, M. VN. Ultramar Veterinary Hospital, Ferrol, A Coruña (Spain).

Gil Cano, F. DVM, PhD. Professor of Veterinary Anatomy, University of Murcia (Spain).

Gorostiza, J. F. DVM, MS. Surgical Consultation Services, Miami, Florida (United States).

Guerrero, T. Dipl ECVS. Surgical Area. St George's University, True Blue (Grenada).

Johnson, K. Professor, MVSc, PhD, FACVSc, Dipl ACVS & ECVS. University of Sydney (Australia).

López Albors, O. DVM, PhD. Professor of Veterinary Anatomy, University of Murcia (Spain).

Luera Carbó, M. DVM, PhD. Dr. Luera Veterinary Clinic, Barcelona (Spain). †

Maestre Antequera, J. Graduate in Nursing. Jesús Usón Minimally Invasive Surgery Center (JUMISC), Cáceres (Spain).

Martí, J. M. DVM. Cert SAO, Dipl ACVS & ECVS, MRCVS. Veterinary Surgical Specialists, Chesapeake, Virginia (United States).

Martínez Gomariz, F. DVM, PhD. Professor of Veterinary Anatomy, University of Murcia (Spain).

Matis, U. Professor, PhD, Dipl ECVS. Ludwig Maximilian University of Munich (Germany). Former president of the European Society of Veterinary Orthopaedics and Traumatology (ESVOT).

Molins de Sas, M. DHM. Doctor at Ferrol Teaching Hospital (CHUF, in its Spanish acronym), A Coruña (Spain).

Montavon, P. Professor. School of Veterinary Medicine, University of Zurich (Switzerland).

Penabad Ott, A. W. DVM. Ultramar Veterinary Hospital, Ferrol, A Coruña (Spain).

Portabales Meijide, E. DVM. Ultramar Veterinary Hospital, Ferrol, A Coruña (Spain).

Ramírez Zarzosa, G. DVM, PhD. Professor of Veterinary Anatomy, University of Murcia (Spain).

Rodríguez Quirós, J. DVM, PhD. Professor at the School of Veterinary Medicine, Complutense University of Madrid (Spain).

Ruiz Pérez, M. DVM. Founding president of the Spanish Society of Veterinary Traumatology and Orthopaedics (SETOV). Mediterráneo Veterinary Clinic, Madrid (Spain).

Sánchez Collado, C. DVM. Professor of Veterinary Anatomy, University of Murcia (Spain).

Sánchez Fernández, J. DVM, PhD. Training Director, Jesús Usón Minimally Invasive Surgery Center (JUMISC), Cáceres (Spain).

Sever Bermejo, R. DVM. Professor at the School of Veterinary Medicine, University of Zaragoza (Spain). Former president of the Spanish Society of Veterinary Traumatology and Orthopaedics (SETOV).

Souto Rey, V. DHM. Head of the Orthopaedic Surgery Service, Ferrol Teaching Hospital (CHUF). Professor at the University of A Coruña (Spain).

Vázquez Autón, J. DVM, PhD. Professor of Veterinary Anatomy, University of Murcia (Spain).

Vela González, F. J. DVM. Research fellow, Microsurgery Department, Jesús Usón Minimally Invasive Surgery Center (JUMISC), Cáceres (Spain).

PROLOGUE

It is enormously satisfying to witness the publication of the book *Orthopaedic pathologies of the stifle joint*. I am convinced that veterinary medical clinical professionals and students will refer to this manual often.

This book has essentially been designed as a practical, effective tool for reference and training to aid in continuous improvement of surgical practice. Its excellent iconography, demonstrative case reports and extraordinary anatomical preparations allow the reader to gain in-depth knowledge of the main conditions affecting the stifle joint in dogs.

Needless to say, in recent years access to information has been completely revolutionised. Still, information is perhaps most useful once it has been processed and refined by experts. This book is organised into 11 chapters in which experts examine the clinical anatomy and functional aspects of the stifle joint in dogs and analyse the different disease processes that affect this joint in detail with explanatory diagrams and videos that describe the aetiopathogenesis, signs and symptoms, and diagnostic methods used in each case, including differential diagnoses and treatment options.

Surgical techniques such as tibial plateau levelling osteotomy (TPLO) and tibial tuberosity advancement (TTA) are specifically analysed with special attention to surgical details, which in turn are supported with high-quality illustrations. Diagnostic examinations with computed tomography and magnetic resonance imaging of ex vivo models have been included to support the monograph with documentary evidence and give it added value despite the limitations inherent in the use of cadavers. This manual includes an annex with photographs of the different surgical approaches to the stifle joint. I find this very wise as the annex serves as an ideal supplement when putting each treatment option into practice.

Finally, I would like to congratulate the authors of and contributors to this innovative monograph, since I believe that it will come to figure among the reference manuals of veterinary clinical professionals and students.

Prof. Jesús Usón Gargallo
Professor of Surgical Pathology and Surgery
Honorary President of the CCMIJU Foundation

PREFACE

This book is a compendium of the most commonly diagnosed orthopaedic diseases and abnormalities in the stifle joint in dogs and cats. It particularly focuses on dogs, since the incidence of such diseases and abnormalities is greater in dogs due to the sporting and work activities in which they often engage.

The book begins with an in-depth review of anatomy. This review is illustrated with images of the different structures that comprise the joint in which every single element is described in detail. It then shows the clinical approach with a description of the clinical dynamics and the different examination manoeuvres that may be performed to detect the origin of the injury or problem. This content is supported by videos of the examination tests of the stifle joint and algorithms that will aid in diagnostic and therapeutic decision-making.

Concerning orthopaedic abnormalities themselves, the book is organised by anatomical and functional structure and by disease entity. The reader will find chapters dedicated to bone fractures, flexors and extensors, dislocations of the stifle joint and patella, injuries of ligaments and menisci, osteochondritis and osteonecrosis, osteoarthritis, and soft tissue diseases. The part dedicated to surgical treatment highlights two techniques: tibial plateau levelling osteotomy (TPLO) and tibial tuberosity advancement (TTA). Both are described step by step with images. From here we would like to thank Dr Juan M. Martí and Dr Tomás G. Guerrero for their collaboration in the preparation of these chapters. The chapter on TTA addresses neither the TTA Rapid technique, recently implemented in the United States and Europe, nor the Porous TTA technique, also increasingly used in Spain. This is because rigorous long-term studies on their outcomes are not yet available, although they seem to be promising since implant rupture is a disadvantage of classic TTA. This exciting topic will no doubt be addressed in future editions; in any case, it is referenced in the bibliography of this book.

The book concludes with an annex featuring the most indicated surgical approaches to resolve diseases that require surgery. The annex shows the different steps through anatomical dissection photographs of high quality and technical clarity.

It would not be right to finish this preface without expressing our most sincere and profound appreciation to Dr Tatiana Blasco, the editor of the publishing company, who was kind enough to publish this book. Surely, this work would not have come into being without her unwavering commitment to it. It must be recognised that coordinating three different working groups (clinicians, anatomists and diagnostic imaging specialists) is no easy task, especially when there are several authors from different disciplines (we can attest to this). We extend to her our most heartfelt appreciation.

It is our hope that the reader is pleased with the end result.

The authors

TABLE OF CONTENTS

CHAPTER 1

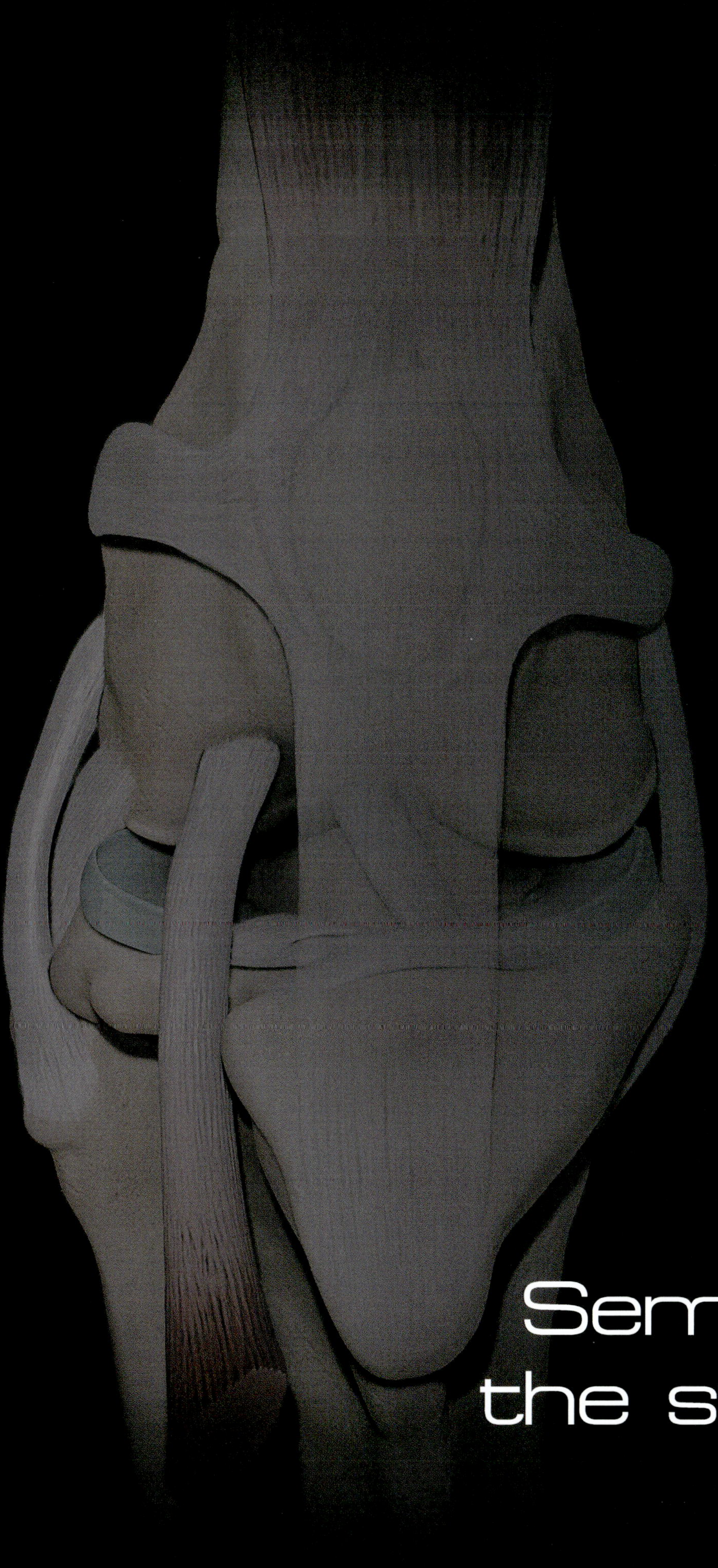

Semiology of the stifle joint

3D drawings of the anatomical structures

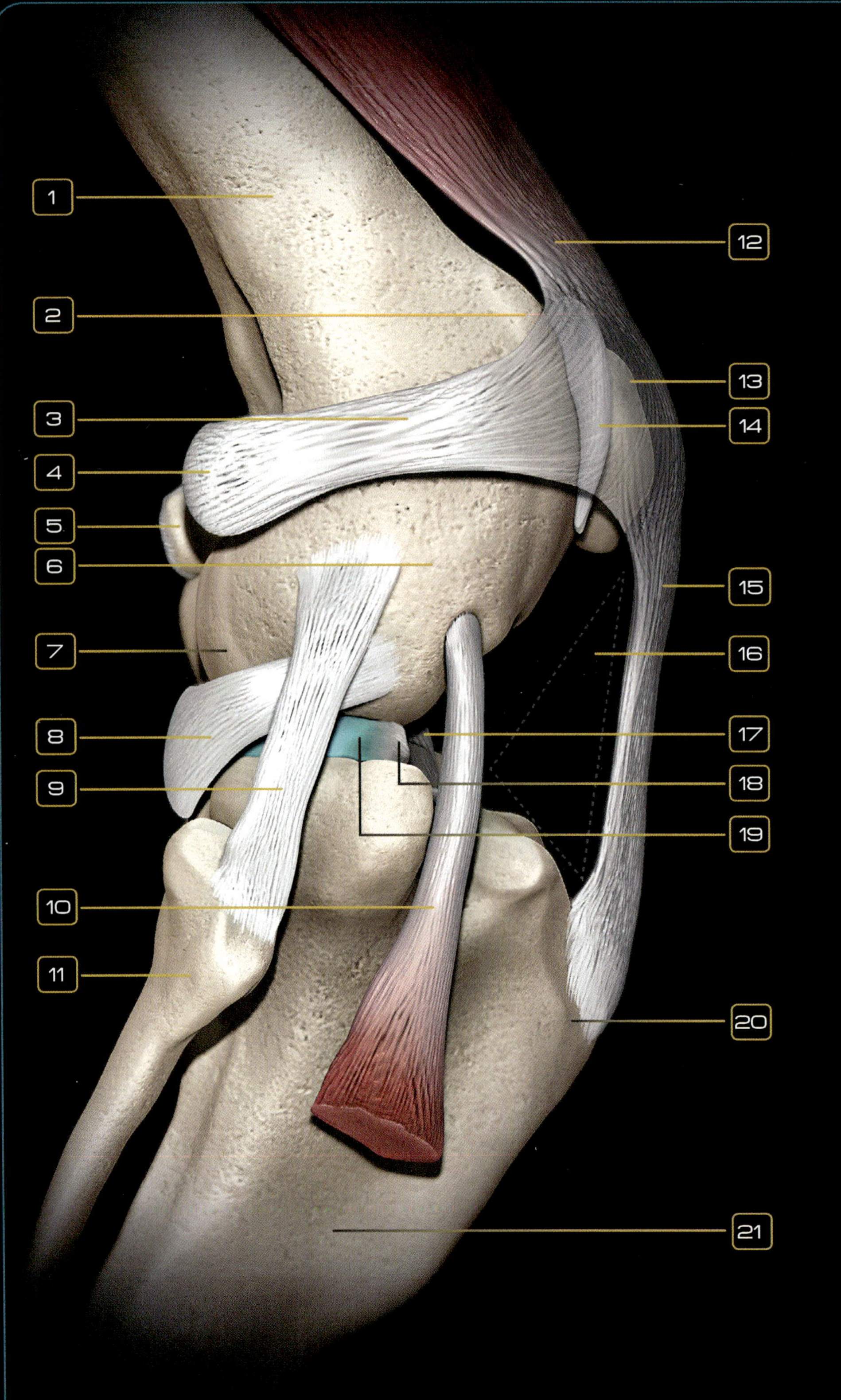

LATERAL VIEW

1 Femur
2 Lateral lip of the trochlea of the femur
3 Lateral femoropatellar lig.
4 Lateral gastrocnemius sesamoid bone
5 Medial gastrocnemius sesamoid bone
6 Lateral epicondyle of the femur
7 Lateral condyle of the femur
8 Tendon of origin of the popliteus muscle
9 Lateral collateral lig.
10 Tendon of origin of the long digital extensor muscle
11 Fibula
12 Tendon of insertion of the quadriceps femoris muscle
13 Patella
14 Lateral parapatellar fibrocartilage
15 Patellar lig.
16 Space occupied by the infrapatellar fat pad
17 Cranial cruciate lig.
18 Lateral cranial meniscal lig.
19 Lateral meniscus
20 Tibial tuberosity
21 Tibia

CAUDAL VIEW

1 Medial femoropatellar lig.
2 Medial gastrocnemius sesamoid bone
3 Medial condyle of the femur
4 Medial collateral lig.
5 Medial meniscus
6 Medial condyle of the tibia
7 Caudal cruciate lig.
8 Caudal meniscal lig.
9 Lateral femoropatellar lig.
10 Lateral gastrocnemius sesamoid bone
11 Lateral condyle of the femur
12 Lateral collateral lig.
13 Meniscofemoral lig.
14 Tendon of the popliteus muscle
15 Popliteal sesamoid bone

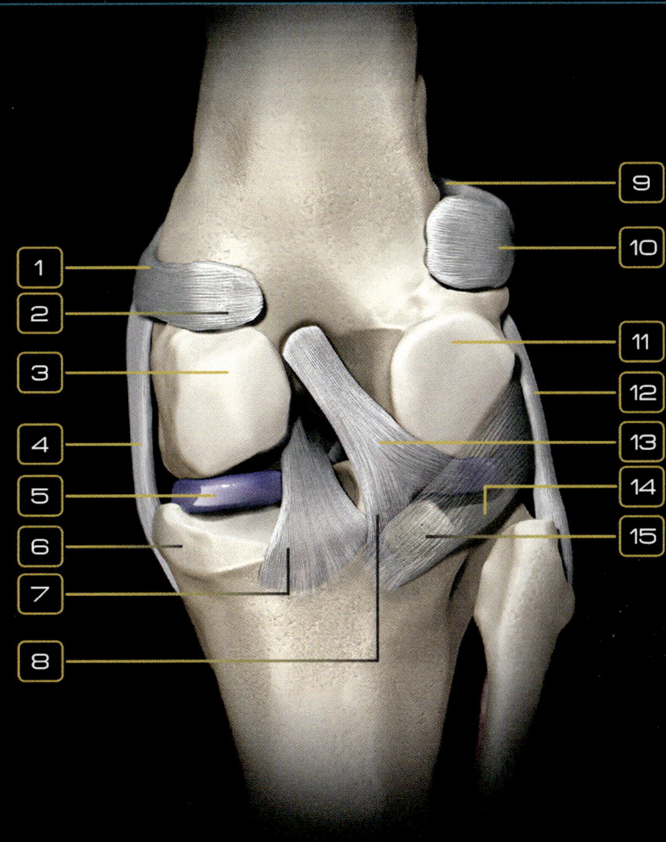

MEDIAL VIEW

1 Tendon of insertion of the quadriceps femoris muscle
2 Patella
3 Medial parapatellar fibrocartilage
4 Medial lip of the trochlea of the femur
5 Medial epicondyle of the femur
6 Patellar lig.
7 Medial cranial meniscal lig.
8 Medial femoropatellar lig.
9 Medial condyle of the femur
10 Medial meniscus
11 Medial condyle of the tibia
12 Medial collateral lig.

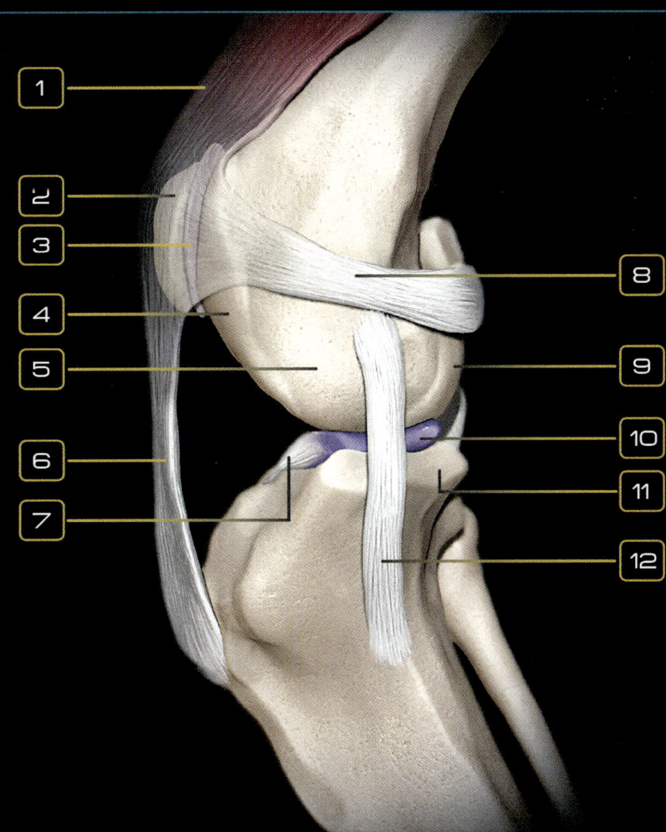

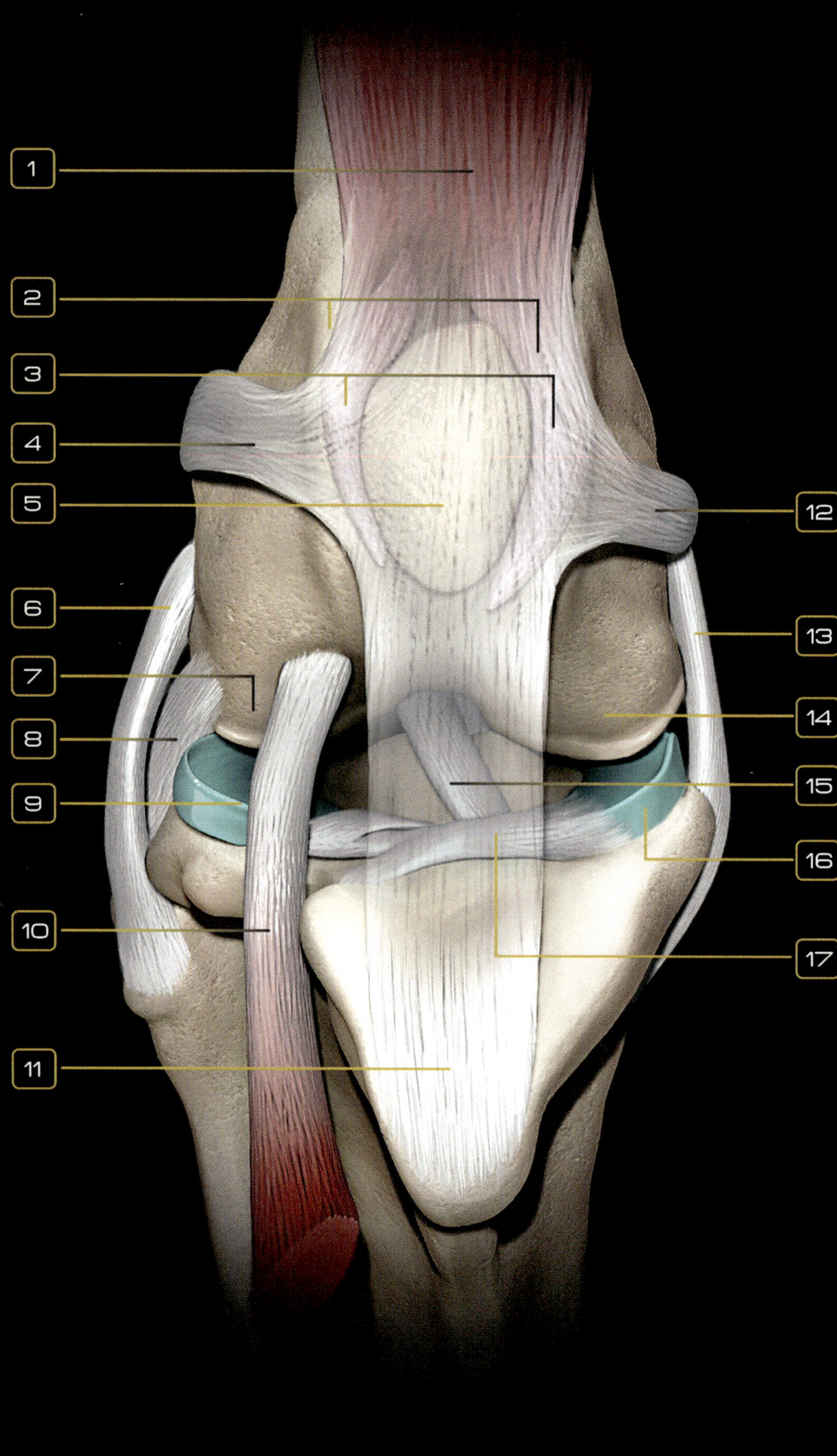

CRANIAL VIEW

1 Tendon of insertion of the quadriceps femoris muscle

2 Trochlea of the femur

3 Parapatellar fibrocartilage

4 Lateral femoropatellar lig.

5 Patella

6 Lateral collateral lig.

7 Lateral condyle of the femur

8 Tendon of origin of the popliteus muscle

9 Lateral meniscus

10 Tendon of origin of the long digital extensor muscle

11 Patellar lig.

12 Medial femoropatellar lig.

13 Medial collateral lig.

14 Medial condyle of the femur

15 Cranial cruciate lig.

16 Medial meniscus

17 Transverse lig. of the stifle joint

Introduction

The stifle joint is the largest synovial joint in the musculoskeletal system. It is a trochlear articular complex with two distinct joints: the femorotibial joint and the femoropatellar joint. The articular menisci enable the congruity of the femorotibial joint and sometimes are the origin of diseases.

The stifle joint has a surface configuration with no protective muscle or adipose tissue, so it is often affected by direct or indirect trauma as well as degenerative or inflammatory joint processes.

The keys to diagnosing conditions in this joint are possessing an in-depth knowledge of its anatomy, performing specific manoeuvres to collect information on potential abnormalities in the different anatomical elements and recognising cytological abnormalities in the synovial fluid. All this must be supported by peripheral clinical data on the animal, which are obtained in the medical history.

Anatomy

The stifle joint consists of bone structures, capsuloligamentous structures, menisci and the musculotendinous system. In addition, the cranial and caudal parts of the joint feature anatomically and clinically significant recesses.

Bone structures

The stifle joint consists of three articular surfaces: the condyles of the femur, the condyles of the proximal end of the tibia and the patella. The articular incongruity between the femur and the tibia is offset by the menisci.

The condyles of the femur diverge distally and cranially. The lateral condyle is slightly wider cranially, and the medial condyle is more or less uniform. On the transverse plane, both condyles are slightly convex. On the sagittal plane, their curvature is accentuated caudally and the radius of the condylar curvature is decreased. The medial condyle also curves inwards around a vertical axis. The condyles are separated cranially by the trochlea and caudally by the intercondylar fossa.

The lateral and medial condyles on the proximal end of the tibia have a flat surface and correspond to the condyles of the femur. They are separated by the intercondylar eminence, which aligns with the intercondylar fossa of the femur. The eminence consists of the lateral and medial intercondylar tubercles. Between these tubercles are the cranial, central and caudal intercondylar areas for attachment of the meniscal and cruciate ligaments. The tibial tuberosity (where the patellar ligament is attached) and the extensor groove for the tendon of the long digital extensor muscle are found cranially. The popliteal notch can be seen caudally.

The oval-shaped patella is located on the cranial aspect of the stifle joint and articulates with the trochlea of the femur. It is incorporated into the tendon of insertion of the quadriceps femoris muscle and gives rise to the patellar ligament.

The head of the fibula, found lateral to the femorotibial joint, articulates with the lateral condyle of the tibia.

Capsuloligamentous structures

Joint capsule

The loose, wide capsule is thin cranially and laterally, and is reinforced by ligaments and tendons. The patella is located relative to the cranial wall of the capsule.

The joint capsule has a fibrous layer that connects to the bone at the edges of the articular cartilage except at three points: first, on the cranial aspect of the femur, where it is attached proximally to the trochlea; second, on its cranial aspect, where it is attached to the patella; and, finally, in the intercondylar area, where it reflects and courses cranially to merge with the cruciate ligaments which are intracapsular and extra-articular. The synovial membrane is inside of the fibrous capsule.

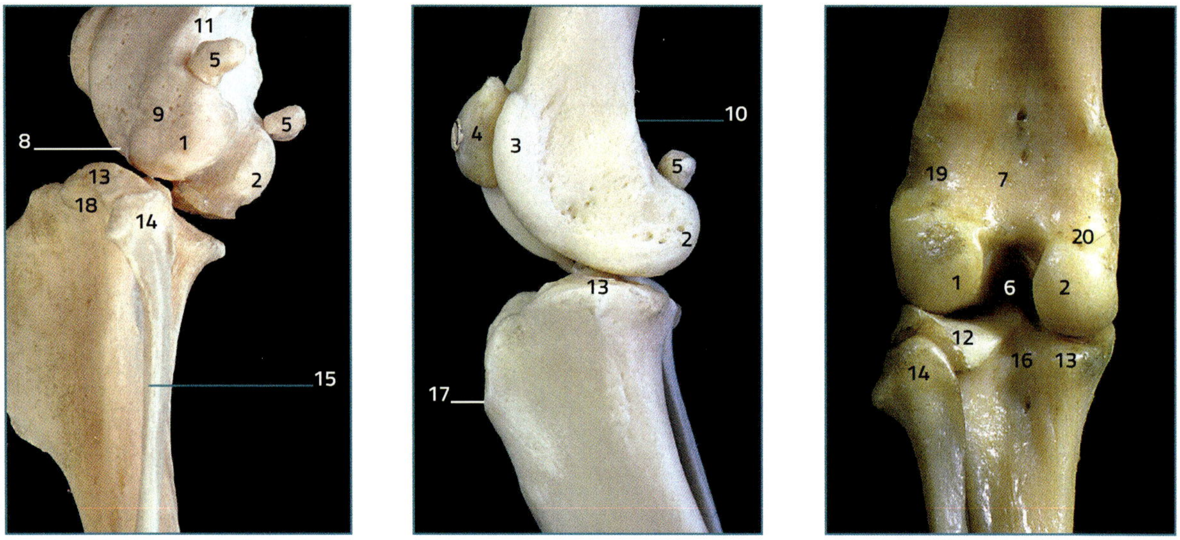

1 Lateral condyle of the femur
2 Medial condyle of the femur
3 Trochlea of the femur: medial lip
4 Patella
5 Sesamoid bones of the gastrocnemius muscle
6 Intercondylar fossa
7 Popliteal aspect of the femur
8 Extensor fossa
9 Popliteal fossa
10 Medial supracondylar tuberosity
11 Lateral supracondylar tuberosity
12 Lateral condyle of the tibia
13 Medial condyle of the tibia
14 Head of the fibula
15 Body of the fibula
16 Popliteal notch
17 Tibial tuberosity
18 Extensor groove of the tibia
19 Lateral sesamoid articular aspect
20 Medial sesamoid articular aspect

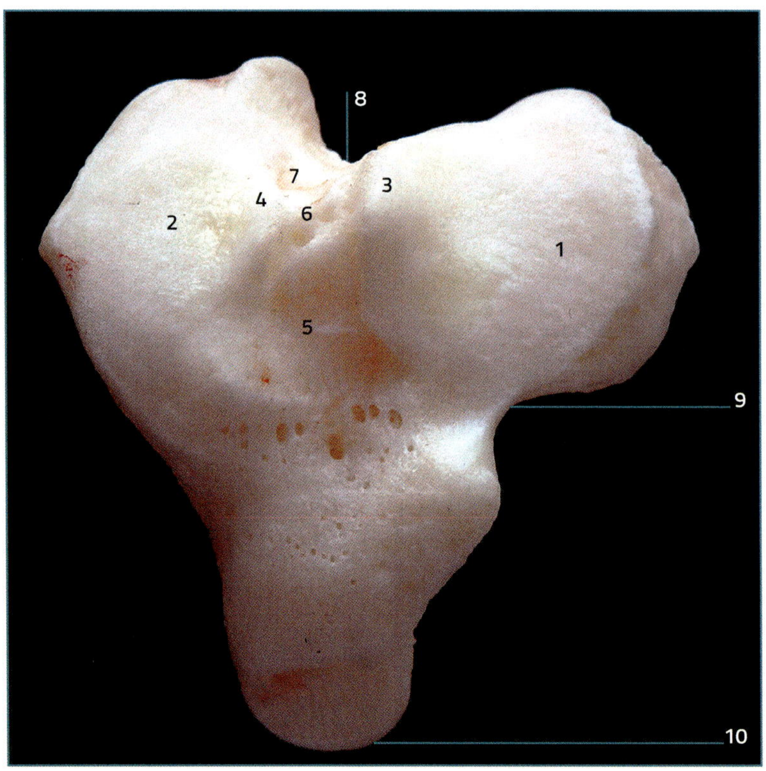

1 Lateral condyle of the tibia
2 Medial condyle of the tibia
3 Lateral intercondylar eminence
4 Medial intercondylar eminence
5 Cranial intercondylar area
6 Central intercondylar area
7 Caudal intercondylar area
8 Popliteal notch
9 Extensor groove of the tibia
10 Tibial tuberosity

The synovial membrane of the femoropatellar sac and the fibrous layer of the capsule are separated by adipose tissue, which on the cranial aspect becomes the infrapatellar fat pad. On the cranial aspect, the synovial membrane starts at the level of the cartilaginous covering, reflects cranially under the quadriceps femoris muscle and gives rise to the supratrochlear recess, the base of the synovial sac which widens the joint cavity. On the caudal aspect, the synovial membrane connects to the femur on the cartilaginous edge of the condyles and conforms to them.

The lateral and medial femorotibial synovial sacs have projections in the form of recesses that distance themselves from the joint cavity, such as the subextensor recess (relative to the tendon of origin of the long digital extensor muscle) and the subpopliteal recess (relative to the tendon of origin of the popliteus muscle). This is clinically significant when accounting for joint injuries caused by apparently distant wounds.

The inner surface of the synovial membrane features large numbers of membranous villi or projections which vary in thickness and size. These greatly increase its actual surface area. Unlike the mucosae, the synovial membrane lacks uninterrupted cellular coverage; the most cellular parts, in relatively protected areas, are responsible for producing the lubricating mucous component of the synovial fluid and aminoglycans. All other components of the synovial membrane come from blood plasma; thus it is a vascular, sensitive membrane.

The ligaments of the stifle joint can be classified as central or peripheral. The central ligaments include the cranial and caudal cruciate ligaments, also known as the anterior and posterior cruciate ligaments, respectively. There are distinct groups of peripheral ligaments on the medial, lateral, cranial and caudal aspects of the stifle joint.

1 Suprapatellar recess of the femoropatellar joint
2 Extensor recess of the femorotibial joint
3 Patella
4 Tibial tuberosity
5 Lateral condyle of the femur
6 Lateral sesamoid bone of the gastrocnemius muscle
7 Lateral condyle of the tibia
8 Head of the fibula
9 Interosseous space of the leg
10 Body of the fibula

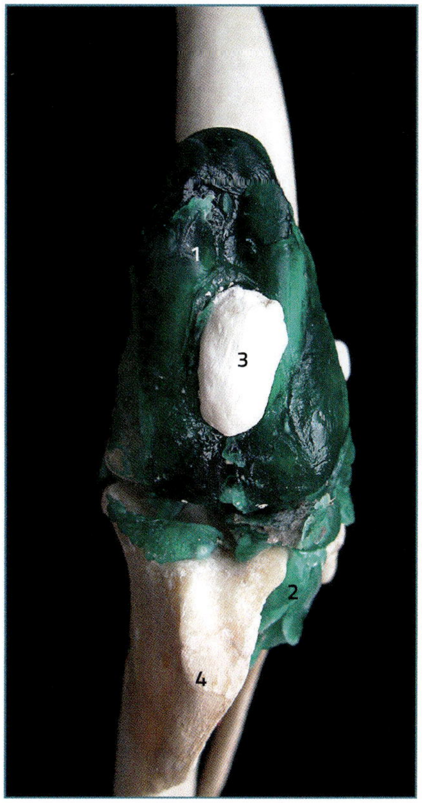

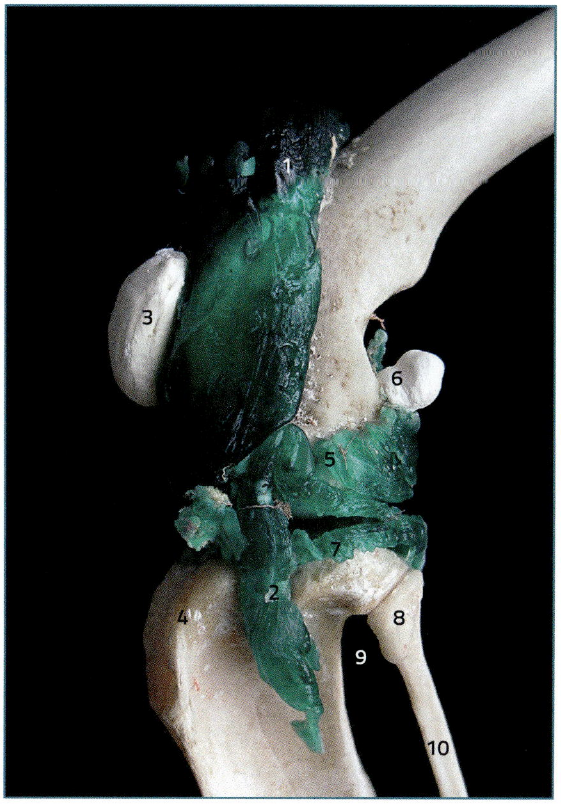

Central ligaments

The **anterior cruciate ligament** (ACL) extends from the internal caudal portion of the lateral condyle of the femur to the central intercondylar area of the tibia, following a cranial path and arranged laterally to the posterior cruciate ligament.

The **posterior cruciate ligament** (PCL) connects the cranial part of the internal aspect of the medial condyle of the femur to the popliteal notch of the tibia. It follows a more vertical path than the other cruciate ligament and courses obliquely in a caudal and medial direction compared to the ACL.

While this book does not discuss the extensive studies that have been conducted on the structure and function of these ligaments, it should be noted that they run inversely to one another. They intersect twice, first in a craniocaudal direction and then in a mediolateral direction. The ACL controls the extension and cranial movement of the tibia. The PCL controls the flexion and caudal movement of the tibia relative to the femur.

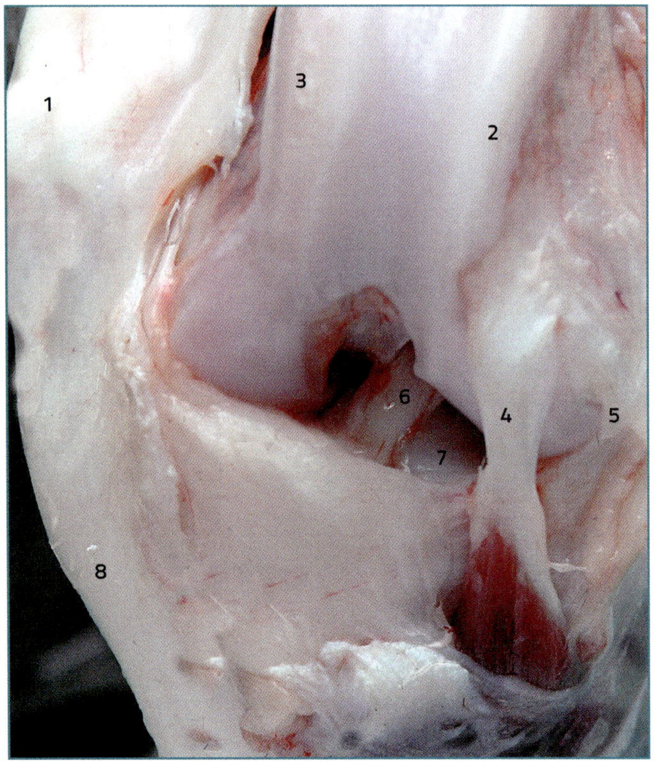

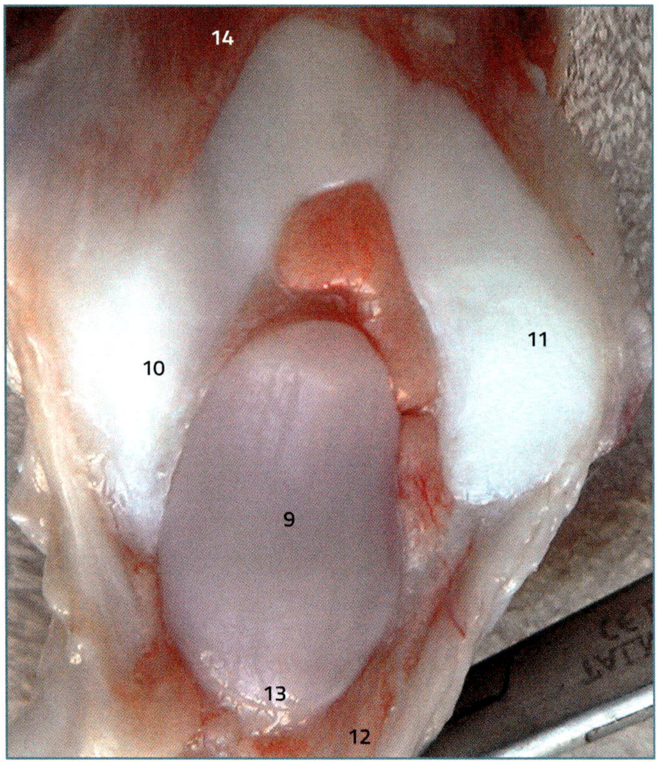

1 Patella
2 Trochlea of the femur: lateral lip
3 Trochlea of the femur: medial lip
4 Tendon of the long digital extensor muscle
5 Tendon of the popliteus muscle
6 Cranial cruciate ligament
7 Lateral cranial meniscal ligament

8 Patellar ligament
9 Articular aspect of the patella
10 and 11 Lateral and medial parapatellar fibrocartilage
12 Infrapatellar fat pad
13 Apex of the patella
14 Tendon of insertion of the quadriceps muscle

Peripheral ligaments

Different peripheral ligaments surround the stifle joint on its various aspects:

- The **patellar ligament** is the continuation of the tendon of insertion of the quadriceps femoris muscle from the patella to the tibial tuberosity.
- The **lateral patellar retinaculum** is a tendinous expansion of the vastus lateralis muscle. The rectus femoris muscle plays a role in its lateral insertion into the tibial tuberosity.
- The **medial patellar retinaculum**, an extension of the vastus medialis muscle, inserts into the tibia in front of the medial collateral ligament.
- The **medial collateral ligament** is a flattened triangular band resulting from the thickening of the fibrous layer of the capsule, which fuses with the medial meniscus. This ligament covers the tendon of insertion of the cranial portion of the semimembranosus muscle. It also features the pes anserinus, which consists of the tendons of insertion of the sartorius, gracilis and semitendinosus muscles.
- The **lateral collateral ligament** does not fuse with the capsule or lateral meniscus, and extends from the lateral epicondyle of the femur to the head of the fibula.
- Finally, the **oblique popliteal ligament** arises from the head of the fibula and courses towards the joint capsule.

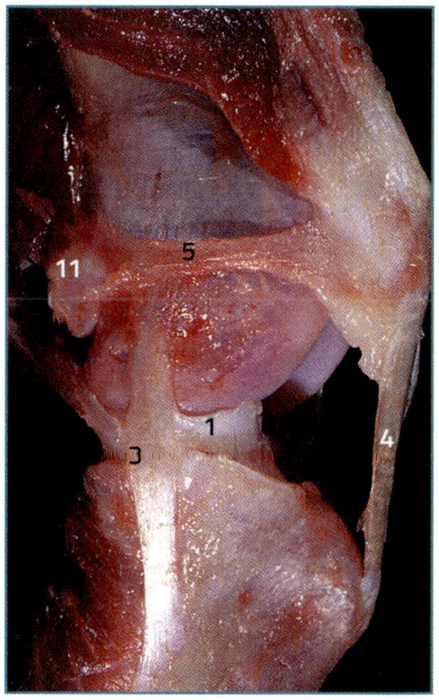

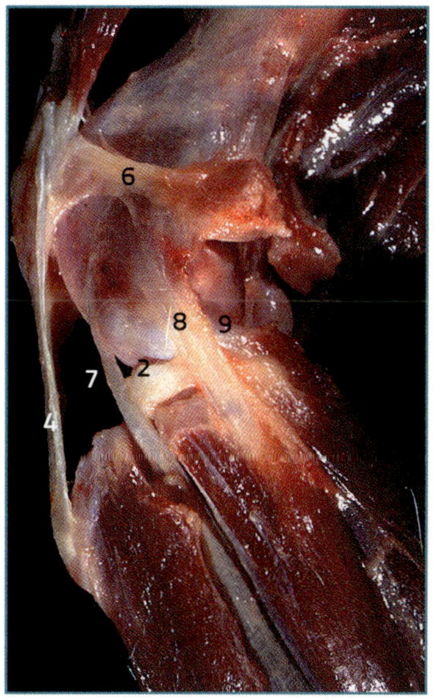

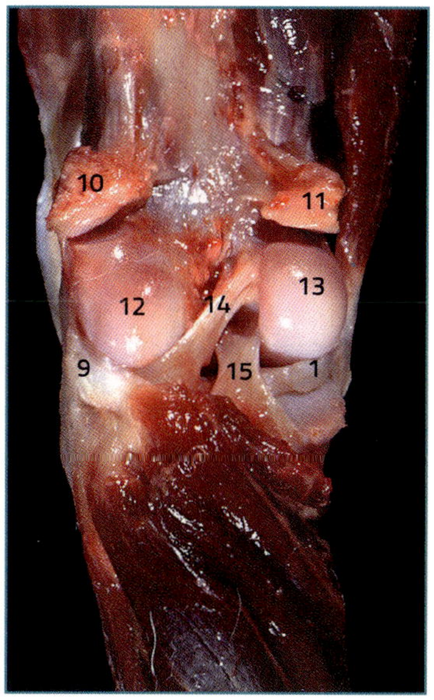

1 Medial meniscus
2 Lateral meniscus
3 Medial collateral ligament
4 Patellar ligament
5 Medial femoropatellar ligament
6 Lateral femoropatellar ligament
7 Tendon of the long digital extensor muscle
8 Lateral collateral ligament
9 Tendon of origin of the popliteus muscle
10 Lateral sesamoid bone
11 Medial sesamoid bone
12 Lateral condyle of the femur
13 Medial condyle of the femur
14 Meniscofemoral ligament
15 Caudal cruciate ligament

Menisci

The menisci consist of connective tissue rich in collagen fibres, with some cells similar to chondrocytes (fibrocartilage). The thickest collagen fibres are arranged longitudinally, and the thinnest collagen fibres are arranged mediolaterally.

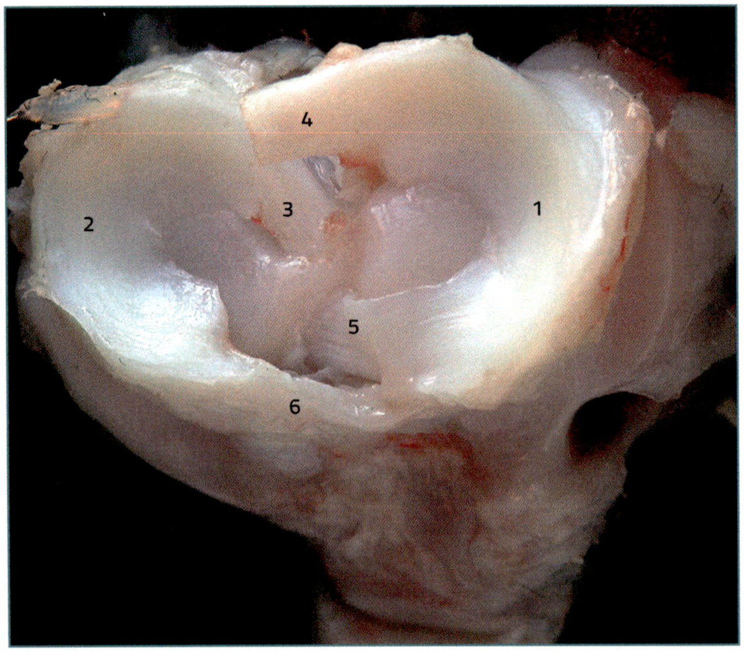

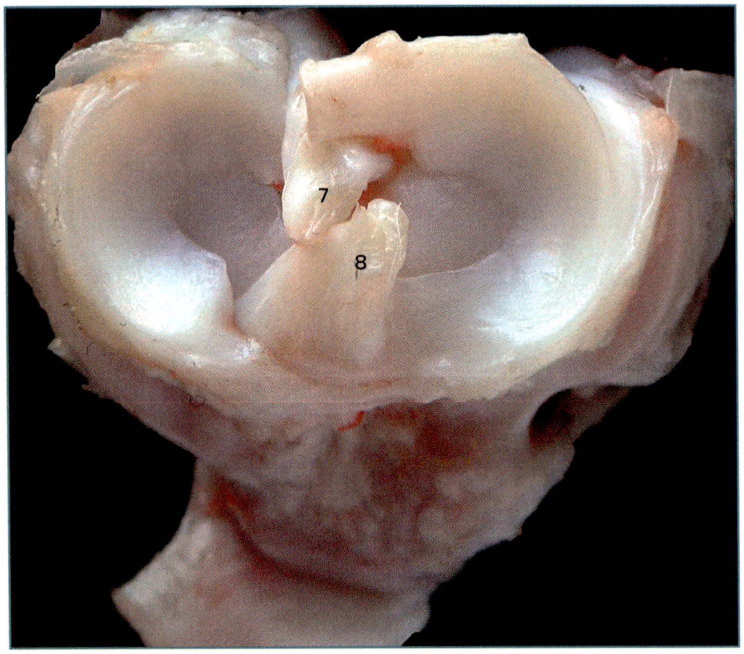

In mediolateral section the menisci are in the shape of a wedge that tapers from the periphery to the centre. The superior aspect of the menisci, which is concave, touches the condyles of the femur. The inferior aspect, which is more or less flat, slides over the tibia. The outer edge of the menisci is fused along the capsule and its cranial horns are connected by the transverse ligament. The menisci are supplied by the medial and distal genicular arteries, which form perimeniscal arches.

The medial meniscus is in the shape of a half-moon or *C*. Its cranial horn is attached to the cranial intercondylar area by the medial cranial meniscal ligament, proximal to the ACL. Its peripheral edge is connected to the joint capsule by the medial collateral ligament. Its caudal horn is attached to the caudal intercondylar area of the tibia by the medial caudal meniscal ligament.

The lateral meniscus is nearly in the shape of a circle or *O* and has a uniform width. Its cranial insertion through the lateral cranial meniscal ligament affects the cranial intercondylar area of the tibia, while its caudal attachment through the lateral caudal meniscal ligament corresponds to the popliteal notch. It is more mobile than the medial meniscus. The craniolateral portion of the capsule is loosely attached to it whereas the caudolateral portion is not. The meniscofemoral ligament arises from the caudal horn of the lateral meniscus.

The menisci stabilise the stifle joint and follow the condyles of the femur in cranial and caudal movement and horizontal rotation. They move cranially in extension and caudally in flexion.

1 Lateral meniscus
2 Medial meniscus
3 Medial caudal meniscal ligament
4 Meniscofemoral ligament
5 Lateral cranial meniscal ligament
6 Medial cranial meniscal ligament
7 Caudal cruciate ligament
8 Cranial cruciate ligament

Musculotendinous system

Few muscles act only in the stifle joint; these originate in the hip and insert into the proximal part of the tibia. The essential movements of the stifle joint are flexion and extension around a mediolateral axis and lateral and medial rotation around a longitudinal axis when the collateral ligaments are lax.

Extension of the stifle joint results almost exclusively from contraction of the quadriceps femoris muscle, which is minimally supported by the tensor fasciae latae muscle and the cranial portion of the sartorius muscle. The quadriceps femoris muscle acts more powerfully on the stifle joint when the hip joint is in extension and thus with the animal standing still.

The semimembranosus, semitendinosus, gracilis and sartorius muscles, which are all located on the medial aspect of the thigh, play a role in the flexion of the stifle joint. The latter three form the pes anserinus by inserting into the medial aspect of the tibial tuberosity, and are very important in tibial plateau levelling osteotomy (TPLO) surgery. These muscles flex the stifle joint and internally rotate the tibia.

The biceps femoris and popliteus muscles are on the lateral aspect of the thigh. These muscles flex the stifle joint. The biceps femoris muscle rotates the tibia laterally, while the popliteus muscle rotates the tibia medially.

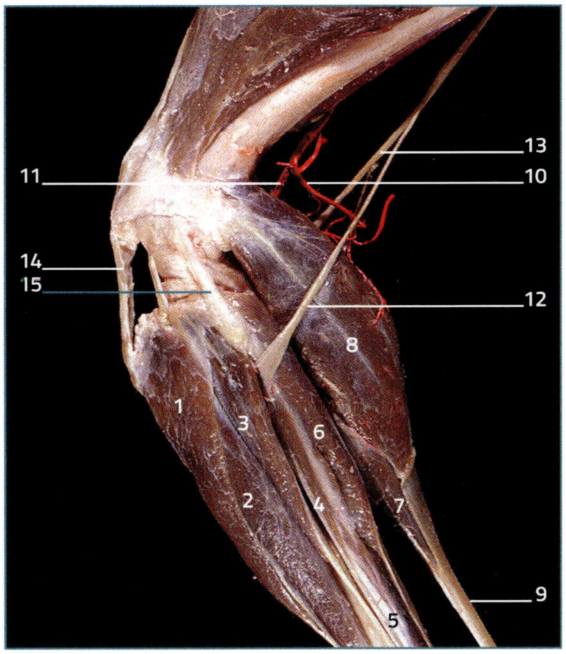

1 Tibialis cranialis muscle
2 Long digital extensor muscle
3 Long peroneal muscle
4 Lateral digital extensor muscle
5 Short peroneal muscle
6 Lateral digital flexor muscle
7 Superficial digital flexor muscle
8 Gastrocnemius muscle: lateral head
9 Common calcaneal tendon
10 Distal caudal femoral artery
11 Popliteal artery
12 Common peroneal nerve
13 Tibial nerve
14 Patellar ligament
15 Lateral collateral ligament

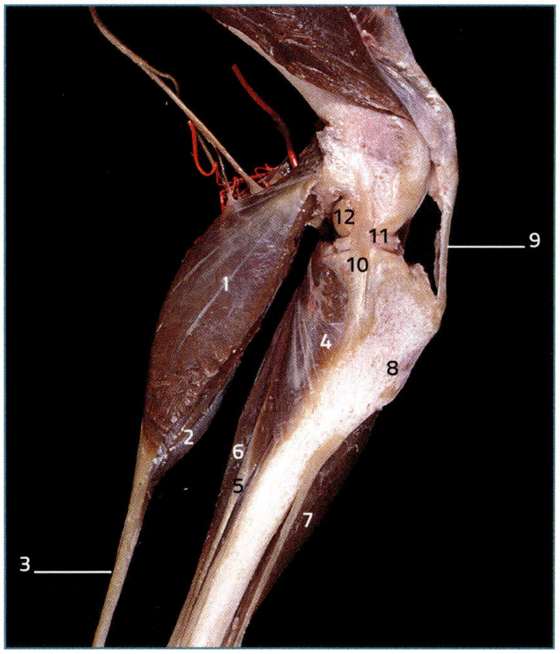

1 Gastrocnemius muscle: medial head
2 Superficial digital flexor muscle
3 Common calcaneal tendon
4 Popliteus muscle
5 Deep digital flexor muscle: medial digital flexor muscle
6 Lateral digital flexor muscle
7 Tibialis cranialis muscle
8 Tibial tuberosity
9 Patellar ligament
10 Medial collateral ligament
11 Medial meniscus
12 Medial condyle of the femur

Clinical examination

Clinical examination of the stifle joint must follow the same guidelines as examination of other joints. In addition, evaluation of the stifle joint is a part of examination of the entire musculoskeletal system. A systematic approach must be taken based on inspection, palpation and a number of manoeuvres intended to demonstrate specific injuries in the different structures of the stifle joint. These manoeuvres can be classified as patellar manoeuvres, meniscal manoeuvres or manoeuvres of stability of the stifle joint.

The approach to abnormalities of the stifle joint differs depending on whether the abnormality derives from genuine trauma or from inflammation of metabolic, infectious or tumoural origin. In the former case, the date of symptom onset and the causative mechanism in particular are crucially important. Trauma may be indirect, such as sudden rotation causing meniscal injuries, or direct. It is also important to delimit acute processes, which manifest more on the topography of the injury than chronic processes. Chronic processes manifest more as general failures in the stifle joint and are accompanied by chronic pain that is sometimes difficult to trace back to its origin. In inflammatory diseases, the mechanism of production is generally a secondary consideration and it is necessary to emphasise the general symptomatic manifestations of the animal in other locations: synovitis in other joints, skin injuries, abnormalities in haematology and blood clinical chemistry, eye impairment, etc.

All professionals who examine animals with musculoskeletal system diseases should bear this dual approach in mind when examining the stifle joint.

Inspection

Inspection must be performed while the patient is walking, bearing weight and at rest on the examination table, in lateral, dorsal and ventral decubitus. Comparing the two stifle joints may reveal unilateral abnormalities, which may be symmetrical or asymmetrical. Initial inspection of the stifle joint provides information on the approach to the joint.

Genu varum (limbs bowing or forming an *O*) tends to be due to single-compartment abnormalities of the stifle joint (medial compartment) and is characteristic of general osteoarthritis of the stifle joint and osteoarthritis deriving from chronic meniscal injuries.

Genu valgum (limbs forming an *X*) is the usual deformity in inflammatory joint diseases with impairment of the three compartments: cranial, lateral and medial.

It is important to attempt to distinguish between deformity of articular origin and deformity due to bone abnormalities, such as malunited fractures leading to angulation and subsequent osteoarthritis, bone or synovial tumours and autoimmune diseases.

Other abnormalities that can be recognised when inspecting the stifle joint, although much less common, are: genu recurvatum, which is a hyperextension deformity common in syndromes of joint hypermobility or muscle paralysis, some of which are secondary to postoperative contractures; and deficient flexion of the stifle joint, which may be detected when the stifle joint has some degree of constant flexion and is incapable of full extension. This is particular to degenerative inflammatory joint diseases and joint diseases following malunited joint fractures, which characteristically make walking difficult.

Gait abnormalities

It is important to note the different gait abnormalities resulting from impairment of the stifle joint. Usually, the stifle joint extends in the stance phase and flexes during the subsequent swing phase. Synovitis of the stifle joint or a pre-existing deformity may make full extension difficult, giving rise to an antalgic gait with short steps. This is a very typical characteristic of animals with acute pain. Fixed extension gives rise to a gait with semicircular movement of the entire limb called circumduction. This may occur in some cases as an undesirable effect of triple pelvic osteotomy (TPO) surgery on the hip.

With the patient in dorsal decubitus, inspection may reveal the presence of localised swelling (conditions of synovial sacs or meniscal cysts) or generalised swelling (intra-articular effusion). Inspection to determine articular effusion is simple yet essential. It is based on comparison with the healthy side and on the disappearance of the lateral and medial patellofemoral depressions on both sides of the patella. Generalised swelling distorts the entire contour of the stifle joint, which tends to be in flexion in major effusion, since the capacity of the stifle joint is greater in this position than in extension.

Localised swelling is particularly found at the level of the patella (prepatellar bursitis), tibial tuberosity (infrapatellar bursitis) and internal aspect of the tibial tuberosity among the muscles of the pes anserinus (pes anserine bursitis).

The quadriceps femoris muscle visibly atrophies if stifle joint disease persists for some time.

> It is useful to quantify atrophy by measuring the perimeter of the leg above the tibial malleolus at the level of the gastrocnemius and also the thigh above the proximal edge of the patella.

The popliteal fossa is inspected in sternal decubitus. The presence or absence of localised swelling is a useful piece of information in preoperative and postoperative radiological examination with the TPLO technique. There may also be localised abnormalities due to vascular conditions resulting from injuries of the popliteal vessels, or nerve abnormalities due to abnormalities of the sciatic nerve or its branches or to local lymphadenopathy following local or general abnormalities in the animal.

Palpation

Examination is performed with the patient in dorsal decubitus and the following are evaluated:

- Temperature.
- Presence of painful points when pressure is applied.
- Presence of effusion, using appropriate manoeuvres.
- Removal of synovial fluid.
- Potential asymmetry.

The back of the hand is used to examine the temperature of the skin above the patella, which tends to be lower than the temperature of the leg and thigh. An increase in the temperature of the stifle joint compared to the contralateral side is extensive and occurs at the suprapatellar level in synovitis of infectious, inflammatory or traumatic origin, but is more localised in bursitis.

Palpation of painful points and anatomical structures

Palpation of painful points is particularly useful in trauma, since they are indicators of meniscal injuries, injuries of specific ligaments and even fractures. Palpation is best performed with the stifle joint in flexion, since some protrusions of the joint cannot be palpated in extension. Palpation of the stifle joint and its painful points can be classified according to the aspect examined: cranial and medial surfaces, lateral surface, trochlear surface and patella, and caudal surface. The bony prominences and corresponding soft tissues on all these aspects are palpated in search of painful points when pressure is applied.

Cranial and medial surfaces

Palpation must be performed such that both hands surround the stifle joint. The thumbs actively palpate while the fingers rest on the caudal surface (popliteal fossa). Pressing on both sides of the patellar ligament reveals some depressions that serve as points of reference for palpation of the femoropatellar joint area.

On the medial aspect the thumb palpates the sharp upper edge of the tibial plateau, which serves as a point of insertion for the medial meniscus. In this area pain is present when pressure is applied if there is a meniscal injury. The painful point becomes more caudal when the limb is flexed and increases when the limb is rotated medially.

The patellar ligament is followed distally up to its attachment to the tibial tuberosity and this attachment is palpated. Medial to this is the subcutaneous surface of the tibia, into which the tendons of the pes anserinus insert.

The medial condyle of the femur is found towards the area proximal and immediately medial to the patella and is palpated with the stifle joint flexed just over 90°. Osteophytes are palpated along this condyle in cases of osteoarthritis and cartilage defects due to osteochondral fragments. The insertion of the adductor muscles, between the vastus medialis and the tendons of the pes anserinus, can be palpated caudally. The insertion of the tendons of the pes anserinus is a painful point when osteoarthritis is present.

In cases of genu valgum there is pain on the lateral aspect of the joint area. By contrast, in the most common cases of genu varum there is greater pain in the medial area.

On the cranial and medial aspect, soft structures, which are key in semiology of the stifle joint, are also palpated. The quadriceps femoris muscle inserts into the proximal and medial edges of the patella. The tendon of insertion of the quadriceps femoris muscle forms the patellar ligament which is attached to the tibial tuberosity. The vastus lateralis and vastus medialis muscles are easily palpated as two masses on both sides of the femur. They are palpated to compare them to the contralateral side and detect any tears or ruptures. The most common findings are observed in the rectus femoris muscle or the vastus intermedius muscle, proximal to the patella. It is also important to evaluate muscle atrophy, especially in the vastus medialis muscle, which occurs early after the onset of synovial effusion or stifle joint surgery. Assessment of atrophy of the quadriceps femoris muscle is discussed above.

The patellar ligament runs distally to the patella, towards the tibial tuberosity. Its insertion is painful in cases of Osgood-Schlatter disease. The infrapatellar fat pad is located distally, on both sides of this ligament. It may increase in volume nonspecifically or become inflamed and painful on palpation (Hoffa's disease).

Clinicians must also be accustomed to palpating the most significant synovial bursae which lie on the cranial and medial aspects. The distal infrapatellar synovial bursa is adjacent to the patellar ligament and may become inflamed with forced movements of the stifle joint. The prepatellar subcutaneous synovial bursa, which covers the cranial portion of the patella, often becomes inflamed in humans, leading to prepatellar bursitis, commonly known as "housemaid's knee" or "coal miner's knee". This bursa allows the skin to slide unimpeded over the patella when the stifle joint is in flexion. The tendons of the muscles of the pes anserinus form an easily accessible jutting which can be palpated in the caudomedial portion of the stifle joint; a subtendinous synovial bursa is found among them. This subtendinous bursa of the pes anserinus is located among the tendons of the sartorius, gracilis and semitendinosus muscles. It may be painful on palpation and sometimes detected as rounded or pyriform swelling.

If the thumb moves caudally along the medial and superior edge of the tibial plateau, it palpates other significant soft structures such as the medial meniscus, the medial collateral ligament and the tendons of the pes anserinus.

As mentioned above, the medial meniscus is attached to the tibia by meniscal ligaments. Tearing of these ligaments leads to pain at the edge of the joint. When the meniscus tears, the medial joint area becomes painful on palpation. The medial meniscus is somewhat mobile, and when the tibia is positioned in internal rotation, its edge is more prominent and palpable.

The medial collateral ligament connects the medial condyle of the femur with the tibia outside of the capsule. The internal portion of the ligament is attached to the medial meniscus. The ligament is not palpated as a separate anatomical unit; however, the area it covers is located proximally to the joint area, which is palpated by sliding the fingers caudally. This ligament becomes injured in forced valgus, and pain and local defects can be detected on palpation.

Lateral surface

If the thumb moves laterally it palpates the dorsolateral edge of the tibial plateau (lateral condyle of the tibia). A prominence corresponding to the tibial tuberosity is palpated distally to the tibial plateau. The lateral condyle of the femur can be detected on proximal palpation. It is partially covered by the patella and less palpable than the medial condyle of the femur. The head of the fibula is palpated caudally and distally to the joint area.

The lateral meniscus can also be palpated at this level, especially with the stifle joint in slight flexion. The lateral medial meniscus, like the medial meniscus, is painful on palpation if there is tearing of the ligaments that attach it to the tibia. The lateral meniscus is more mobile than the medial meniscus as it is separated from the collateral ligament by the tendon of origin of the popliteus muscle. It incurs fewer injuries than the medial meniscus due to this greater mobility.

On this aspect the lateral collateral ligament and the tendon of insertion of the biceps femoris between the tibia and the fibula, as well as the iliotibial band, are palpated for evidence of disease demonstrable by palpation. The iliotibial band is a distal expansion of the fascia lata which stabilises the patella and the vastus lateralis muscle.

The lateral collateral ligament connects the lateral epicondyle of the femur with the head of the fibula. It is an extracapsular ligament. It is best palpated with the stifle joint in 90° of flexion and the hip in abduction and external rotation (with the limb crossed). Tearing of this ligament causes local pain on palpation; however, it incurs fewer injuries than the medial collateral ligament. The cranial and caudal ligaments of the head of the fibula are found between the tibia and the head of the fibula. These are rarely a site of disease but have semiological significance as they must be cut when performing cranial transposition of the head of the fibula to treat ACL rupture. With the stifle joint in 90° of flexion, the tendon of the biceps femoris is palpated where it inserts into the head of the fibula. It may be torn away from the fibula in cases of severe trauma to the stifle joint.

Trochlear surface and patella

The trochlea of the femur, on which the patella moves, is covered in articular cartilage. Over this trochlear groove the patella is stationary in flexion and mobile in extension. The dorsal aspect of the patella is best palpated during extension. The trochlear groove and its walls can be palpated during extension; its lateral aspect is higher than its medial aspect. Osteoarthritis injuries and chondromalacia can be primarily evaluated on the articular aspect of the patella.

Caudal surface

The caudal surface of the stifle joint is defined by the popliteal fossa, which is delimited proximally by the tendons of the semimembranosus and semitendinosus muscles in the medial portion and laterally by the tendon of insertion of the biceps femoris muscle. Distally, the popliteal fossa is delimited by the heads of the gastrocnemius muscle. There are three very important vascular and nerve elements in the popliteal fossa:

- The tibial nerve (sciatic branch), which superficially crosses the fossa.
- The popliteal vein, which is immediately distal to the tibial nerve.
- The popliteal artery, which is deeper and runs along the joint capsule.

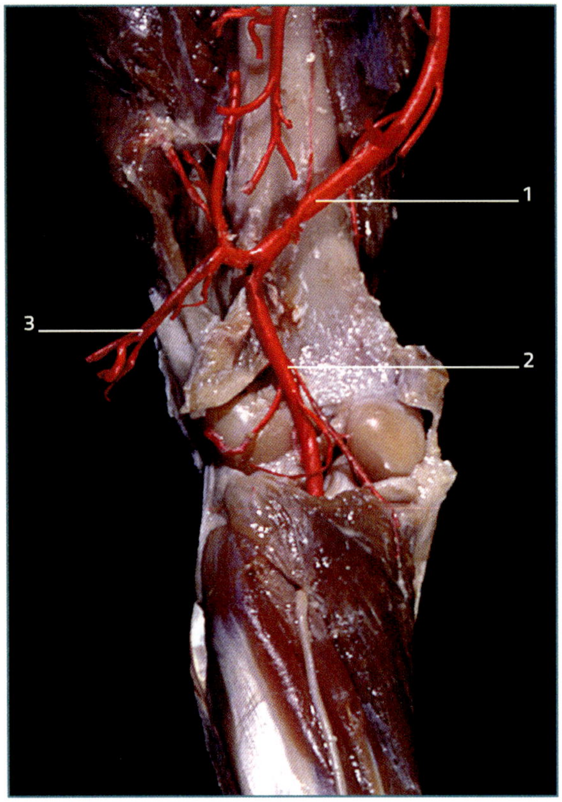

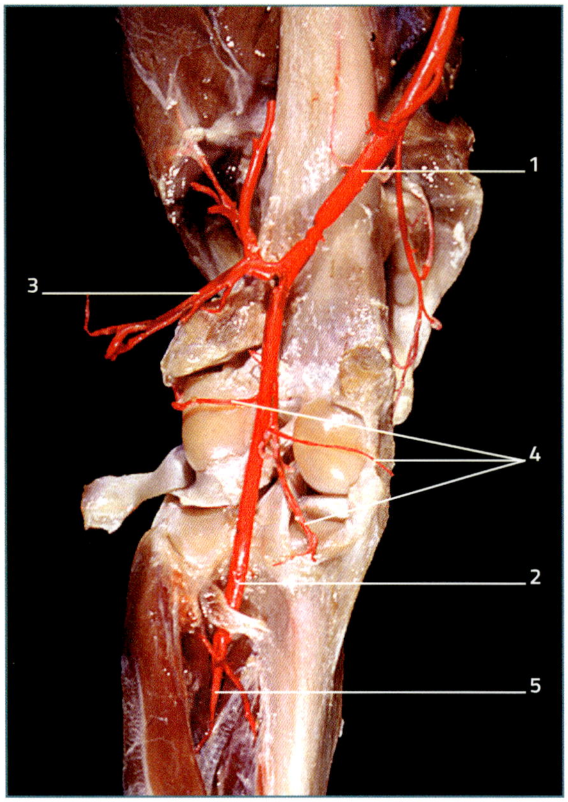

1 Femoral artery
2 Popliteal artery
3 Distal caudal femoral artery
4 Arteries of the stifle joint
5 Caudal tibial artery

It is not possible to palpate any structure in the popliteal fossa with the stifle joint in extension. It is possible to palpate the pulse of the popliteal artery with the stifle joint in flexion, although it is unlikely as the artery is very deep. As mentioned above in reference to inspection of the popliteal fossa, well defined swelling may be found at this level and requires a differential diagnosis between vascular and nerve injuries (usually of iatrogenic origin) and long-standing osteoarthritis problems.

Manoeuvres to detect intra-articular fluid

In addition to basic clues that inspection may provide to detect articular effusion, certain manoeuvres detect it more reliably.

Bulge sign

This detects small amounts of fluid which are not necessarily abnormal. In expert hands, this manoeuvre is very sensitive to detect synovial effusion. The palm of one hand is used to sweep over the medial aspect of the stifle joint from bottom to top and front to back with the intention of emptying the joint of fluid at that level. With the palm of one hand above the medial condyle of the femur and the back of the other hand flexed, pressure is applied to the lateral aspect of the stifle joint from top to bottom and back to front. If effusion is present, the displaced fluid instantly forms a bulge on the medial aspect. When synovial effusion is moderate or taut, the bulge sign is no longer valid and other manoeuvres are required.

Balloon sign

One hand is positioned with the thumb on the medial edge of the patella and the index and middle fingers on the lateral edge. The other hand repeatedly applies pressure to the suprapatellar recess. If there is effusion, the fingers holding the patella detect tapping and even movement each time pressure is applied. This is considered to be one of the most specific tests to detect synovial effusion.

Patellar ballottement

This is only considered to be useful when significant effusion is present. It is also detected when there is abundant fat in the infrapatellar fat pad or in front of the femur. This sign is performed by extending the stifle joint and using both index fingers to press on the dorsal surface of the patella. When there is effusion, the patella sinks into the synovial fluid and strikes the femur before rising again.

Manoeuvres to evaluate mobility

As noted above, there are three types of movement of the stifle joint: flexion, extension and internal and external rotation. Flexion and extension result from movement between the femur and the tibia. The quadriceps muscle is responsible for extension and influences the importance and action of the hamstring muscles during flexion. Rotation occurring when the stifle joint is in some degree of flexion includes movement of the menisci over the tibia and movement of the tibia over the femur. This rotation is performed by different muscles on the medial and lateral side.

Usually only passive mobility is examined and maximum degrees of flexion and extension are evaluated. It is very important to compare the ranges of motion of the two stifle joints.

Flexion of the stifle joint

The stifle joints must be flexed symmetrically. In passive examination both hands are used to perform maximum flexion. Maximum flexion of the stifle joint is approximately 135° from the position of extension (neutral zero method). During maximum flexion, the angle between the leg and the thigh is approximately 30°.

Extension of the stifle joint

In examination, the stifle joints are fully extended and observed to determine whether full extension is achieved with both joints. The limbs are also stretched in alternation. Extension is examined passively by checking that the popliteal fossa touches the surface of the examination table.

> If full extension is not achieved, it is advisable to regularly measure degrees of flexion in order to subsequently evaluate treatment response.

Internal and external rotation

The animal is able to perform 10° of rotation in both directions. Passive rotation is examined by using one hand to hold the femur, using the other hand to hold the tarsus and rotating the tibia inwards and outwards.

During passive range of motion testing, friction may be palpated and crunching may be heard. This is common in long-standing degenerative or inflammatory abnormalities. Pain may also be detected in extreme movements of the joint.

The specific manoeuvres for the diagnosis of rupture of the anterior cruciate ligament are explained in their respective sections below.

Arthrocentesis of the stifle joint

Detection of synovial fluid by means of inspection or different specific manoeuvres is only prudent if that fluid is subsequently drawn to be thoroughly examined and classified. With this simple manoeuvre the disease causing synovial effusion (septic or aseptic arthritis) may be diagnosed or, depending on the type of synovial fluid, the diagnosis of the disease may be informed.

Arthrocentesis of the stifle joint may be performed internally or externally (laterally or medially) with the animal in dorsal decubitus. To perform it, the patella is divided into three parts by palpation. The puncture site is where the middle third meets the upper third. The needle is positioned perpendicularly or cranially depending on whether infrapatellar puncture (lateral or medial femorotibial synovial sac) or suprapatellar puncture (femoropatellar sac) is to be performed. It is very useful to use the contralateral hand to apply pressure to the medial edge of the patella (or the lateral edge if puncturing internally) and attempt to open the patella like a book, thereby enlarging the puncture site.

Puncture may also be performed by placing the stifle joint in flexion and inserting the needle into the cranial area.

CHAPTER

2

Clinical evaluation of the stifle joint and decision-making

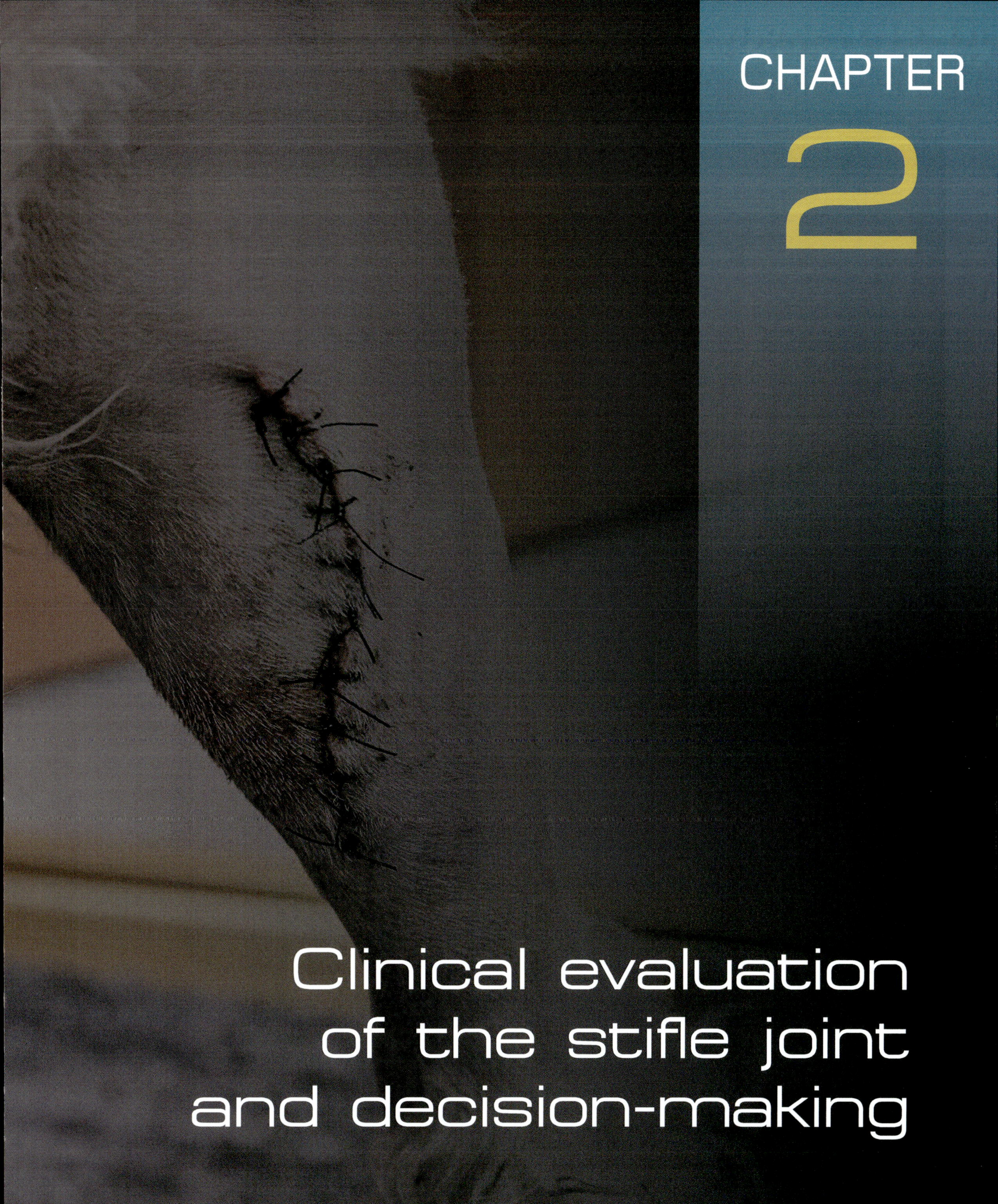

Advanced complementary diagnostic methods such as arthroscopy and magnetic resonance imaging (MRI) are very useful to definitively confirm and evaluate ligament and meniscal injuries. However, their use is justified in a limited number of cases, since in many cases a proper medical history and physical examination are sufficient to make an accurate diagnosis of injury. This chapter analyses the different aspects of the approach to clinical diagnosis of diseases of the stifle joint and describes the examination manoeuvres that may be used to determine the structure of origin in question.

The end of the chapter includes diagnostic algorithms summarising the clinical and therapeutic approach to the main diseases of the stifle joint. These are:

1. Recent injury of the stifle joint.
2. Instability of the stifle joint.
3. Chronic swelling of the stifle joint.
4. Dislocation of the stifle joint.
5. Suspected distal fracture of the femur.
6. Suspected meniscus injury.
7. Suspected fracture of the patella.
8. Dislocation of the patella.

Medical history

As always, the medical history should include as much information as possible to best delimit the problem that the animal is experiencing. Once it has been focused on the stifle joint, the most important aspects of the medical history are as follows:

- **History of prior trauma:** it must be borne in mind that the current episode may correspond to a new defect in a prior injury or a worsening of a pre-existing partial rupture.
- **Presence and rate of onset of articular effusion:** if this is significant and taut with an onset less than 24 hours ago, in many cases it indicates a serious ligament injury (of the ACL in 70 % of cases). However, it may also accompany disinsertion of the vascularised area of the menisci, osteochondral fractures, dislocations of the patella or pinching of the synovial membrane. Injuries of the avascular area of the menisci (which are more common than disinsertion), chronic femoropatellar syndromes and ligament instability which has been present for some time generally cause hydrarthrosis of slower onset.
- **Suspension of activity:** 80 % of animals that experience serious ligament injuries cannot continue their sporting activity (e.g. racing, hunting and agility events). The injury may occur while they are engaging in routine physical activity and render them unable to continue this activity; however, they are able to leave walking on all four legs with ostensible signs of lameness in the affected leg. This may be observed even in animals that suffer from locking due to meniscal folding and exhibit an antalgic gait the next day.
- **Age:** Young animals are more resistant to ligament and meniscal injuries, but not growth plate injuries, which translate to different fractures clinically classified according to the Salter–Harris system from Type I to Type V. In young animals an epiphysiolysis is more common than a ligament injury. By contrast, ligament injuries occur more often in adult animals for obvious reasons. Such injuries occur in both athletic and sedentary animals; in the latter they are due to metabolic reasons. Meniscal injuries of traumatic origin are more common in athletic animals. An overwhelming percentage of secondary meniscal injuries are due to prior ACL injuries.

Clinical examination

Examination of the patient proceeds as usual, with an organised, systematic review allowing the clinician to detect any abnormality or clinical sign that may aid in diagnosis. Once the problem has been localised in the stifle joint, this joint is comprehensively inspected.

Visual inspection

First of all, prior to physical examination, the patient is observed so that the following matters may be evaluated:

- Type of gait, presence of contracture in flexion, claudication and degree of disability.
- Bony prominences and deformities: disappearance of parapatellar grooves, lateral movement of the patella, dislocation of the stifle joint, etc.
- Ecchymosis or bruising: bleeding of immediate onset is due to direct contusion and its location may provide information on the mechanism of injury. Bleeding of late onset denotes extravasation of haemarthrosis and therefore significant capsule tearing.

Matters and signs to be evaluated in the physical examination

In the acute phase, the condition of the joint (effusion, pain, contracture, etc.) precludes full examination with tests and manoeuvres specific to ligaments and menisci. Incidentally, the former must precede the latter, since meniscal injuries are less therapeutically urgent and more difficult to reliably diagnose in the acute phase. What is most important in terms of physical examination in this acute phase is to determine the presence and amount of articular effusion and to identify specific pain points.

Articular effusion

Mild effusion, up to 10 ml, is detected by manually applying pressure to the fluid of the femoropatellar synovial sac and of the lateral and medial parapatellar groove. This produces a bulge (as the fluid protrudes) which must be attributed to effusion in the absence of oedema or significant prior infiltration. Moderate effusion, of 10–20 ml, creates resistance to pressure which is transmitted from the base of the sac to the opposite side. The patellar ballottement or tap sign is observed: the patella is separate from the lips of the trochlea of the femur due to the tension created by the fluid, and so it may sink until it touches the condyles when the examiner applies pressure to it with the fingers, then float again when the examiner releases this pressure. Severe effusion, which exceeds 20 ml, causes severe pain and functional limitation of the affected limb. An antalgic gait is observed and the joint, which is visibly bulky and swollen, remains in approximately 30° of flexion. The effusion volumes designated as moderate (10–20 ml) or severe (more than 20 ml) apply to medium-sized breeds; it must be borne in mind that these data vary depending on the size of the dog.

Pain

The absence of severe pain may be seen in the initial stages; this does not rule out the presence of a serious injury, since, for example, extensive capsuloligamentous rupture prevents the accumulation of intra-articular fluid, thereby reducing the severity of pain, and the meniscal fold itself does not lead to locking until the joint cools.

Injury diagnosis is guided by the presence of pain in specific anatomical areas, which are indicated in the part of this chapter on clinical examination manoeuvres. These manoeuvres are essential both to locate the injury and to make the prognosis.

Crepitation

A popping sound heard when the injury occurs tends to be indicative of ACL injury. If such an assessment by the owner is accompanied by articular effusion of immediate or rapid onset, the sign is pathognomonic. In serious trauma not accompanied by bone injuries, such popping with immediate severe effusion may correspond to bilateral meniscal injury. It is even possible for a horn to break free and occupy the intra-articular space. This is less common, but it cannot be ruled out. It may also correspond to dislocation of the patella or even full or partial dislocation of the stifle joint in the worst-case scenario.

Temporary joint locking

This is common in meniscal injuries and may even be observed in chronic ligament injuries, although to a lesser extent. Locking is caused by a fold in the affected part of the meniscus which, without surgery, invades the articular space and prevents free joint movement. It is accompanied by severe pain that causes an antalgic gait as the animal is unable to bear weight on the paw due to the pain caused by any movement of the stifle joint. If the clinician detects loose movement of the articular surfaces whilst examining the sedated animal, this indicates a concomitant serious ligament injury. Joint locking of meniscal origin in a patient whose owner decides against a meniscectomy may be resolved by subjecting the animal to deep sedation and analgesia and then restoring movement to the joint by repairing the fold, thereby eliminating joint locking.

Radiological examination

Usually craniocaudal and lateral X-rays of the stifle joint are taken in order to identify fractures of the patella, proximal tibia or distal femur, as well as traumatic osteochondral loose bodies or osteoligamentous avulsions. Axial X-rays may also be taken to examine the femoropatellar joint and to verify patellar or parapatellar injuries.

X-rays also provide information on osteophytes on the tibial tuberosity in ACL rupture or on the posterior tibial rim (popliteal notch) in chronic joint injuries and PCL injuries, as well as osteophytes on the trochlea of the femur and on the condyles of the femur in osteoarthritis injuries secondary to ACL ruptures. Of course, a differential diagnosis must be made in cases of concomitant stifle joint disease and patellar disease.

Therapeutic approach to soft tissue injuries

Most soft tissue injuries do not require immediate surgery and planned surgery can eventually be performed. Therefore, a puncture is initially performed to drain as much intra-articular effusion as possible as a preliminary step to relieve discomfort in animals with severe effusion. In mild cases, drainage has more disadvantages than conservative treatment due to its potential subsequent complications, deriving from infections, etc. In any case, a Robert Jones compression bandage without an accompanying posterior splint must be used, cold or similar (methyl bromide) must be applied and the patient must rest, but not be inactive, since walking within a space of 2 m^2 is considered to be ideal to maintain muscle tone, both before and after surgery.

Examination of the synovial fluid removed reveals the presence of haemarthrosis. If an intra-articular fracture is also present, within a few seconds, a fatty supernatant is observed on the surface of the blood deposited in the tube.

Examination in the acute phase

Although in theory an examination can be performed under anaesthesia at the clinic in the acute phase of the process, the authors prefer to perform the tests referred to here in this acute phase, since are more informative than tests performed under anaesthesia. The authors prefer to perform tests under anaesthesia a few days later as a final diagnosis phase, which has the value of certainty. These tests under anaesthesia confirm the prior clinical diagnosis. The prior clinical diagnosis is the important one, having provided the most reliable information based on the animal's responses, which derived from acute symptoms and were not masked by either anti-inflammatory treatments or the anaesthesia administered to the patient.

Exploratory tests of the stifle joint

This chapter shows the reader a number of clinical procedures to diagnose the different diseases that may be found in the stifle joint. It goes well beyond presenting solely the well known "anterior drawer" clinical test to describe various tests in detail, specifying the mechanical procedure to be performed by the clinician or veterinary orthopaedic surgeon, the clinical evaluation merited by the specific behaviour of the animal and the reading to be done by the clinician depending on how the animal responds to the proposed manoeuvres. Furthermore, in order to make this evaluation easier and more objective, it sets out those things to which the clinician must be attentive when performing the manoeuvres to evaluate potential disease.

The chapter is divided into two major sections: one to evaluate patellar disease and another to evaluate joint disease, strictly speaking, which focuses on examination of meniscal and ligament injuries.

Patella

Premature hardening of the femoropatellar joint is commonly observed in patellar chondropathy, patellar chondromalacia and retropatellar osteoarthritis. Unfavourable mechanical overloads on the femorotibial surface can occur due to abnormalities in the shape of the patella (dysplasia) or the surface of the femur (flattening of the lateral lip of the trochlea of the femur and trochlear hypoplasia — it is important to bear this disease in mind in straight-limbed animals whose limbs become crooked as a result of this abnormality) or malposition of the patella (elevation and medial or lateral deviation). Such unfavourable mechanical overloads can cause osteoarthritis. This must be associated with other cases inherent to the process of animal ageing and cartilage injuries (fractures and contusions), including distal fractures and premature growth plate closure not surgically treated and ultimately not orthopaedically resolved.

Therefore, recurring dislocations of the patella, inflammation associated with such dislocations and dislocations consecutive to trauma represent additional factors that can cause osteoarthritis.

Clinically, animals display retropatellar discomfort, pain due to bearing weight during forced flexion of the stifle joint and when climbing a hill or, preferably, a staircase (this objective element is essential in clinical examination); they even display discomfort when the limb itself is raised due to a feeling of instability. This is a key clinical element when making a differential diagnosis with diseases of the coxofemoral joint, which consistently also feature this antalgic gait. Such a gait is an uncommon diagnostic element in stifle joint injuries and clearly initially draws the clinician's attention to the hip.

From a clinical perspective, symptoms of patellar injury can manifest with various signs: the patella may move slightly or pain may be observed when pressure is applied to the patella, when the patella is moved or along the edges of the patella. Most of the time the apprehension test is positive. This test, which is described in detail below, involves moving the patella laterally while flexing the stifle joint. The test is positive if the animal attempts to stop the examination, generally by attempting to bite the examiner, since the pain is very severe. This test indicates not only chondropathy but also potential dislocation of the patella.

Abnormalities in the shape of the patella and the articular surface of the femur often lead to medial dislocation of the patella in small animals and lateral dislocation of the patella in large animals.

Elevation, axis abnormalities (*genu valgum*), rotational movement disorders of the tibia and capsuloligamentous weakness may also promote dislocation of the patella. In some cases these abnormalities are congenital and in other cases they are due to a lack of surgical resolution, depending on the universal orthopaedic principles of: anatomical reduction, rigid stability and early restoration of function in growth plate fractures or injuries, of both the distal femur and the proximal tibia.

"Dancing patella" test

This test is used in the diagnosis of articular effusion of the stifle joint. The clinical procedure is performed with the animal in dorsal decubitus or even standing still. One hand presses the base of the suprapatellar sac from above or from the dorsal part (depending on the position of the patient), and the other hand presses the patella from the distal part against the femur or moves it medially and laterally with gentle pressure.

The patella moves somewhat against elastic resistance and rebounds against the force applied by the clinical veterinary surgeon (thereby earning the name "dancing patella"). This can be affirmed to be a pathognomonic sign of articular effusion or synovitis, whose origin must be investigated by evaluating ligaments, menisci, etc. Obviously, there are several causes of articular effusion, but this is the most basic method of diagnosing stifle joint disease which the generalist clinical veterinary surgeon must know.

Patellar displacement test

For this test the animal is placed in dorsal decubitus; the clinician stands near the stifle joint of the patient and positions the thumb and index finger of each hand on the upper and lower half of the patella, respectively (by the dorsal and ventral area). To cause lateral movement, both thumbs move the patella above the lateral lip of the trochlea of the femur. Alternatively, the index finger moves the patella laterally. To cause medial movement, both index fingers move the patella in the opposite direction. The posterior surface of the patella can be palpated with the index fingers. If an increase in lateral movement is suspected, the same test is performed with the quadriceps muscle tense to check stability.

With the hand in the same position, traction can be applied to the patella by elevating the condyles.

Evaluation: physiologically, painless bilateral movement of the patella occurs with no crepitation or

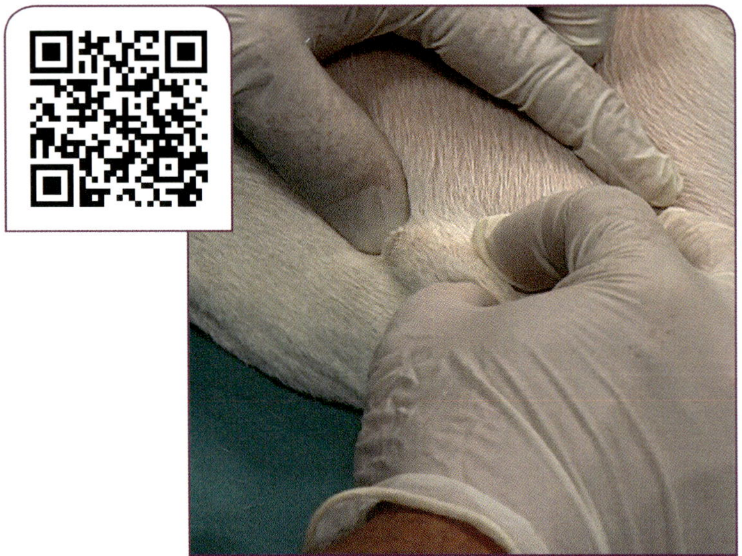

"DANCING PATELLA" TEST.

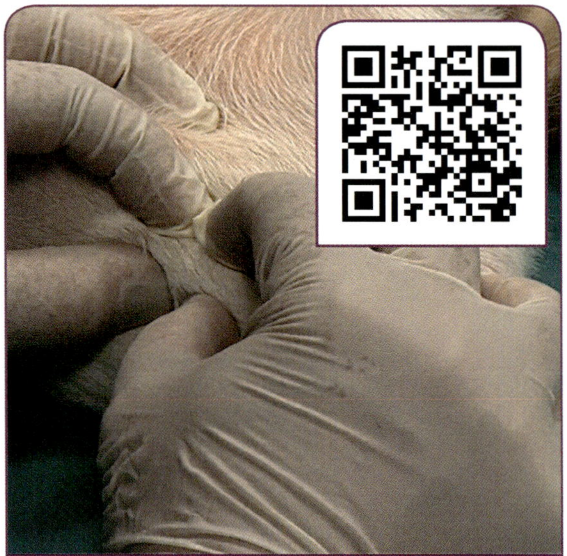

PATELLAR DISPLACEMENT TEST.

tendency towards dislocation. An increase in lateral or medial movement suggests ligament laxity, subluxation of the patella or a tendency towards dislocation. Crepitation on patellar movement indicates patellar chondropathy or retropatellar osteoarthritis.

Observation: with the hands in the same position, the test can be extended by moving the patella distally. Limited distal movement of the patella indicates shortening of the rectus femoris muscle or elevation of the patella.

Apprehension test

This test is used to evaluate dislocation of the patella. The animal is placed in dorsal decubitus, with the stifle joint extended and the thigh musculature tense. The clinician attempts to simulate dislocation by pressing the patella laterally with both thumbs and then tries to flex the stifle joint.

Evaluation: if the patella has dislocated, the animal exhibits severe pain and fear of experiencing another dislocation in extension as well as flexion.

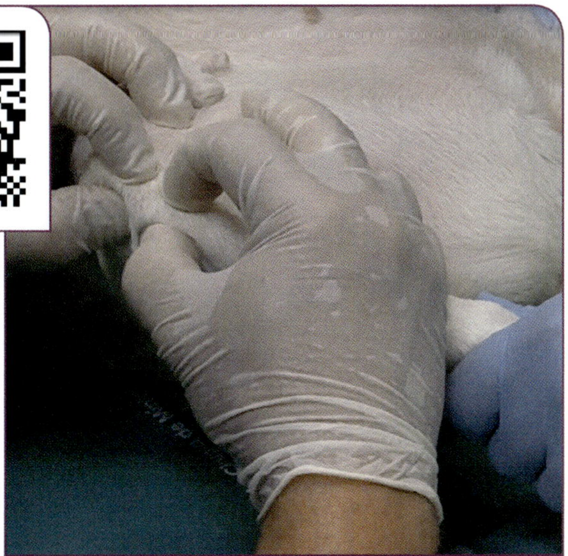

APPREHENSION TEST.

Menisci and ligaments

The menisci play an important role in joint functioning and stability; they also enable pressure to be transmitted and distributed between the femur and the tibia, thereby cushioning contusion. Meniscal injuries involve tearing or displacement of these cartilaginous discs. The medial meniscus is much more commonly affected than the lateral meniscus due to anatomical reasons.

Meniscal injuries may be degenerative or traumatic. In degenerative tissue disorders, which may occur even in young animals, injuries may be observed with day-to-day movement of the joint, with no prior history of trauma or discomfort. In stifle joint injuries, the clinician should always consider not only a meniscal abnormality but also combined injuries affecting the collateral and cruciate ligaments. All poorly treated ligament abnormalities, with instability of the stifle joint, as well as untreated hip injuries, can trigger meniscal injuries. The main symptoms of injuries of the meniscus are progressive pain depending on weight-bearing, which decreases with movement, and irritative phenomena.

There are a number of diagnostic indications for meniscal injuries. Function tests are based on causing pain by pressure, traction or pinching of the meniscus.

Performing a single test to evaluate the menisci is rarely useful; in general, a combination of several tests is required to make a diagnosis.

Rotation test

The patient is placed in dorsal decubitus and both the stifle joint and the hip joint are fully flexed. With the stifle joint in one hand and the paw in the other, the clinician rotates the thigh externally or internally, holds the limb in this position and extends it to 90°.

Evaluation: pain that occurs during extension of the stifle joint in external rotation and in abduction of the thigh indicates an injury of the medial meniscus. By contrast, pain in internal rotation indicates an injury of the lateral meniscus. When elevation is present due to a bucket-handle tear of the posterior horn, a jutting or popping in the joint is detected in pronounced flexion. Right-angle jutting indicates an injury of the middle portion of the meniscus.

Observation: full flexion of the limb to 0°, external rotation and slow extension of the stifle joint are used to observe the condition of the medial meniscus.

Payr's test

The patient is placed in dorsal decubitus. The clinician holds the stifle joint in place with the left hand and uses the thumb to palpate the lateral aspect of the joint and the index finger to palpate the medial aspect of the joint. The clinician holds the tarsal joint in place with the right hand. With the stifle joint in maximum flexion, the clinician performs external rotation of the limb as far as possible and then gentle adduction (varus movement).

Evaluation: pain in the medial and dorsal joint interline indicates a disorder of the medial meniscus (of the posterior horn, which can be compressed with the movement manoeuvre). In addition, the posterior horn of the lateral meniscus may be examined by performing internal rotation and abduction of the limb (valgus movement).

Steinmann I sign

The patient is placed in dorsal decubitus. The clinician uses the left hand to hold the flexed stifle joint in place and the right hand to hold the limb, then quickly forcibly rotates the limb inwards and outwards.

Evaluation: pain in the medial joint interline during sudden external rotation suggests a disorder of the medial meniscus; such pain occurring in the lateral joint interline during internal rotation indicates an abnormality of the lateral meniscus.

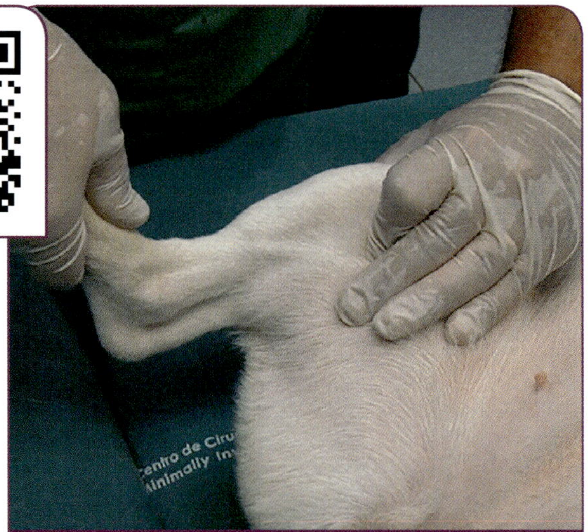

ROTATION TEST.

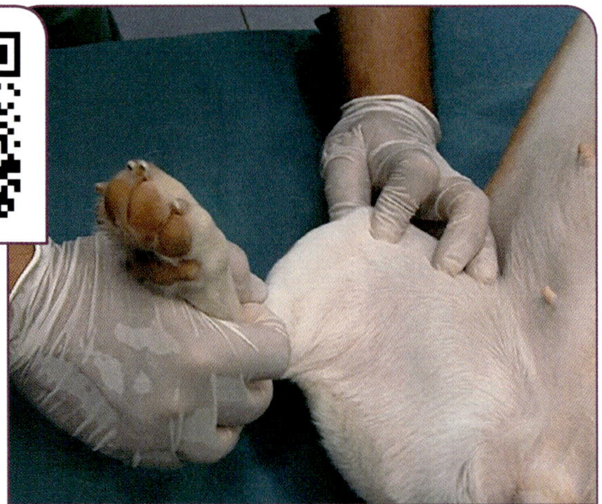

PAYR'S TEST.

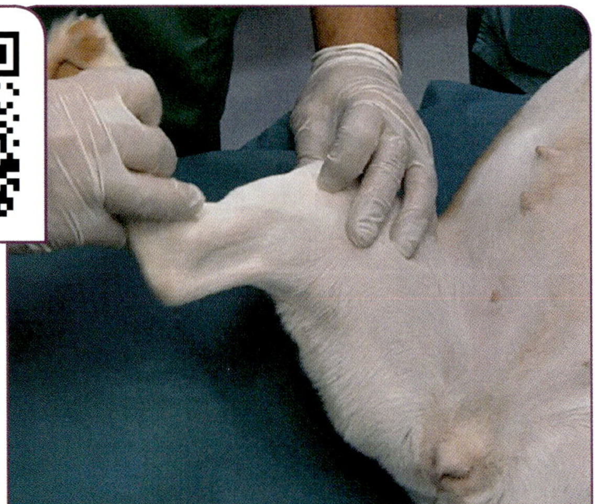

STEINMANN I SIGN.

Steinmann II sign

The patient is positioned in dorsal decubitus. The left hand of the clinician holds the stifle joint while palpating the interarticular line. The right hand holds the limb above the lateral and medial malleoli. The clinician performs external rotation and internal rotation of the limb with the thigh held in place, and flexes and extends it axially on a slight incline.

Evaluation: pain on the internal or external aspect of the joint interline indicates an injury of the meniscus. When pressure is applied to the interline, pain moves towards the medial and dorsal part up to the medial collateral ligament during flexion and slight external rotation of the stifle joint, and moves forwards during extension of the stifle joint. With internal rotation of the limb, if an abnormality of the lateral meniscus is suspected, pain when pressure is applied moves forwards in extension of the stifle joint and backwards in flexion.

Observation: although the test can be used to detect injuries of the lateral meniscus, it is particularly informative in injuries of the medial meniscus.

Finochietto's sign (jump sign)

This method is used to confirm a simultaneous injury of the ACL and meniscus. It consists of the anterior drawer test with the stifle joint in 90° of flexion.

Evaluation: in ACL rupture, the anterior drawer test in 90° of flexion involves distal movement of the tibia. During the anterior drawer movement the condyle of the femur rises up to the posterior horn of the medial meniscus due to a lack of ligament suspension. A positive Finochietto's test involves audible crunching and/or palpable jutting. When the tibia is pressed dorsally, the femoral condyle slides back downwards from the posterior horn of the medial meniscus. Sometimes, after a positive Finochietto's sign has been elicited, the dislocation of the meniscus must be reduced; in this case, complete posterior detachment of the medial meniscus and/or a longitudinal ("bucket handle") tear must be suspected.

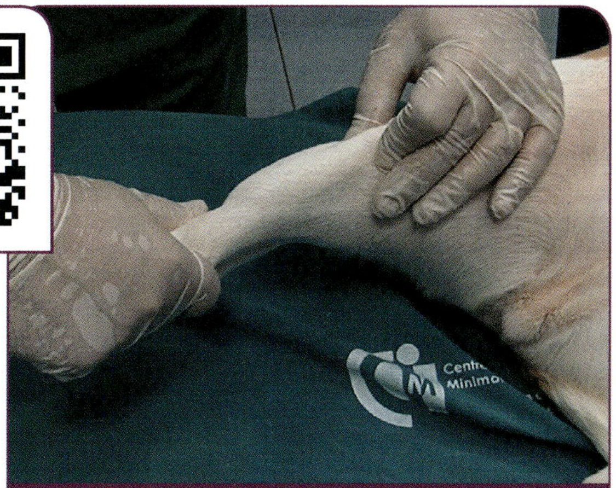

STEINMANN II SIGN.

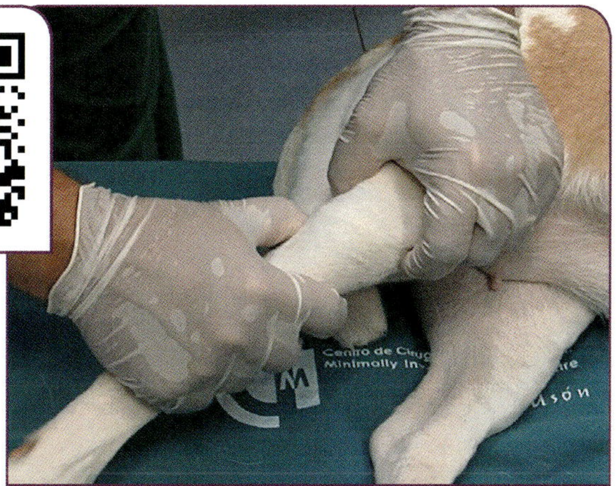

FINOCHIETTO'S SIGN.

Observation: an abnormality in the posterior horn of the medial meniscus or its capsular suspension (which is less flexible and loose than that of the lateral meniscus) in relation to an ACL insufficiency involves an abnormality in the rolling–sliding mechanism of the stifle joint, which occurs following rupture of the cruciate ligament. That rupture and that failure in the mechanism lead to a tear in the posterior horn of the medial meniscus.

In summary, in the anterior drawer test the clinician places the thumb of the right hand on the lateral sesamoid bone of the condyle of the femur and the index finger of the same hand on the patella to stabilise the femur. At the same time, the clinician places the thumb of the left hand caudal to the head of the fibula and the index finger of this same hand on the tibial crest, then attempts to move the tibia cranially.

Other structures

Osteochondritis dissecans test: pressure and flexion of the stifle joint

This test is used to detect osteochondritis dissecans in the medial condyle of the femur. The clinician holds the stifle joint above the patella with one hand while palpating the internal joint interline.

Evaluation: in osteochondritis dissecans joint discomfort may occur when pressure is applied to the joint by means of flexion (20°–30°) or local palpation with the fingers; this discomfort is reduced when the limb is rotated externally.

Observation: osteochondritis dissecans is characterised by aseptic necrosis limited to the area of subchondral bone of the articular surface, with abnormality of the cartilage covering it. In more advanced stages, the cartilage and adjacent bone detach; this produces an arthrolith (a loose body in a joint), also known as a "joint mouse". The joint cavity in which the fragment of bone and cartilage is housed is called a "mouse bed". The presence of this condition in young animals, articular effusion and pain in the stifle joint indicate osteochondritis dissecans.

Slocum's test

The animal is placed in lateral decubitus on the healthy side, with the hip and stifle joints in flexion, and the injured limb is held in extension with slight internal rotation of the paw. In this position, the weight of the limb exerts slight valgus pressure (abduction). The clinician remains behind the patient and uses one hand to hold the thigh and the other hand to hold the head of the tibia while palpating the head of the fibula with the thumb or index finger.

The authors have decided to include this test not only due to its clinical value but also as a small posthumous tribute to Dr Slocum Jr, the inventor of the TPLO technique described in a chapter of this book. The test referred to here, however, was invented by his father, Dr Slocum Sr, a renowned human orthopaedic surgeon in the United States.

Evaluation: if the ACL is affected, the head of the femur subluxates forwards in a position close to extension. Flexion of the femur of approximately 30° reduces subluxation of the head of the tibia dorsally.

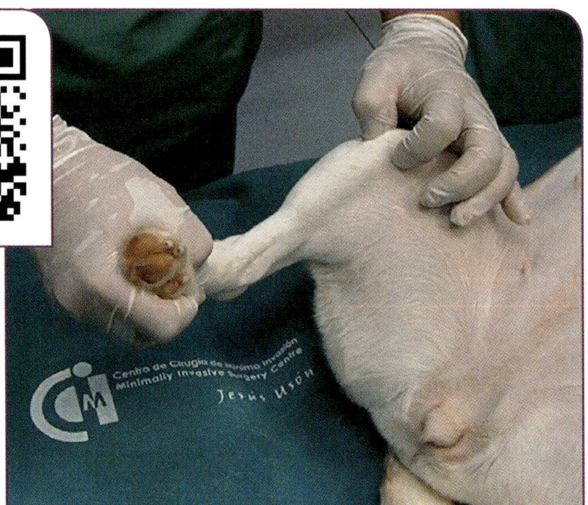

OSTEOCHONDRITIS DISSECANS TEST.

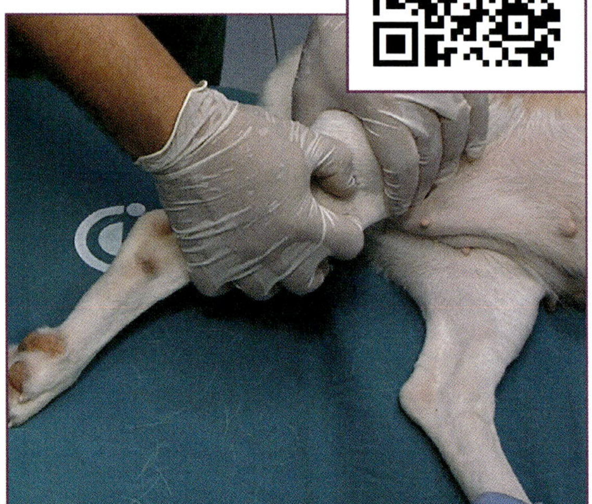

SLOCUM'S TEST.

Henderson and Milton's test: tibial thrust

This is a tibial compression test: with one hand, the stifle joint is held in place with the index finger on the tibial crest; with the other hand, the tarsus is flexed to attempt to demonstrate cranial movement of the tibia.

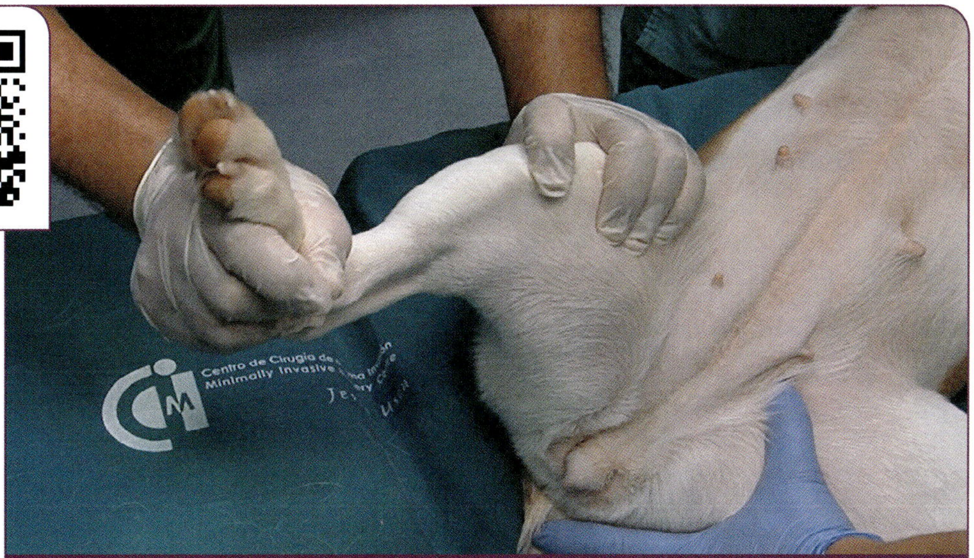

HENDERSON AND MILTON'S TEST: TIBIAL THRUST.

Algorithms for decision-making

A number of algorithms for clinical examination of the stifle joint are presented below. Some mechanisms of action considered most practical for the clinician examining the stifle joint are explained. Each is performed to arrive at an accurate diagnosis of the injury (Fig. 1).

These are:

1. Recent injury of the stifle joint.
2. Instability of the stifle joint.
3. Chronic swelling of the stifle joint.
4. Dislocation of the stifle joint.
5. Suspected distal fracture of the femur.
6. Suspected meniscus injury.
7. Suspected fracture of the patella.
8. Dislocation of the patella.

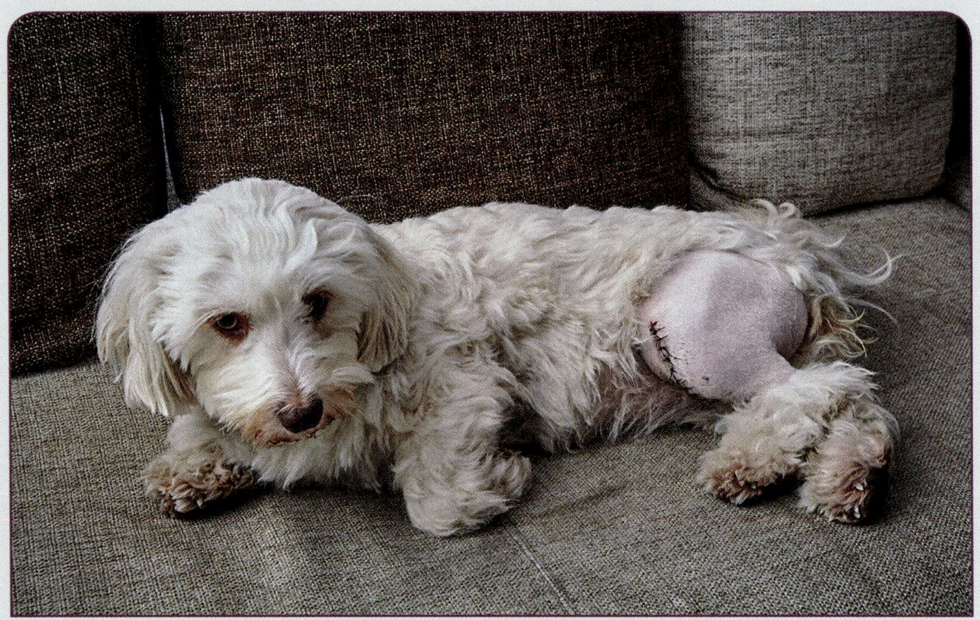

FIGURE 1. Havanese dog having undergone surgery for dislocation of the patella in the left stifle joint (Peter Mayer Photos, Shutterstock.com).

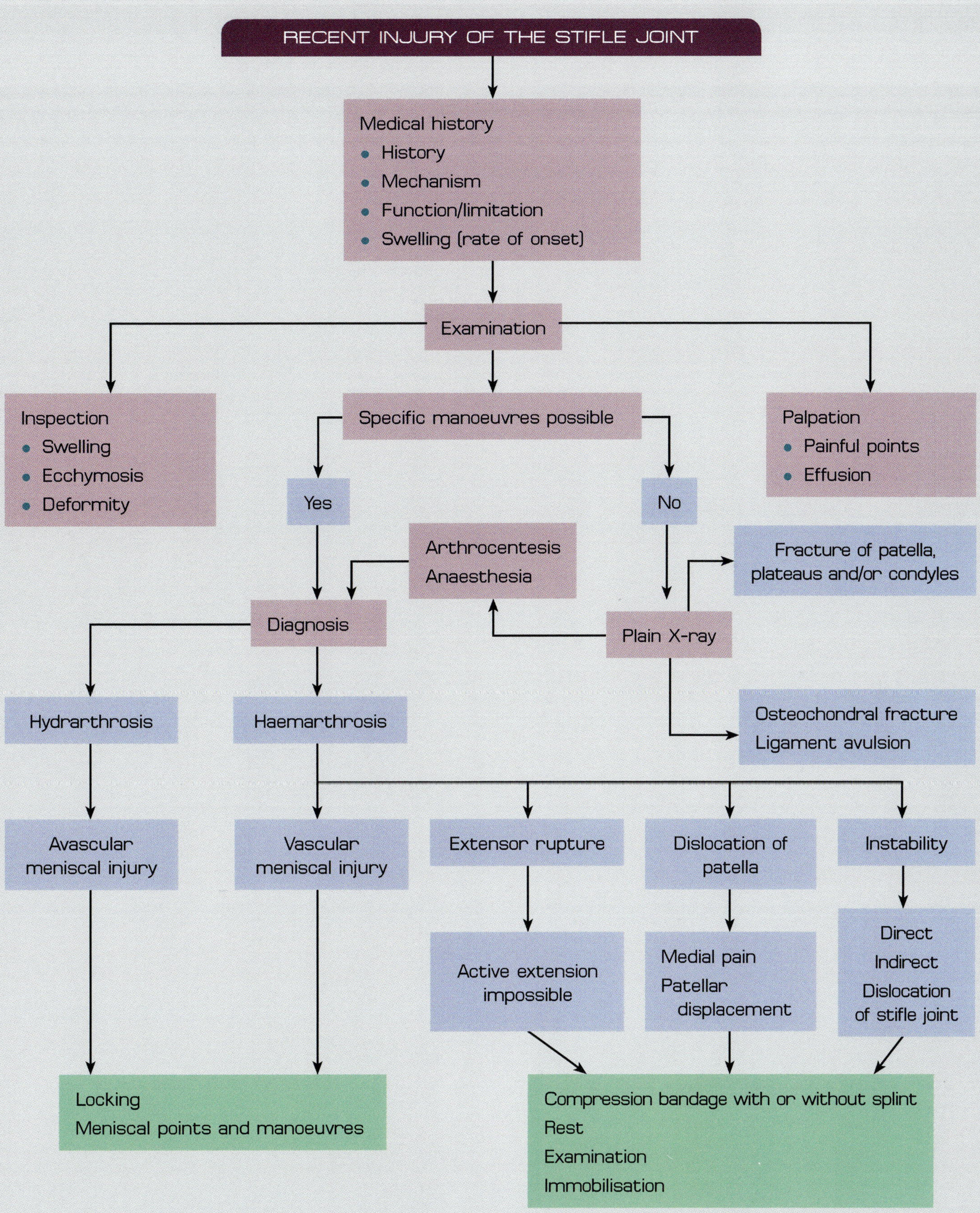
RECENT INJURY OF THE STIFLE JOINT
Medical history
History
Mechanism
Function/limitation
Swelling (rate of onset)
Examination
Inspection
Swelling
Ecchymosis
Deformity
Specific manoeuvres possible
Palpation
Painful points
Effusion
Yes
No
Arthrocentesis
Anaesthesia
Fracture of patella, plateaus and/or condyles
Diagnosis
Plain X-ray
Hydrarthrosis
Haemarthrosis
Osteochondral fracture
Ligament avulsion
Avascular meniscal injury
Vascular meniscal injury
Extensor rupture
Dislocation of patella
Instability
Active extension impossible
Medial pain
Patellar displacement
Direct
Indirect
Dislocation of stifle joint
Locking
Meniscal points and manoeuvres
Compression bandage with or without splint
Rest
Examination
Immobilisation

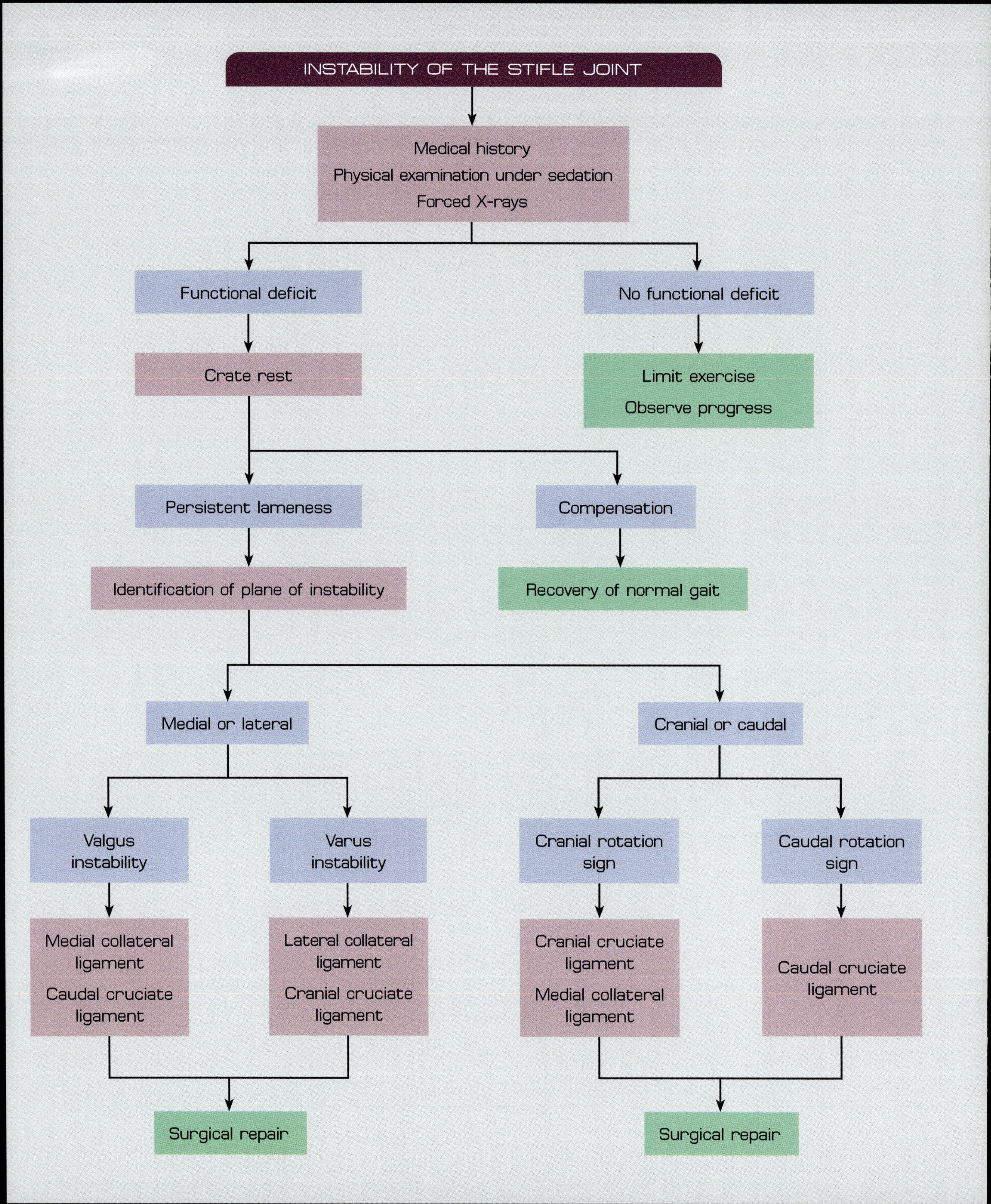
INSTABILITY OF THE STIFLE JOINT
Medical history
Physical examination under sedation
Forced X-rays
Functional deficit
No functional deficit
Crate rest
Limit exercise
Observe progress
Persistent lameness
Compensation
Identification of plane of instability
Recovery of normal gait
Medial or lateral
Cranial or caudal
Valgus instability
Varus instability
Cranial rotation sign
Caudal rotation sign
Medial collateral ligament
Caudal cruciate ligament
Lateral collateral ligament
Cranial cruciate ligament
Cranial cruciate ligament
Medial collateral ligament
Caudal cruciate ligament
Surgical repair
Surgical repair

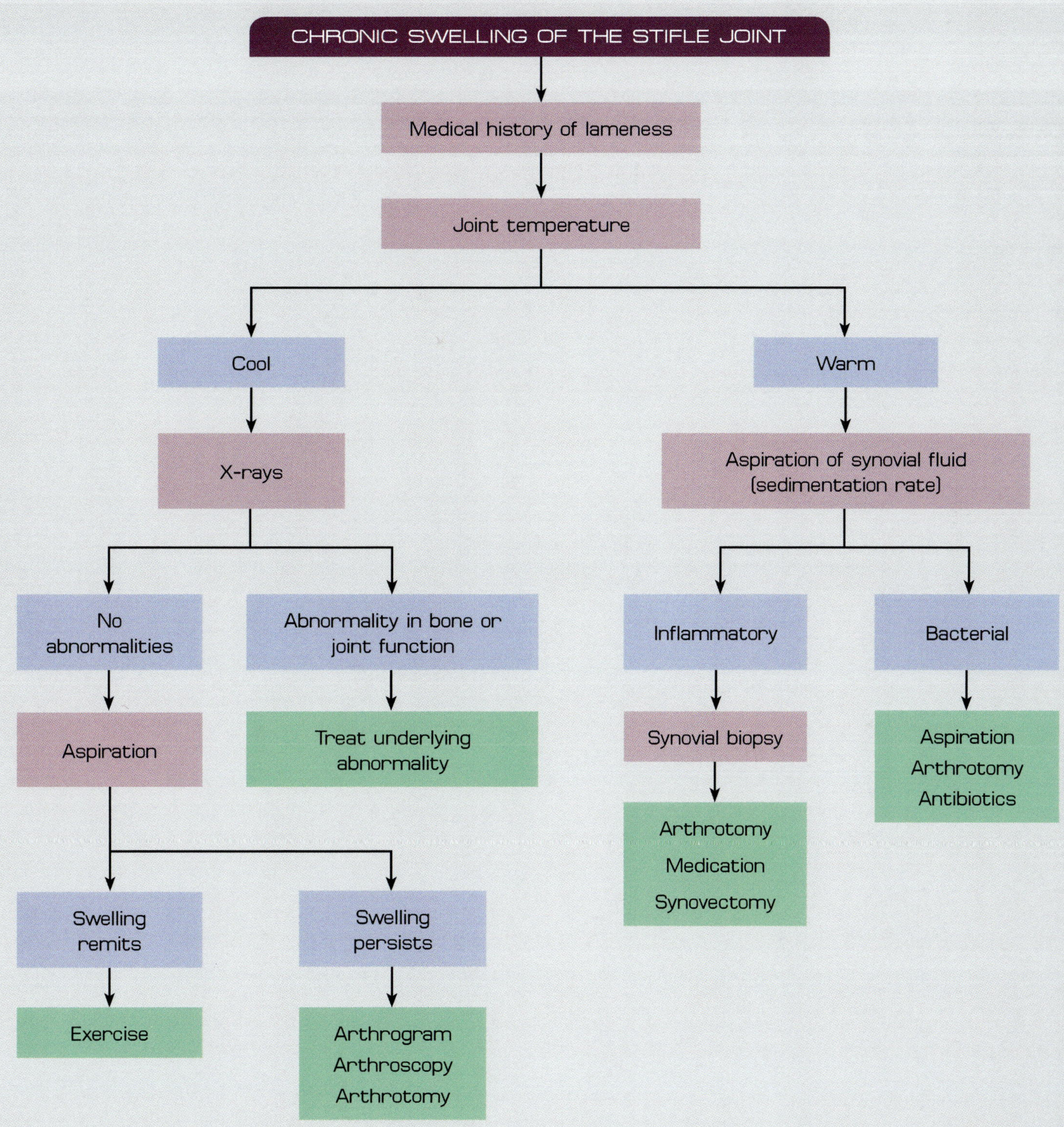
CHRONIC SWELLING OF THE STIFLE JOINT
Medical history of lameness
Joint temperature
Cool
Warm
X-rays
Aspiration of synovial fluid (sedimentation rate)
No abnormalities
Abnormality in bone or joint function
Inflammatory
Bacterial
Aspiration
Treat underlying abnormality
Synovial biopsy
Aspiration
Arthrotomy
Antibiotics
Arthrotomy
Medication
Synovectomy
Swelling remits
Swelling persists
Exercise
Arthrogram
Arthroscopy
Arthrotomy

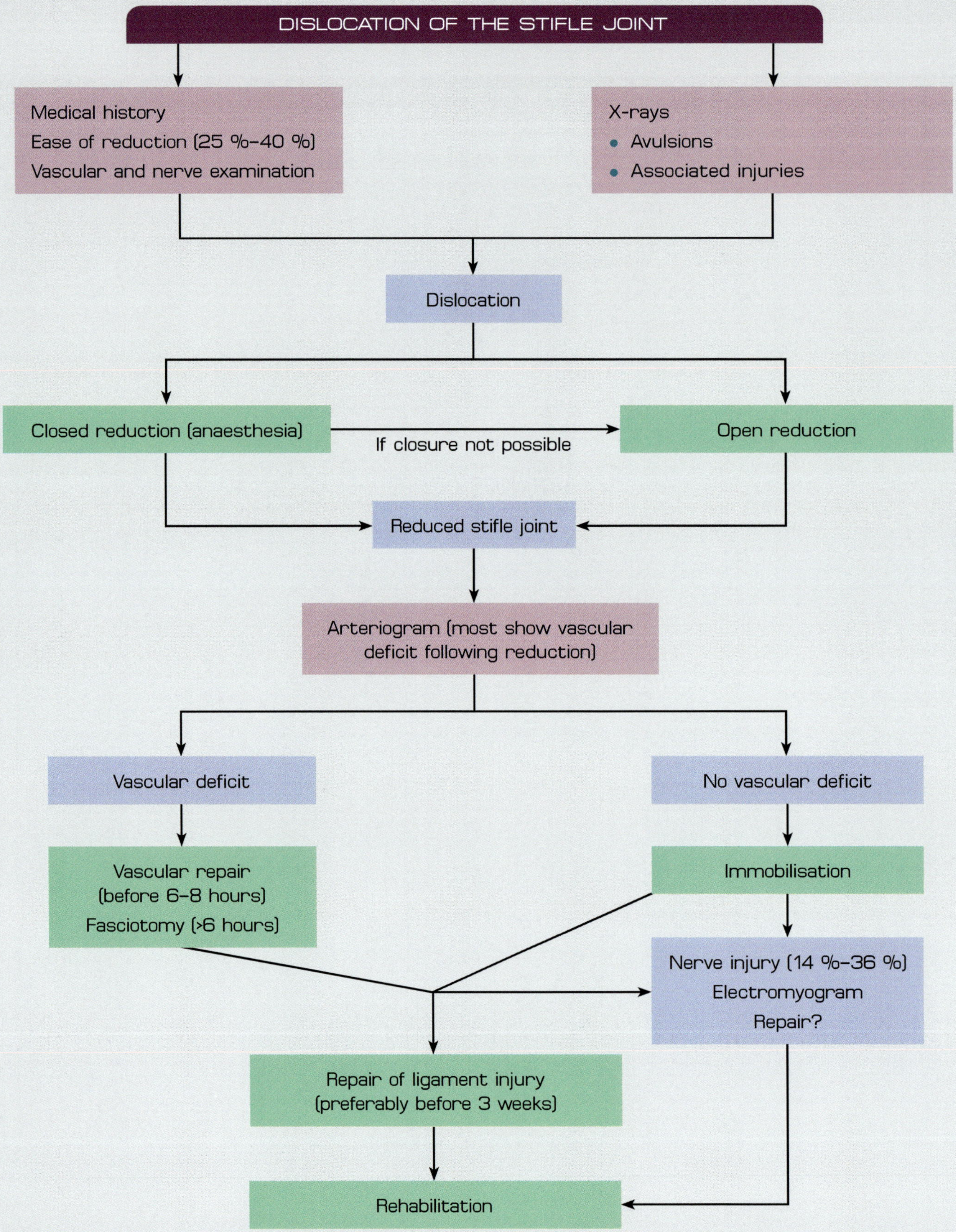
DISLOCATION OF THE STIFLE JOINT
Medical history
Ease of reduction (25 %–40 %)
Vascular and nerve examination
X-rays
Avulsions
Associated injuries
Dislocation
Closed reduction (anaesthesia)
If closure not possible
Open reduction
Reduced stifle joint
Arteriogram (most show vascular deficit following reduction)
Vascular deficit
No vascular deficit
Vascular repair (before 6–8 hours)
Fasciotomy (>6 hours)
Immobilisation
Nerve injury (14 %–36 %)
Electromyogram
Repair?
Repair of ligament injury (preferably before 3 weeks)
Rehabilitation

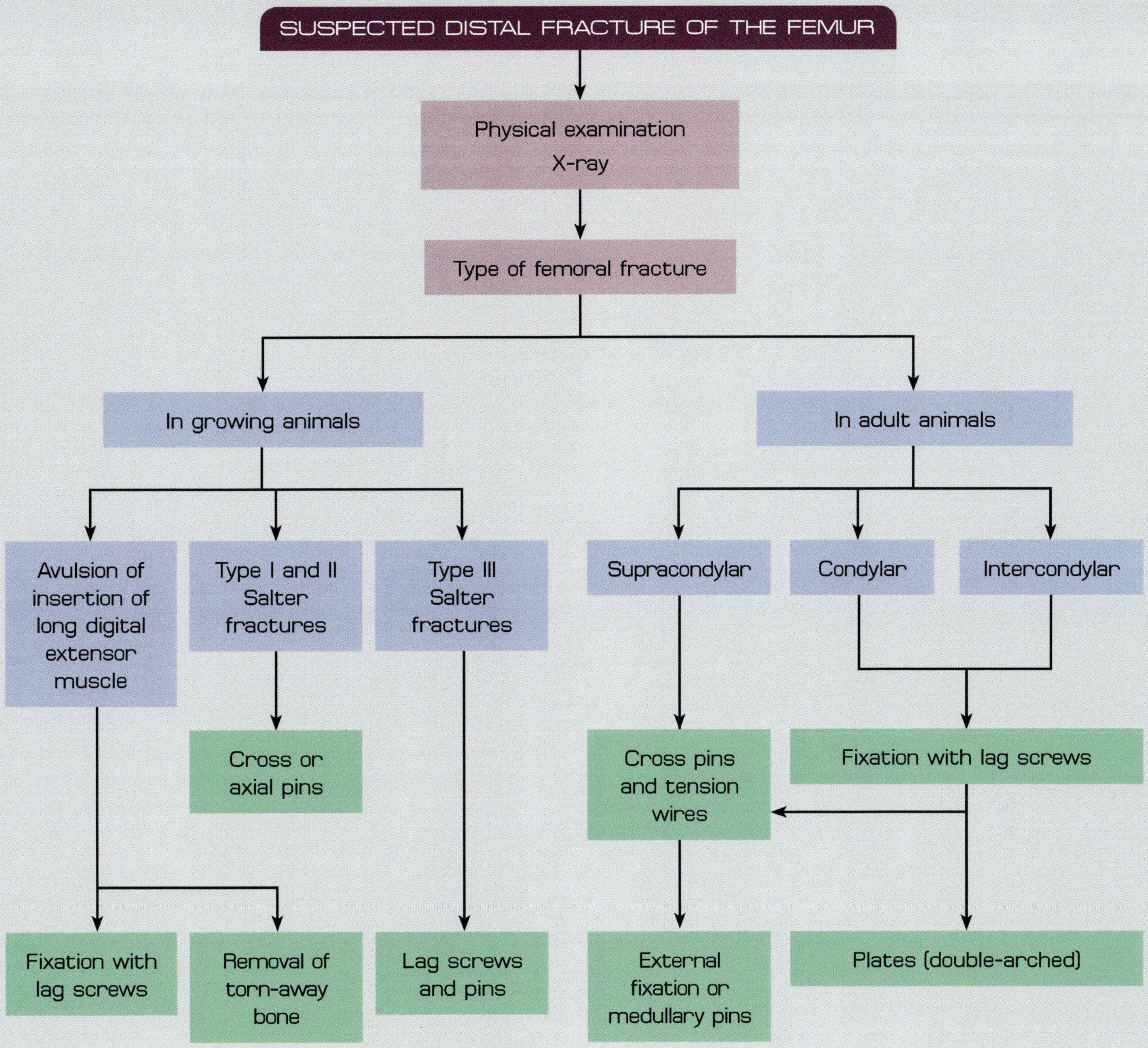
SUSPECTED DISTAL FRACTURE OF THE FEMUR
Physical examination X-ray
Type of femoral fracture
In growing animals
In adult animals
Avulsion of insertion of long digital extensor muscle
Type I and II Salter fractures
Type III Salter fractures
Supracondylar
Condylar
Intercondylar
Cross or axial pins
Cross pins and tension wires
Fixation with lag screws
Fixation with lag screws
Removal of torn-away bone
Lag screws and pins
External fixation or medullary pins
Plates (double-arched)

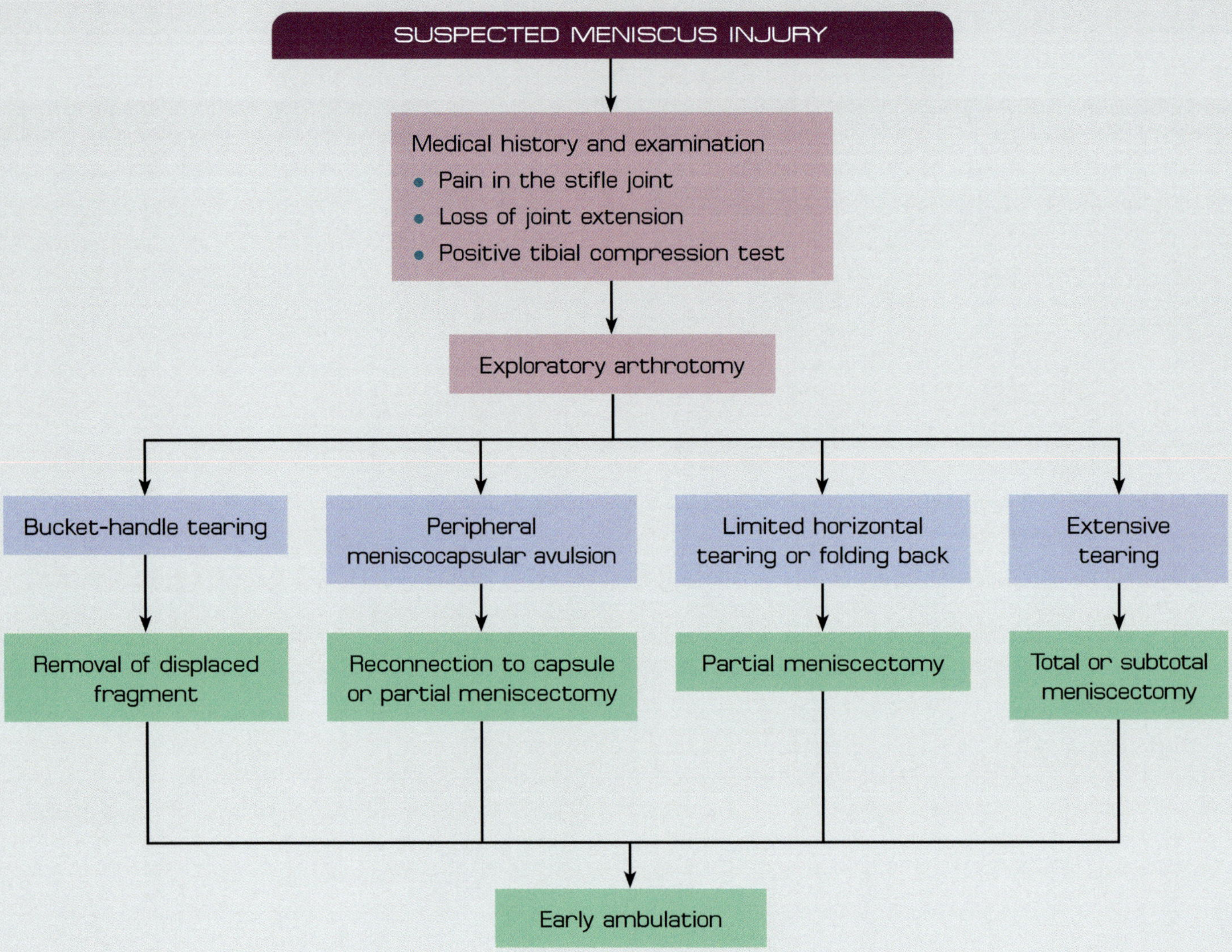
SUSPECTED MENISCUS INJURY
Medical history and examination
Pain in the stifle joint
Loss of joint extension
Positive tibial compression test
Exploratory arthrotomy
Bucket-handle tearing
Peripheral meniscocapsular avulsion
Limited horizontal tearing or folding back
Extensive tearing
Removal of displaced fragment
Reconnection to capsule or partial meniscectomy
Partial meniscectomy
Total or subtotal meniscectomy
Early ambulation

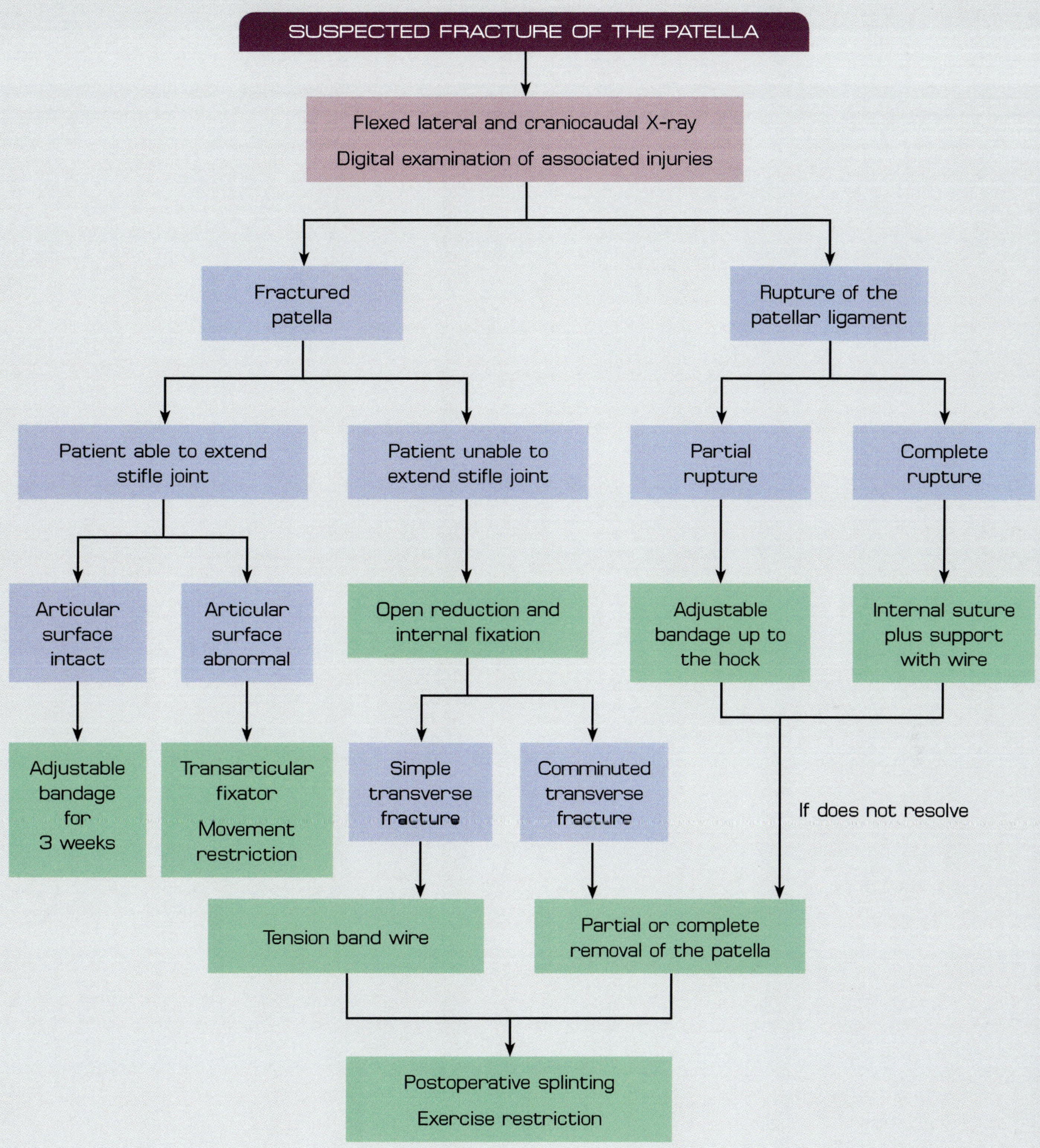
SUSPECTED FRACTURE OF THE PATELLA
Flexed lateral and craniocaudal X-ray
Digital examination of associated injuries
Fractured patella
Rupture of the patellar ligament
Patient able to extend stifle joint
Patient unable to extend stifle joint
Partial rupture
Complete rupture
Articular surface intact
Articular surface abnormal
Open reduction and internal fixation
Adjustable bandage up to the hock
Internal suture plus support with wire
Adjustable bandage for 3 weeks
Transarticular fixator
Movement restriction
Simple transverse fracture
Comminuted transverse fracture
If does not resolve
Tension band wire
Partial or complete removal of the patella
Postoperative splinting
Exercise restriction

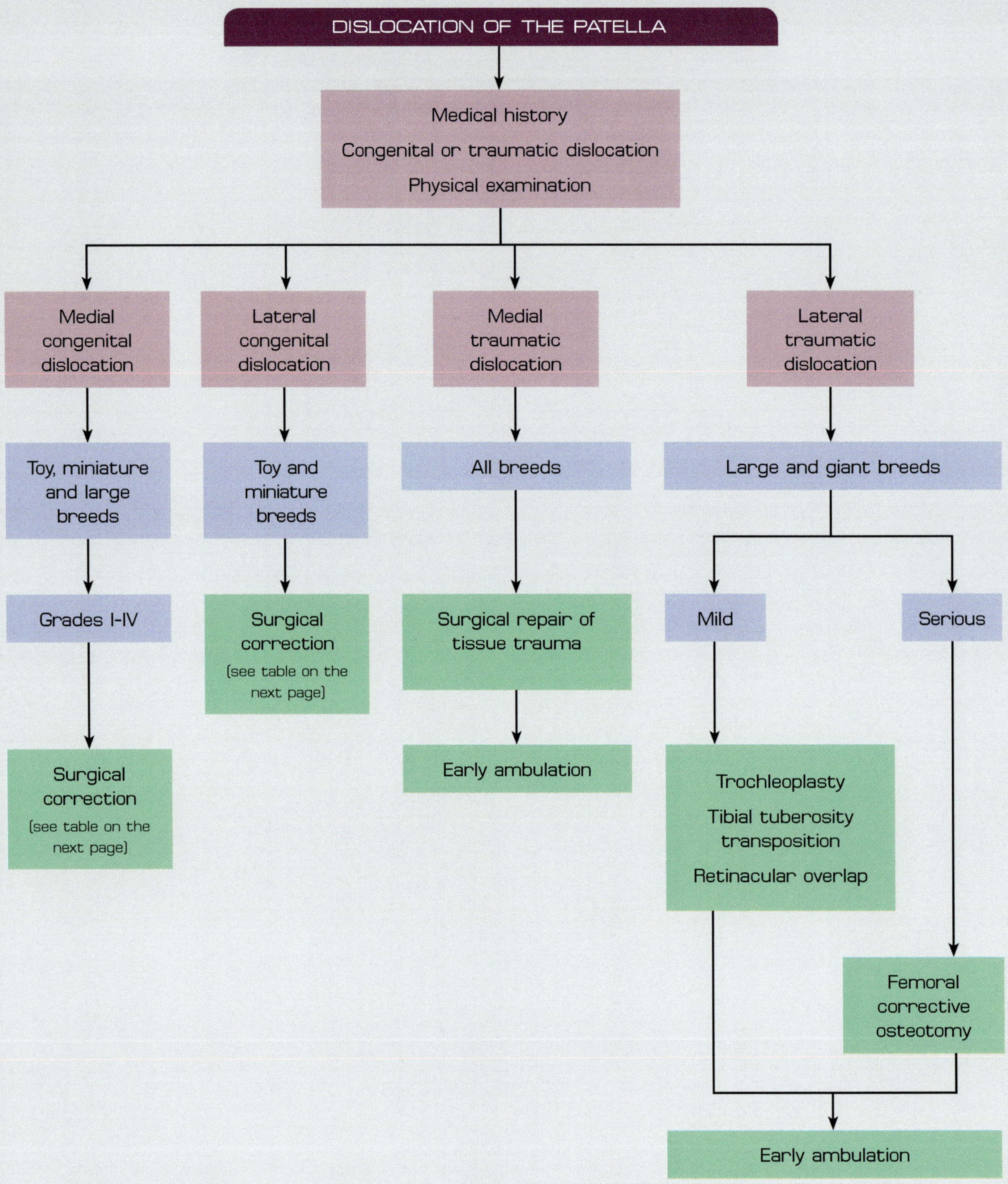
DISLOCATION OF THE PATELLA
Medical history
Congenital or traumatic dislocation
Physical examination
Medial congenital dislocation
Lateral congenital dislocation
Medial traumatic dislocation
Lateral traumatic dislocation
Toy, miniature and large breeds
Toy and miniature breeds
All breeds
Large and giant breeds
Grades I-IV
Surgical correction (see table on the next page)
Surgical repair of tissue trauma
Mild
Serious
Surgical correction (see table on the next page)
Early ambulation
Trochleoplasty
Tibial tuberosity transposition
Retinacular overlap
Femoral corrective osteotomy
Early ambulation

Surgical correction of medial congenital dislocation and lateral congenital dislocation

Grade	Medial congenital dislocation	Lateral congenital dislocation
Grade I	• Medial retinacular release. • Lateral retinacular overlap. • Fixation of the tibial tuberosity to the lateral sesamoid bone to prevent rotation of the tibia (lateral antirotational suture).	• Medial retinacular overlap. • Fixation of the tibial tuberosity to the medial sesamoid bone to prevent rotation of the tibia (medial antirotational suture).
Grade II	• Lateral tibial tuberosity transposition. • Medial desmotomy. • Medial retinacular release. • Lateral retinacular overlap. • Trochleoplasty, if the patella is unstable.	• Medial tibial tuberosity transposition. • Lateral desmotomy. • Medial retinacular overlap. • Trochleoplasty. • Medial antirotational sutures.
Grade III	• Tibial tuberosity transposition. • Medial desmotomy. • Trochleoplasty. • Lateral retinacular overlap. • Medial antirotational sutures.	As in Grade II.
Grade IV	As in Grade III together with: • Release of the quadriceps muscle. • Osteotomy of the tibia and femur.	—

CHAPTER

3

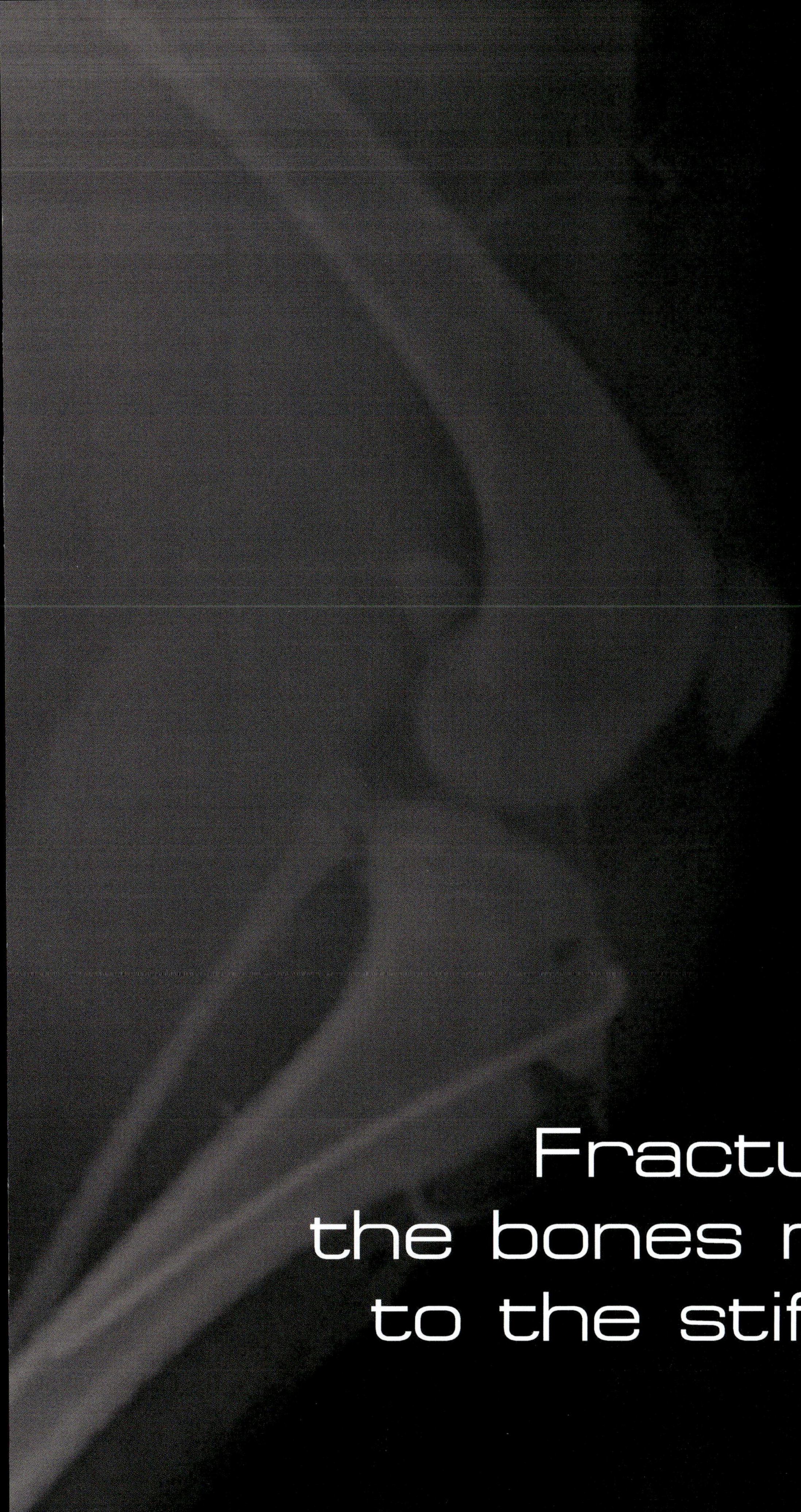

Fractures of the bones related to the stifle joint

Fractures of the distal end of the femur

These include injuries in the distal or condylar epiphyseal area and in the metaphyseal or supracondylar area, and account for approximately 7 % of all femoral fractures. The bone structures in this area are very strong, although they may weaken with age or in young animals that experience high-energy trauma with bone deformity due to bone elasticity and growth plate weakness.

The condyles, which project caudally relative to the diaphysis of the femur, widen caudally and appear asymmetrical in profile. Thus the articular plane is on a slight incline (around 24°) relative to the horizontal plane. On the cranial aspect of the joint, the suprapatellar recess separates the tendon of the quadriceps muscle from the femur. This allows them to properly slide over one another to ensure flexion and extension of the stifle joint.

The action of the quadriceps femoris muscle and the hamstring muscles tends to shorten fractures, while the gastrocnemius muscles, which originate in the supracondylar tubercles, cause the distal fragment to rotate in flexion, thereby increasing deformities. When the condyles are separated by the fracture line, they also tend to rotate independently of one another.

Classes of distal femoral fractures

Depending on the fracture line, these injuries are categorised according to the classification system of the *Arbeitsgemeinschaft für Osteosynthesefragen* (AO), an association for the study of internal fixation. However, in daily clinical practice the classification proposed here is more extensive, perhaps less academic but more intuitive and practical.

Fractures of the femur close to the stifle joint are as follows:

- Supracondylar fractures.
- Fractures in the growth plate area (Salter–Harris Types I-V).
- Intercondylar fractures (*T* or *Y*).
- Fractures of the femoral condyle (unicondylar).

Aetiology of the injury

The most common injuries (75 %) are due to high-energy trauma, accidents, falls, etc. The remaining 25 % are due to low-energy injuries in older animals. In the former group, greater joint impairment and a high number of injuries associated with vascularisation, musculature and tendons of insertion are observed. Such injuries of this joint are quite common.

Clinical examination

In patients with multiple trauma that come to the clinic with a great deal of commotion and shock, clinical examinations and complementary X-rays of the distal femur (for example the hip), the stifle joint itself and the proximal femur must be performed, both to evaluate osteoarticular integrity and to rule out potential vascular injuries and compartment syndromes.

Compartment syndrome is a serious condition that occurs when structures (mainly muscle structures) housed in a compartment delimited by a fascia become inflamed due to trauma. This leads to an increase in pressure inside of this muscle space since the fascia is almost entirely unable to expand and accommodate the inflamed structures. When the increase in pressure is high and prolonged over time, it may end up injuring structures housed in this compartment such as nerves and muscles. It may also end up causing problems in muscle perfusion. Similarly, if immediate measures are not taken, the muscle or muscle group of the affected compartment may end up developing a contracture and losing its function. Amputation may even be necessary.

This is especially important in high-energy injuries in young animals. It is also of particular importance to remember that during a reparative surgical procedure soft tissues must be treated with extreme care and their function must be checked before they are closed in layers.

Radiological examination

Radiological evaluation of distal fractures of the femur is traditionally done with plain X-rays in the usual craniocaudal and laterolateral projections (Fig. 1). As a general rule, oblique projections must be taken if fractures affect the intercondylar area. In these cases, ideally, a computed tomography (CT) scan should be performed.

As a first sign, it must be borne in mind that any widening of the articular space relative to the contralateral stifle joint may be considered to be pathological.

CT scanning, which has already been implemented to a certain extent at veterinary centres specialising in orthopaedic surgery and all university hospitals, is useful in preoperative evaluation of fractures and aids enormously in properly planning surgical treatment.

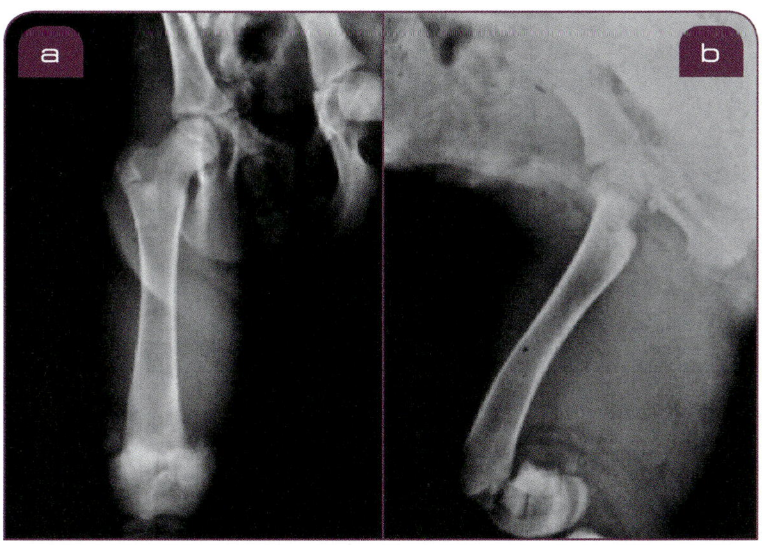

FIGURE 1. Distal growth plate fracture of the femur in craniocaudal projection (a) and laterolateral projection (b).

Treatment

As always, the objectives of treatment are to preserve the limb and recover its function and, more specifically in this case, the function of the stifle joint. This requires:

- Prior detection and treatment of vascular and nerve injuries and complications.
- Suitable alignment of the affected bone elements to restore the relationship between the mechanical and anatomical axes as well as the 24° incline of the interline so that the biomechanics of the joint are the same as they were before the fracture.
- Anatomical reconstruction of the articular surface to prevent excessive stress on the cartilage which would end up eroding it and causing post-traumatic osteoarthritis.
- Prevention of the onset of stiffness due to capsuloligamentous fibrosis or adhesions, and limitation of cartilage impairment by means of monitored and early restoration of function.

Ultimately, the characteristics of any osteosynthesis — anatomical reduction, rigid stability and early restoration of function — must be achieved.

Due to special anatomical features in terms of muscle action and fragment morphology, although it may be more or less easy to achieve alignment of the focal point of the fracture, it is not so easy to achieve maintenance in rigid stability, especially in *T* fractures.

In elderly patients, ossification is slow and not always satisfactory. In any case, clinical experience has shown that surgical treatment by means of stable internal fixation that is properly indicated and performed and allows early mobilisation yields better functional results than the conservative treatments currently rejected by the scientific community.

Although these fractures do not represent an emergency if no vascular or nerve complications are present, the

Osteosynthesis indications and contraindications

Absolute indications

- Associated vascular injury.
- Other ipsilateral or contralateral osteoarticular injuries.
- Open fractures (external fixation).
- Nonreducible displaced fractures:
  - Supracondylar fractures.
  - Fractures in the growth plate area (Salter–Harris Types I-V).
  - Intercondylar fractures (*T* or *Y*).
  - Fractures of the femoral condyle (unicondylar).

Contraindications

- Patients with a very high surgical risk.
- Fractures with serious rupture in which direct arthrodesis must be considered.
- Lack of resources, experience or both.

best results are obtained within the first 24 to 48 hours, once the animal has been biomechanically stabilised and all other injuries, if any, have been brought under control. The principles of osteosynthesis in these fractures are:

- Preoperative analysis by superimposing the implants to be used on an X-ray of the fracture and performing simultaneous comparison to the healthy side: this aids in planning the surgery, in particular when osteosynthesis plates are used as it is helpful in shaping them before and after sterilisation.
- Careful handling of soft tissues, particularly connections among bone fragments, to prevent loss of their vascularisation which would lead to necrosis and subsequent sequestering of the affected fragment.
- Anatomical reduction of the articular surfaces.
- Reduction by indirect procedures such as traction from the diaphyseal part of the femur, thereby minimising direct handling for purposes of alignment in case multiple fragments are present. Maximum accuracy in reduction must not be pursued at the expense of excessive handling which may cause thrombosis in related vessels with soft tissue fixation.
- Use in certain cases of an autologous spongy bone graft to maintain the reconstruction of the collapsed subchondral spongy bone and increase the intrinsic stability of the focal point through contact among fragments.
- Complementation of this fixation by intrinsic support with stable osteosynthesis, ideally a plate in tall animals. Screws and pins are also useful and may be combined in several ways depending on the type of fracture.
- In any case, osteosynthesis must allow a regimen of early mobilisation to be immediately established. This regimen must consist first of passive mobilisation with the help of clinical rehabilitation, then of active mobilisation with no weight-bearing, partial weight-bearing and full weight-bearing, as the clinical course of the fracture permits, with more or less short walks at the discretion of the canine physiotherapist.

In summary, bearing in mind that distal fragments may be rather small, suitable reduction clearly cannot be achieved without a surgical approach, and so conservative treatment does not provide sufficient stability.

The most commonly used methods to treat these fractures are Kirschner wires, which may be combined with cerclage, screws and even plates in tall animals (Fig. 2).

Fractures with multiple fragments in the metaphysis should be fixed with a plate (Figs. 3 and 4).

In any case, surgeons must be aware of their limitations, experience and surgical resources.

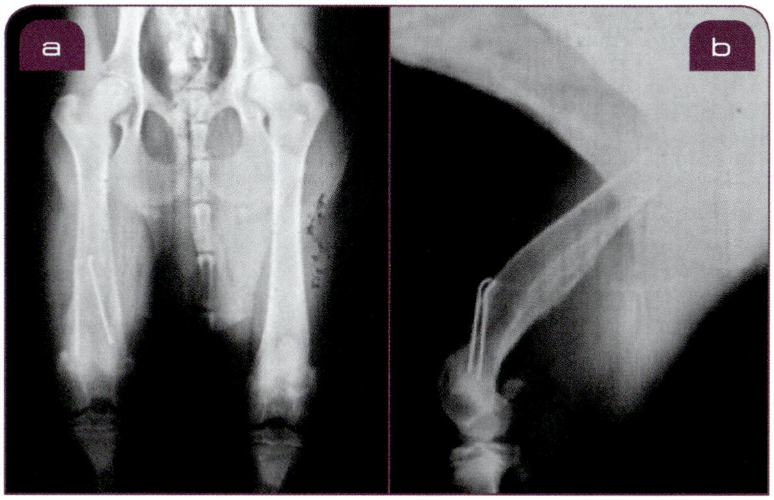

FIGURE 2. Craniocaudal projection of the case in Figure 1 resolved with parallel Kirschner wires (a). Lateral projection (b).

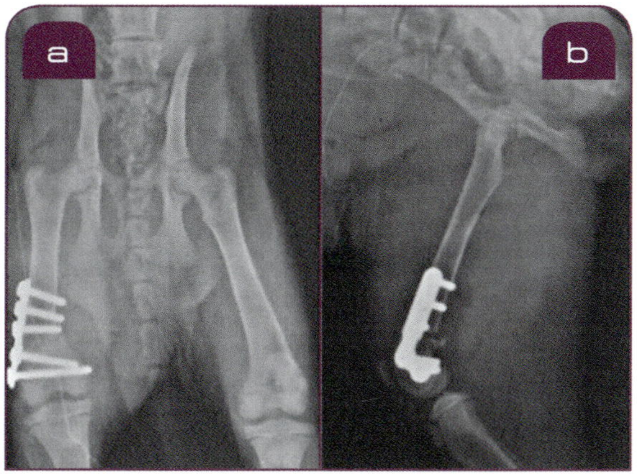

FIGURE 3. Resolution of a distal metaphyseal fracture with an osteosynthesis plate in craniocaudal projection (a) and laterolateral projection (b).

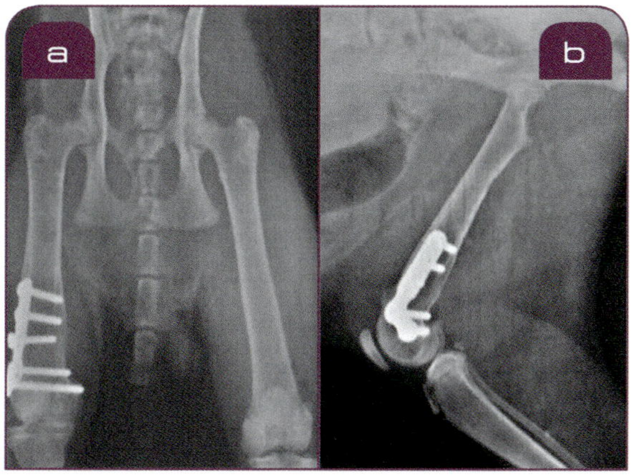

FIGURE 4. Above case with osteosynthesis achieved in craniocaudal projection (a) and laterolateral projection (b).

Good initial conservative treatment while the patient is being referred to a specialist centre is always better than insufficient or incorrect surgery. Secondary reconstruction following conservative treatment is safer and less complex than secondary reconstruction following improper surgery.

Associated injuries that must be borne in mind are as follows:

1. Ligament injuries are usually treated on a secondary basis, when functional recovery allows immobilisation to the extent and for the duration required.
2. Floating stifle joint due to direct impact on the stifle joint, which causes a fracture of the distal femoral end associated with another fracture of the proximal third of the tibia, must be treated by immediate fixation of both injuries to facilitate rehabilitation.
3. Associated ipsilateral fractures also require fixation of all injuries to allow early mobilisation.
4. If a nerve injury does not improve following reduction, a direct examination must be performed in the course of fixation and repair, if applicable, or clinical and electromyographic (EMG) monitoring must be performed if the injury is persistent, as is often the case.

Complications

The results depend on the type of fracture, although overall they are satisfactory thanks to modern osteosynthesis techniques. As mentioned above, the success of the results depends to an extent of more than 80 % on the experience of the surgical team; the success rate is around 60 %–70 % according to most authors consulted.

Stiffness is the most common complication. It may originate in bone due to improper ossification or result from persistent injuries of related soft tissue. As a rule, such stiffness limits flexion and extension of the stifle joint and, depending on the cause, must be surgically corrected. Cases of malunion with formation of bony bridges limiting movement are treated by filing away the bony bridges. Limitation due to persistent failure of mechanisms of soft tissues (ligaments and tendons) must be corrected.

Articular adhesions may be seen with some frequency at the base of the suprapatellar synovial recess due to capsuloligamentous retraction scarring or muscle fibrosis. These adhesions must be gradually combatted by means of manipulation under anaesthesia, arthroscopic arthrolysis (sectioning of adhesions) or even release of the muscle bellies attached to the cortex of the femur by scar tissue. Lengthening of the tendon of the quadriceps muscle by means of a tenotomy in the shape of an inverted *V* may also be attempted. The results may improve flexion and extension in cases with an already acceptable range of motion. However, the prognosis is poor in serious cases with a contracture of all quadriceps muscle bellies.

Infection and nonunion are uncommon and occur in around 5 % of cases as the area is well vascularised. Conversely, other distal fractures such as those of the radius have a high rate of nonunion or at least delayed union as the area is poorly vascularised.

Varus or valgus malunion particularly depends on the quality of the surgery and must be treated with the appropriate osteotomies. If these are not done then, without fail, both the proximal and distal joints become impaired in the medium and long term as the biomechanical axis of the affected limb changes.

Fractures of the proximal end of the tibia

Unlike fractures of the distal end of the femur, in the tibia the fracture line directly affects the articular surfaces themselves and is associated with some frequency with injuries of the ligaments and menisci of the stifle joint (Fig. 5).

As in distal fractures of the femur, associated neurovascular injuries determine the prognosis and stiffness. Secondary deviations caused by defective union are precursors to secondary osteoarthritis.

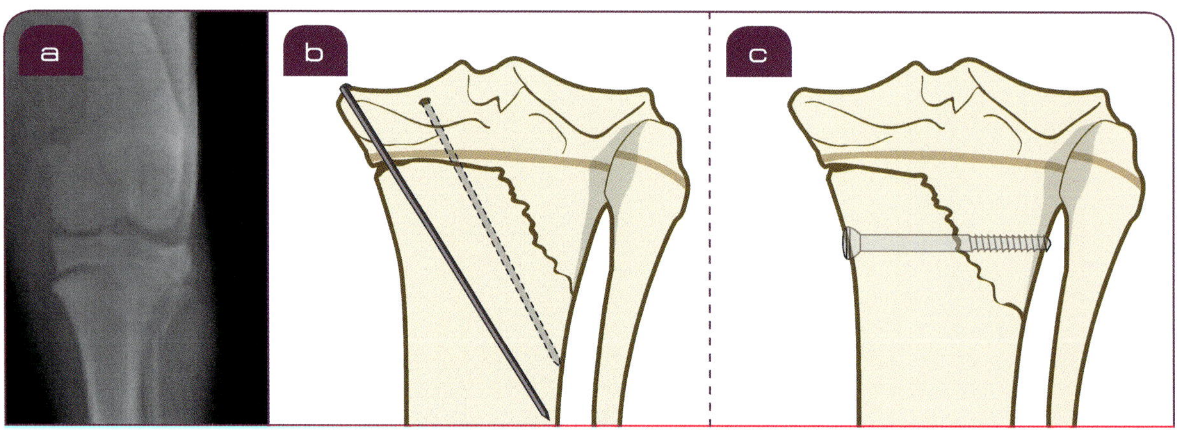

FIGURE 5. Craniocaudal X-ray of a Type II Salter–Harris fracture of the proximal growth plate of the tibia (a). Possibility of resolution with a Kirschner wire placed as indicated in the diagram (b). Possibility of resolution with a compression screw in the metaphyseal area (c). In the authors' opinion, although both methods are valid, the age of the animal must be taken into account when the screw is used, since in very young animals the cortices are excessively soft and the screws will end up loosening and failing to fulfil their function.

Aetiopathogenesis

As in the femur, the type of fracture depends on the quality of the bone structure (determined by the age of the animal), the energy of the trauma and the direction of the force of the trauma (forced movement of the joint towards varus, towards valgus or both; compression; etc.). Tibial plateau fractures require high-energy trauma as this area of the tibia has a stronger trabecular structure. They also tend to involve associated ligament and meniscal injuries.

The multiple classifications of these injuries deal with two essential fracture lines: the vertical line, which separates one of the plateaus and combines them with one another, and the horizontal line, which may or may not involve the growth plate.

Classification of fractures of the proximal tibia

- Tibial tuberosity fractures.
- Tibial plateau fractures.
- Fractures in the growth plate area (Salter-Harris Types I-V).
- Metaphyseal fractures.

Clinical examination

Pain, functional disability, deformity with abnormal mobility and crepitation alert the clinician to the possibility of a fracture. A proper examination must be performed to rule out associated injuries such as:

- **Neurovascular injuries**: these may affect the tibial nerve and, depending on their severity (neurotmesis, axonotmesis or neurapraxia), cause different degrees of abnormality in the tibial neuromuscular system, thereby limiting extension of the tarsus and flexion of the toes. If the affected nerve is the peroneal nerve, this neuromuscular system is altered such that flexion of the tarsus and extension of the toes becomes limited.
- **Muscle injuries**: these are less common in this area and are accompanied by pain caused by passive mobilisation of the muscles and tension in the popliteus and tibialis cranialis muscle bellies in particular.
- **Injuries of the collateral ligaments** of the femorotibial joint: these are associated with mechanisms in varus or valgus; however, their presence does not typically provide much clinical information beyond pain on palpation, which is generalised throughout the area and therefore cannot be attributed to this injury. A stress radiological examination may be useful for diagnosing a complete rupture, while ultrasound is useful for diagnosing a sprain and determining its grade. In a sprain of any grade, capsuloligamentous fibrosis is sufficient to restore stability if appropriate anatomical reduction is achieved between bone surfaces. They may be suspected if pain is present along their path and insertions, and can be confirmed with X-rays in forced varus or valgus.

Radiological examination

Sometimes plain X-rays must be taken in oblique and stress projections in addition to the usual projections (craniocaudal and laterolateral).

As mentioned in the section on fractures of the distal end of the femur, it must be borne in mind that any widening of the articular space compared to the contralateral stifle joint may be considered to be pathological.

CT scanning is also useful in these cases during preoperative fracture evaluation and aids enormously in properly planning surgical treatment.

Treatment

Immediate treatment of these injuries involves immobilising the injury with a Robert Jones bandage, holding the stifle joint in place in slight flexion (approximately 30°) and administering anti-inflammatory drugs parenterally to slow down the inflammatory process, decrease pain and provide comfort to the animal, which must remain in a cage until surgery.

Surgery is planned to provide a definitive treatment which meets the objectives of restoration of joint function, and therefore mobility, as well as stability in order to prevent subsequent osteoarthritis. Malalignment will lead to stiffness, articular incongruity and ultimately osteoarthritis, and so it must be prevented.

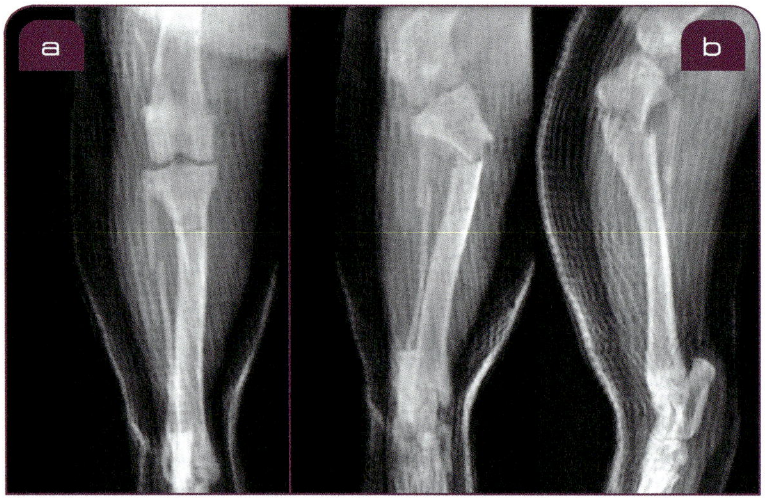

FIGURE 6. Nondisplaced fracture in the proximal metaphysis of the tibia (a). It was decided to use conservative treatment by immobilisation with a fibreglass bandage. Displacement is observed at the focal point of the fracture (b).

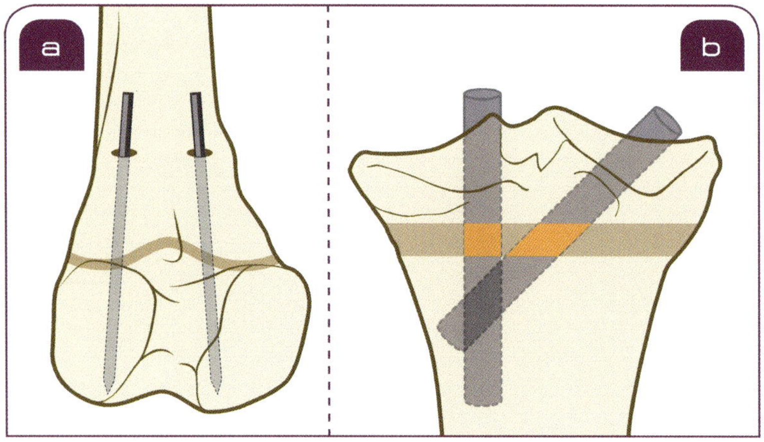

FIGURE 7. Proper way to use Kirschner wires in metaphyseal fractures (a). The portion of growth plate affected when these wires are placed on an inclined plane is substantially larger than when they are placed straight, as seen in the drawing (b). As a result, in the latter case growth plate damage is minor.

The principles for achieving the objectives are the same as the classic principles of osteosynthesis:

- Anatomical reduction within acceptable limits.
- Fixed stability of the focal point of the fracture which allows early mobilisation, thereby preventing subsequent muscle and joint stiffness. Such mobility tends to promote articular cartilage nutrition.
- Passive movements and prolonged rehabilitation to protect cartilage tissue and prevent secondary bone collapse during union.
- These rehabilitation principles can and must also be applied in cases in which conservative treatments have been chosen in Salter–Harris fractures or collateral ligament injuries.

Conservative treatment

Conservative treatment is indicated in:

- Salter–Harris fractures with minimal displacement.
- Elongation or rupture of the collateral ligaments without excessive loss of stability.
- Fractures so severe due to comminution or skin impairment that surgery is impossible.

The definition of "minimal displacement" is a matter of ongoing debate. It is accepted that both Type I and Type V Salter–Harris fractures must undergo conservative treatment; in all other cases conservative treatment would not be optimal with displacement in excess of 3 mm.

Conservative treatment methods that can be used are as follows:

- Minimal displacement: immobilisation with a fibreglass bandage for four weeks, followed by a Robert Jones bandage in slight flexion for progressive mobilisation for another four weeks (Fig. 6).
- Displaced fractures: Kirschner wires and physiotherapy mobilisation starting from the third week (Fig. 7).

Surgical treatment

This is indicated in all fractures not included in the conservative treatment group, that is to say, 70 % of fractures with separation in excess of 3 mm at the focal point of the fracture, 24 % of compressions and nearly all fractures due to collapse, as well as 65 % of *T* and *V* fractures. Fractures with a distal metaphyseal or diaphyseal line require surgical stabilisation. Fractures with associated vascular injuries must also be surgically stabilised.

Osteosynthesis methods that can be used are as follows:

- In fractures with separation, fixation of the fragment with pins tends to be sufficient (Fig. 8).
- In all other fractures, especially metaphyseal fractures in large dogs, a buttress plate must be used. A buttress plate is intended to support the metaphyseal cortex and prevent it from moving in muscle activity and weight-bearing.
- External saucer fractures of the tibial plateau due to shearing have been reported in Dachshunds. Given that this is a common breed throughout Europe, the authors have had the opportunity to observe this type of fracture and witness its long-term postoperative clinical course, and thus can affirm that the best possible treatment in this particular breed involves properly repositioning the focal point of the fracture and fixing it with a traction screw.
- In metaphyseal and diaphyseal fractures, a compression or neutralisation plate must be used so that osteosynthesis achieves one of these effects (Fig. 9).
- Tibial tuberosity injuries are treated with a tension band that physically functions as a brace. Tibial tuberosity fractures in growing animals are always accompanied by proximal displacement of the patella ("patella alta"). Due to the anatomy of the growth plate in this epiphyseal area, in most cases detachment is not complete but partial.

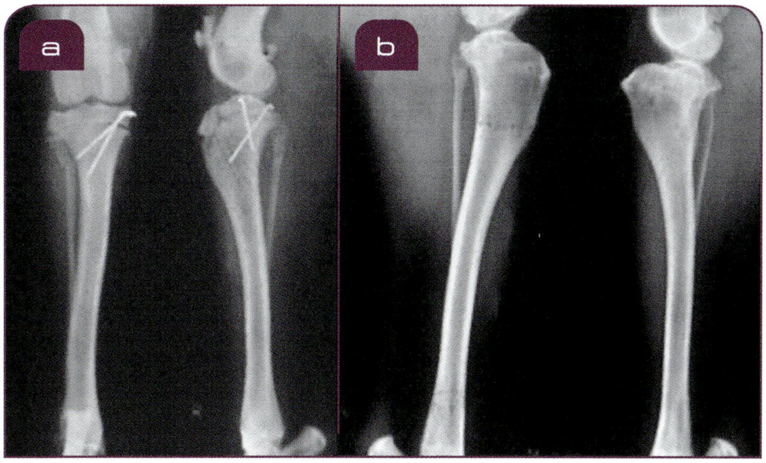

FIGURE 8. Metaphyseal fracture resolved with Kirschner wires (a). Image after 20 weeks with implants removed (b). Ideally, implants should always be removed in periarticular fractures.

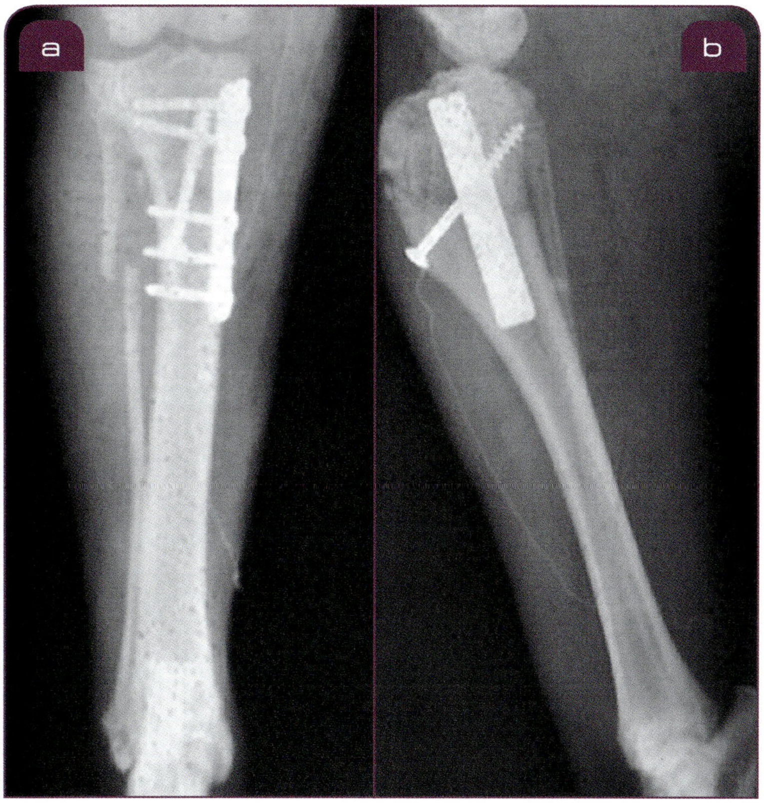

FIGURE 9. Another case of proximal metaphyseal fracture resolved with a compression screw and a buttress plate. Craniocaudal projection (a) and laterolateral projection (b).

Therefore, after proper anatomical repositioning, in most cases fixation with a Kirschner wire that does not reach the opposite cortex is sufficient. This allows the growth of the epiphyseal cartilage and the continuous movement of the tibial tuberosity (Fig. 10). If the attachment of the patellar ligament moves distally, musculoskeletal disorders are very likely to ensue.

- Growth plate fractures are treated according to the same principles set out for fractures of the femur. In Type II Salter–Harris fractures of the tibia, which are very common, conservative treatment is possible. As mentioned, conservative treatment does not achieve satisfactory results in such fractures of the femur.

Metaphyseal fractures are more problematic, as it is very common for a new fragment dislocation to occur. Serious joint complications such as dislocation of the patella and deforming joint disease occur if this new dislocation is not diagnosed early.

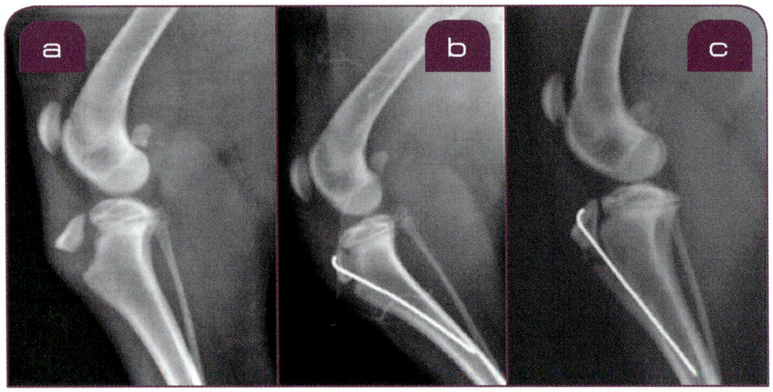

FIGURE 10. Fracture due to avulsion of the tibial tuberosity in a puppy (a). Postoperative image (b) and image eight weeks after surgery (c).

Traumatic injuries of the patella

Contusion

This is quite common due to the superficial location of this bone. It can cause haemarthrosis and some degree of osteochondral collapse, which usually goes unnoticed. It sometimes causes prolonged residual pain.

Dislocation

Traumatic dislocation of the patella is rare, unless the animal is anatomically predisposed to such an event. It is accompanied by tearing of both the capsule and the vastus medialis muscle. If it does not occur spontaneously it is easy to diagnose, but if it does occur spontaneously then on examination it can evoke signs and symptoms consistent with injury of the meniscus or medial collateral ligament. Traumatic dislocations are often accompanied by osteochondral fractures with intra-articular loose bodies. Their treatment involves reducing the dislocation and immobilising the stifle joint for two to three weeks in order to facilitate the healing of the torn structures.

Fracture

The patella may fracture by two mechanisms:

- **Fractures by indirect mechanism** occur when there is sudden, severe contraction of the quadriceps femoris muscle in the course of a fall; this causes a transverse fracture due to traction, with or without tearing of the patellar retinacula (displaced or nondisplaced, respectively). This same mechanism may cause tearing of the tendon of insertion of the quadriceps femoris muscle (sometimes including a small fragment of the proximal end of the patella) or rupture of the patellar ligament (sometimes with the distal end of the patella adhered).
- In dogs, **fractures by direct mechanism** tend not to occur. Such fractures are common in humans due to traffic accidents. Their mechanism of action derives from the impact of the knee against the

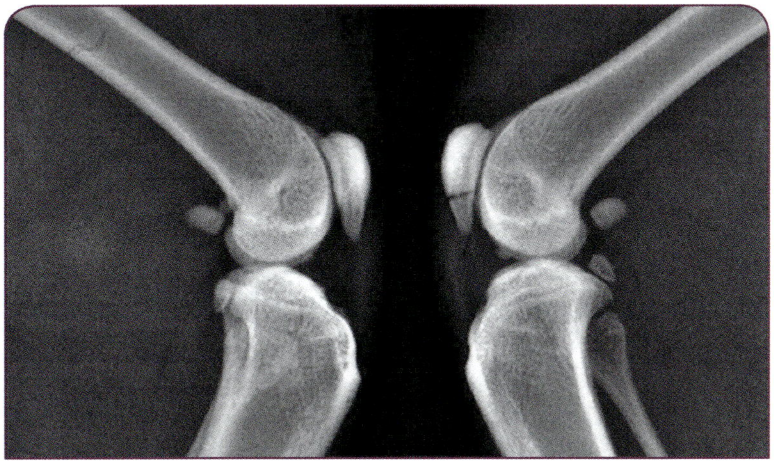

FIGURE 11. Fracture of the patellar apex or vertex.

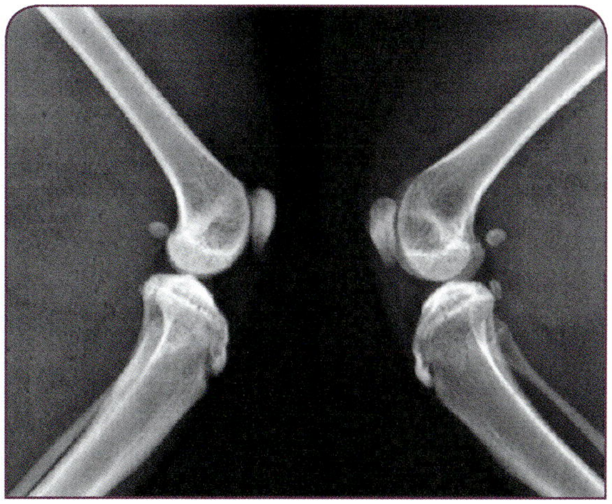

FIGURE 12. Fracture of the patellar edge in laterolateral projection. Nothing more than radiotransparent spaces are seen. These, consistent with the findings of the physical examination, cause the clinician to suspect a patellar injury, which is confirmed with a tangential X-ray.

dashboard of the vehicle. They can occur in dogs due to the impact of the stifle joint against the front seat or the dashboard of the vehicle if their owners irresponsibly transport them without a restraint. They may also be observed in animals that ride in vehicles with open windows and are ejected through them during sudden braking. These events tend to result in a generally comminuted fracture with associated osteochondral injury; this always has a serious prognosis (Fig. 11).

Clinical examination

A fracture of the patella is suspected in a traumatic event with skin injury in the patellar region accompanied by pain, swelling and articular effusion. Crepitation is uncommon due to the limited displacement that occurs at the focal point of the fracture.

The ability of the animal to fully actively extend the stifle joint must be evaluated, since this depends on the integrity of the patellar retinacula which use the action of organised flexion and extension by the quadriceps femoris and hamstring muscles.

Radiological examination

The fracture line may be seen on X-ray. The appropriate projection for the focal point of the fracture is the craniocaudal projection, and the appropriate projection to evaluate the movement and impairment of the patellar cartilage is the laterolateral projection. The tangential projection is very useful to diagnose fractures of the edge of the patella (Figs. 12-14).

Treatment

Fractures with displacement require surgical treatment, which involves repair of the tearing in the patellar retinacula and synthesis of the fracture, generally with Kirschner wires and wire, to form a tension band. In comminuted fractures the largest fragment should be preserved and the continuity of the extensors should be restored (partial patellectomy). However, in cases of serious comminution the only option is a total patellectomy. Common sequelae include development of post-traumatic osteoarthritis and, in patellectomies, loss of extensor force.

The best method to stabilise a transverse fracture of the patella is synthesis of the fracture (generally with or without Kirschner wires and surgical wire) to form a tension band that, as stated, functions as a brace. It has the advantage of allowing immediate mobilisation of the stifle joint.

Wire cerclage on the cranial aspect of the patella, if chosen, neutralises all traction forces and turns them into pressure forces. The wire cerclage is passed

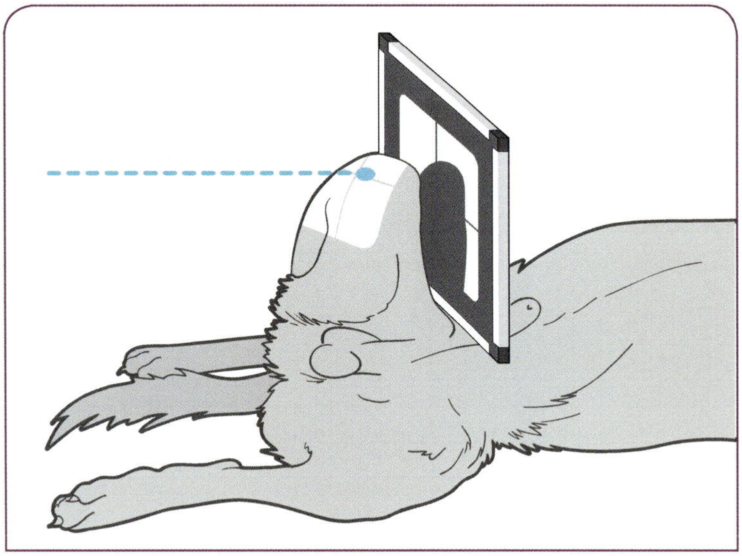

FIGURE 13. The tangential projection is very useful to diagnose fractures of the patellar edge (Fritz technique). The angle should range from 60° to 80° to evaluate the patella in different positions.

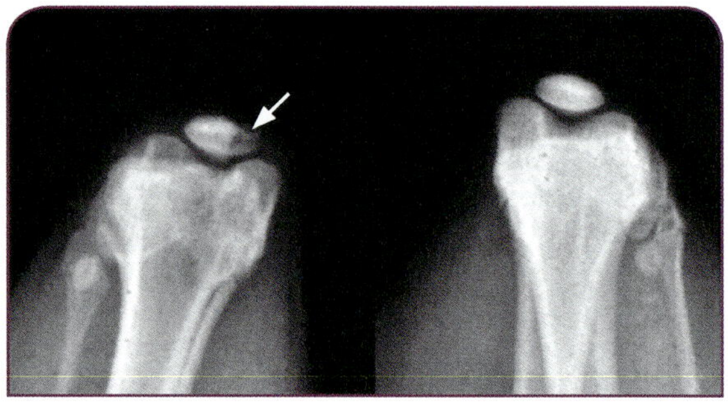

FIGURE 14. The tangential projection reveals an injury on the edge of the patella.

proximally and distally to the patella through the patellar ligament, or better yet through two transverse holes in the patella, and crossed on the cranial aspect. The wire is then adjusted to create slight hyper-reduction. All transarticular fixation with cerclage is performed as described to repair rupture of the patellar ligament.

Another option for fixation is to use one or two Kirschner wires, then place the wire cerclage and support it with them (Figs. 15 and 16). To ensure stability through relaxation of the patellar ligament, a safety cerclage is generally secured to a transverse screw on the tibial tuberosity. The authors have observed that in most cases this cerclage wears out and breaks after five to six weeks; however, these first few weeks are decisive in fracture healing. These forces can also be offset by placing a transarticular external fixator.

This chapter concludes with CT and MRI scans of dog cadavers showing different fractures (Figs. 17-22).

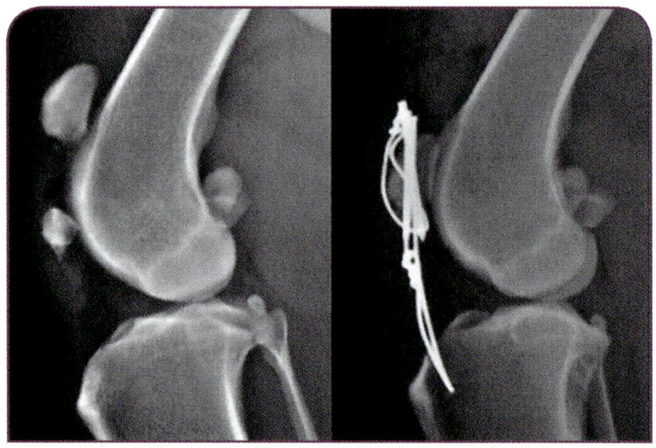

FIGURE 15. Repair of a patellar fracture. One or two Kirschner wires are used, then a wire cerclage is placed and supported with them.

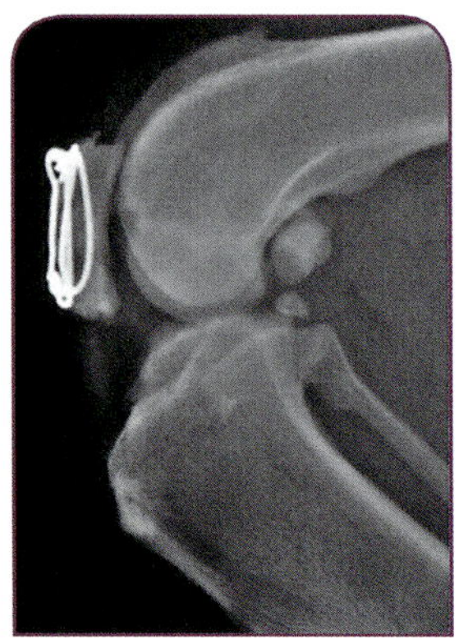

FIGURE 16. Image 18 months after removing the fixator.

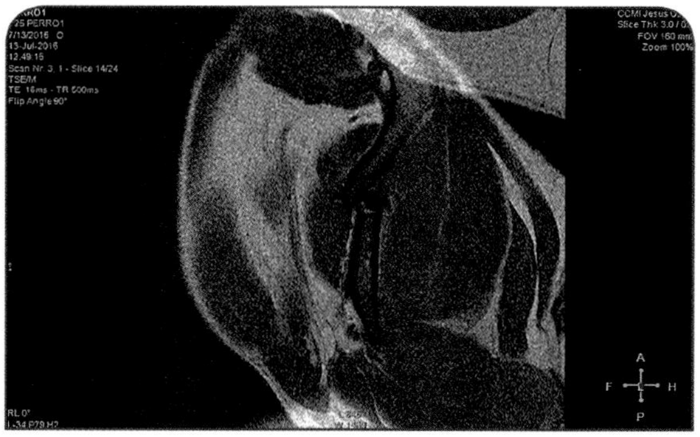

FIGURE 17. MRI scan (sagittal slice). Fracture of the right femur. Sequence: T1 TSE.

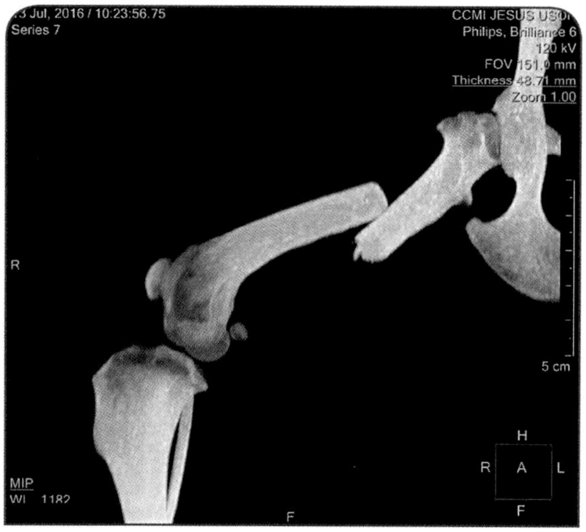

FIGURE 18. CT scan (multiplanar reconstruction). Fracture of the right femur in the same patient shown in the previous figure.

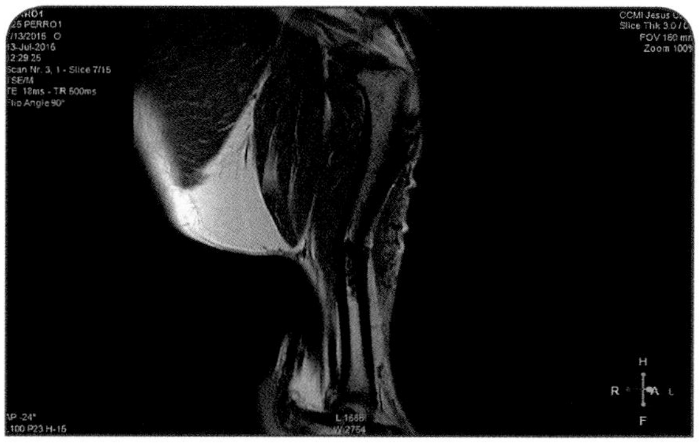

FIGURE 19. MRI scan. Fracture of the left tibia. Sequence: T1 TSE.

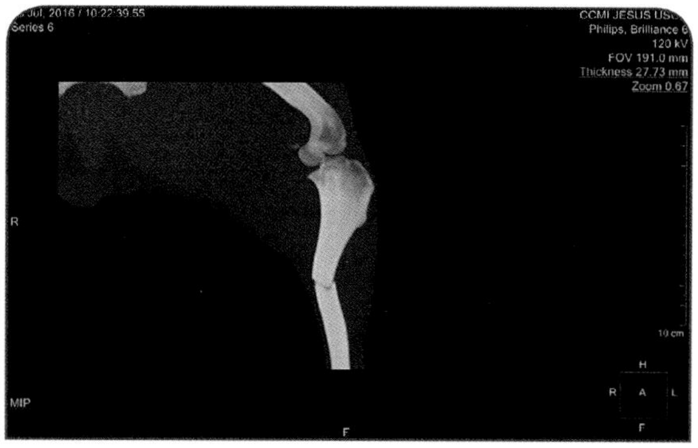

FIGURE 20. CT scan (multiplanar reconstruction). Fracture of the left tibia in the same patient shown in the previous figure.

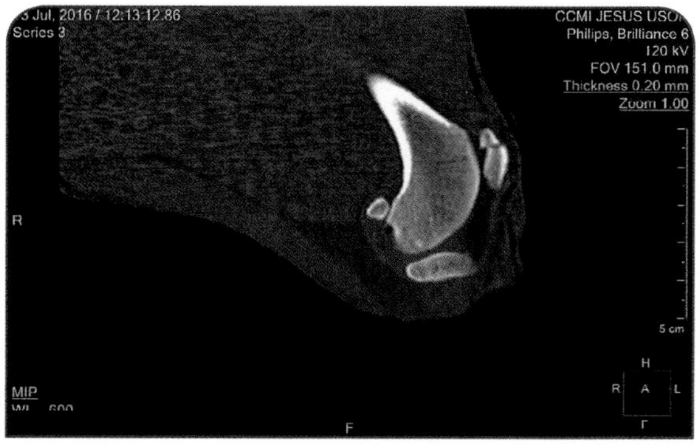

FIGURE 21. CT scan. Fracture of the left patella.

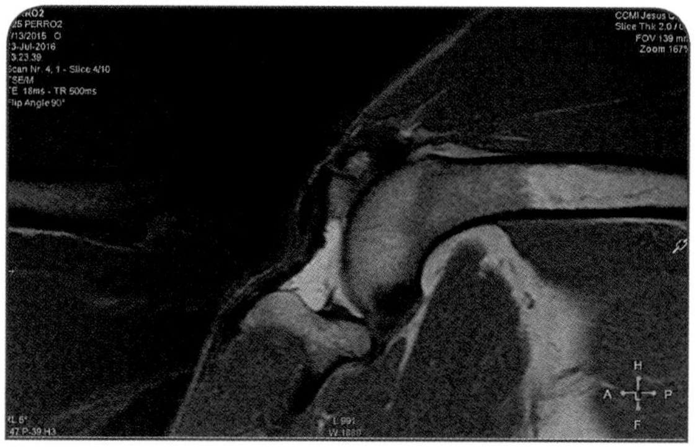

FIGURE 22. MRI scan. Fracture of the left patella in the same patient shown in the previous figure. Sequence: T1 TSE.

CHAPTER

4

Injuries of the flexors and extensors of the stifle joint

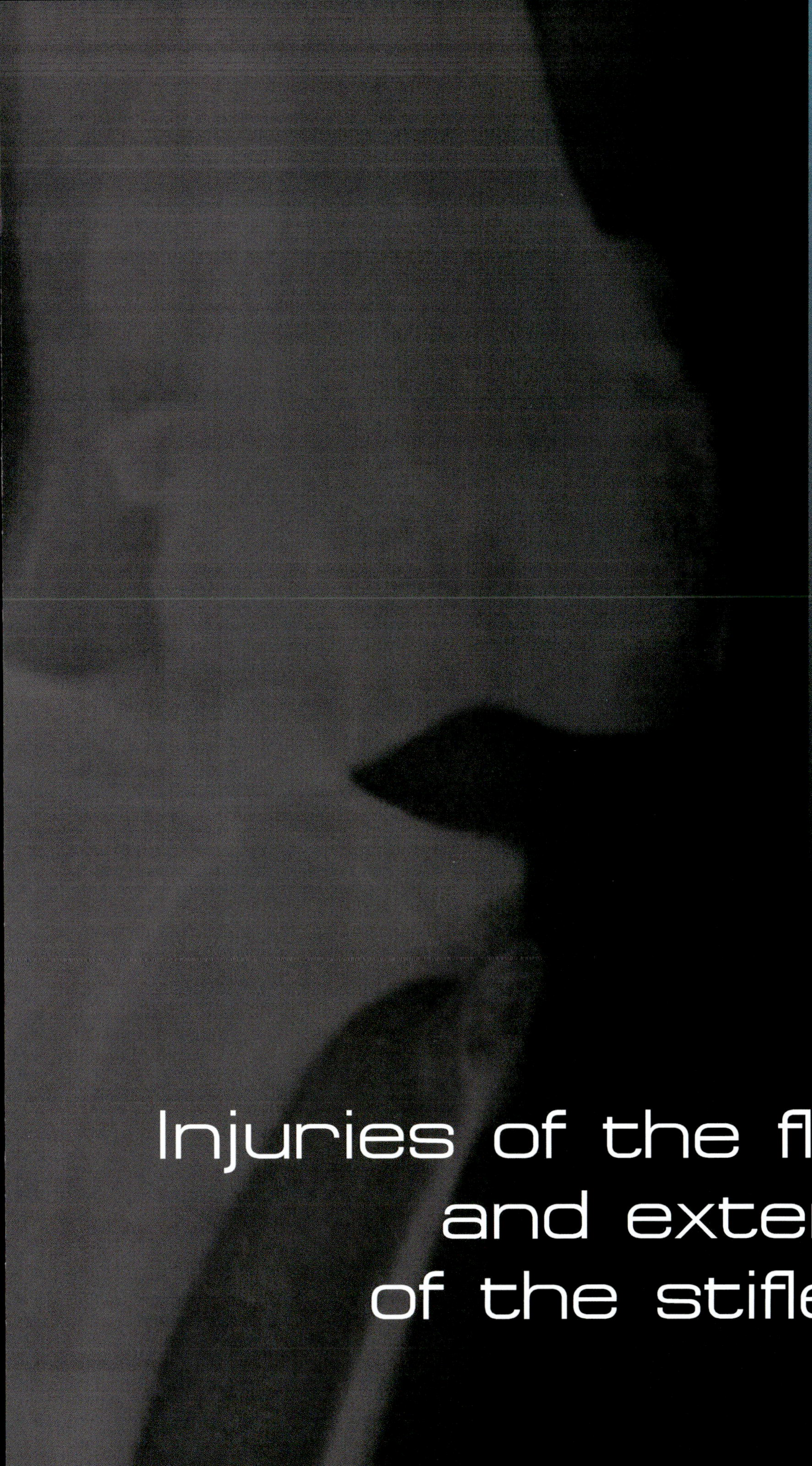

Anatomy and biomechanics of the extensors

The quadriceps femoris muscle and its tendon of insertion

This muscle consists of four muscle bellies: the vastus medialis, the vastus lateralis, the vastus intermedius and the rectus femoris. The three vastus muscles originate proximally on the cortical surface of the femur, while the rectus femoris muscle does so on the ventral iliac spine and in a small lateral area. The vastus medialis muscle belly plays the most important role in stabilising the patella, especially through its medial portion.

The tendon of insertion of the quadriceps muscle is formed by the distal confluence of the four bellies and consists of several layers: a superficial layer, which mainly comes from the rectus femoris muscle and passes in front of the patella to proceed as part of the patellar ligament; a middle layer, which is formed by the insertion of the vastus medialis and vastus lateralis muscles into the dorsal part of the patella; and a deep layer, which comes from the vastus intermedius (cruraeus) muscle and reaches the base of the patella.

The patella

This bone lies within the tibial insertion of the quadriceps femoris muscle. Some authors have considered it to be a sesamoid bone of the extensors. This concept is valid insofar as it confirms that patellar disease depends in part on the alignment of the extensors and abnormalities therein. However, it is inadequate in light of the important biomechanical functions attributed to the patella.

The articular surfaces of the stifle joint do not provide a great deal of craniocaudal stability. In this regard, the patella, connected to the tibia by an elastic tendon, is capable of preventing the femur from sliding cranially. In addition, its connection with the quadriceps femoris muscle serves to cushion the forces created by rapid changes in acceleration due to movements. It achieves this by distributing the loads of the stifle joint, first by absorbing compression loads from the femur and then by transforming them into tensile forces towards the tendon of the quadriceps femoris muscle and the patellar ligament in a dynamic way that depends on the angle of the stifle joint at all times (Fig. 1).

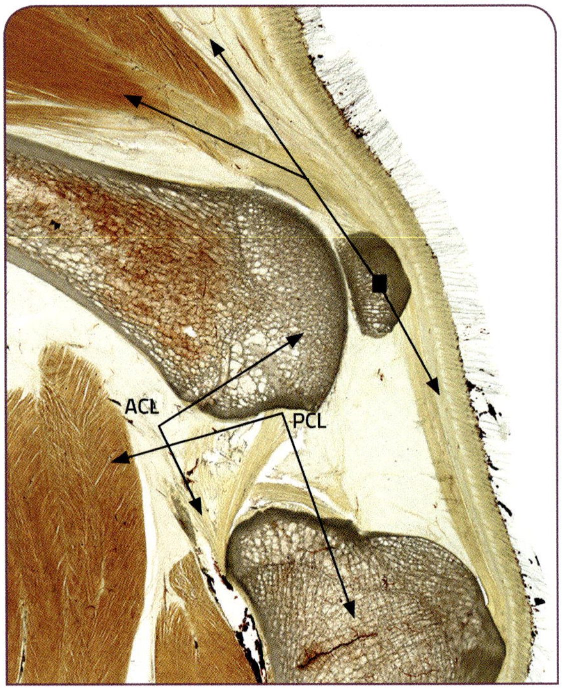

FIGURE 1. Transparent plastinated sagittal section of a stifle joint. ACL: anterior cruciate ligament; PCL: posterior cruciate ligament.

The patella is a sharp, oval-shaped bone. It has a convex, coarse cranial aspect and an articular caudal aspect, with an articular facet or surface. The mechanisms of patellar stabilisation attempt to limit the tendency of the patella to move laterally. This is achieved by means of bone and tendon elements:

- The bone elements include the congruity between the patellar crest and the femoral groove as well as the greater height of the femoral facet over which the narrower facet of the patella slides.
- The tendon and ligament elements include the lateral and medial patellar retinacula, which correspond to the lateral and medial femoropatellar ligaments. The lateral femoropatellar ligament ends on the lateral

gastrocnemius sesamoid bone, and the medial femoropatellar ligament ends on the medial epicondyle of the femur and the medial gastrocnemius sesamoid bone.

There is no clear correlation between patellar morphology and onset of chondromalacia. However, the larger the patellar facet, the stronger the observed tendency to subluxation or dislocation. Hence, chondromalacia is more common in large animals. In addition, the central groove is not as deep in patients with patellar instability, so this condition, by contrast, occurs in small animals.

The main biomechanical function of the patella is to improve the mechanical efficacy of the quadriceps femoris muscle. It achieves this by causing cranial movement of the patellar ligament, which increases leverage when rotating the stifle joint. In fact, a patellectomy (excision of the patella) leads to a 40 % loss of the mechanical effectiveness of the extensor mechanism of the stifle joint in dogs. In addition, the patella centralises the divergent tendons of the quadriceps femoris muscle, improves the capacity for sliding of the extensors and protects the distal portion of the femur.

The area of femoropatellar contact gradually increases with flexion up to 90°, beyond which the quadriceps muscle touches the femur. During flexion, the part of the patella that touches the femur varies: at 20° the lower third of the articular surface touches the femur, at 60° the middle third touches the femur and at 90° the upper third touches the femur. From a clinical perspective, joint contact pressures are greatest at 60°–90° of flexion, and so they must be prevented particularly in animals with diagnosed patellar chondromalacia.

Joint reaction forces

Joint reaction forces vary depending on the capacity of the patella for sliding activity. Most authors consulted have agreed that they represent 0.5 times the animal's body weight while it is walking, but increase up to 3.3 times when the animal is going up or down stairs and as high as 6.5 times when the animal is engaging in counter-resistance extension, that is to say, when the animal must repeatedly jump to catch an object. It is useful to call attention to the clinical relevance of these figures, since exercises involving counter-resistance extension worsen femoropatellar disease and as a result they must be avoided or at least not taken too far.

The patellar ligament and the infrapatellar fat pad

The patellar ligament is a strong structure, the length of which determines the vertical position of the patella. Some patients have patella alta or a shallow femoral trochlea; both of these conditions promote femoropatellar instability.

The infrapatellar fat pad, or Hoffa's fat pad, has a great deal of functional importance with respect to patellar vascularisation. In fact, one author has called it a patellar vascular hilum. As explained later on, this structure may be responsible for signs and symptoms of pain under certain circumstances.

The biomechanics of the different forces acting on stifle joint movement are described in Figures 1-5 in Chapter 6.

Main disorders

The diseases that tend to affect the structures of the flexors and extensors of the stifle joint are:

- Rupture of the collateral ligaments.
- Rupture of the patellar ligament.
- Tearing and ossification of the tendon of origin of the long digital extensor muscle.
- Dislocation of the tendon of origin of the long digital extensor muscle.
- Osgood-Schlatter disease.
- Chondropathy or chondromalacia of the patella.
- Dislocation of the stifle joint.
- Fat pad abnormalities (Hoffa's disease).
- Tumours.

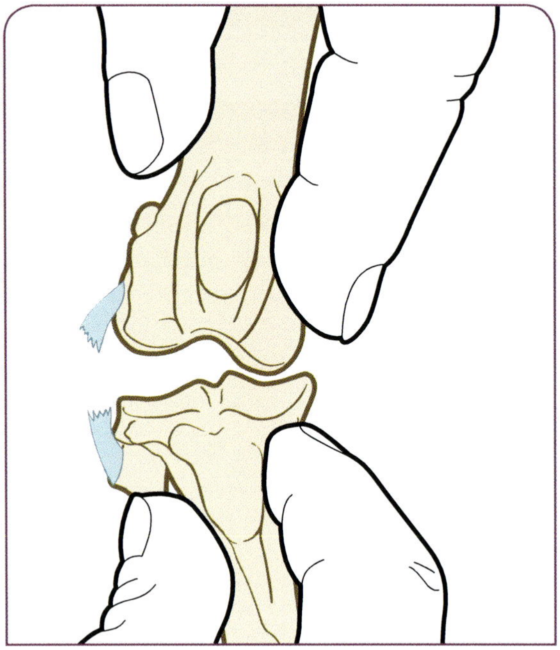

FIGURE 2. Mechanism of rupture of the lateral collateral ligament.

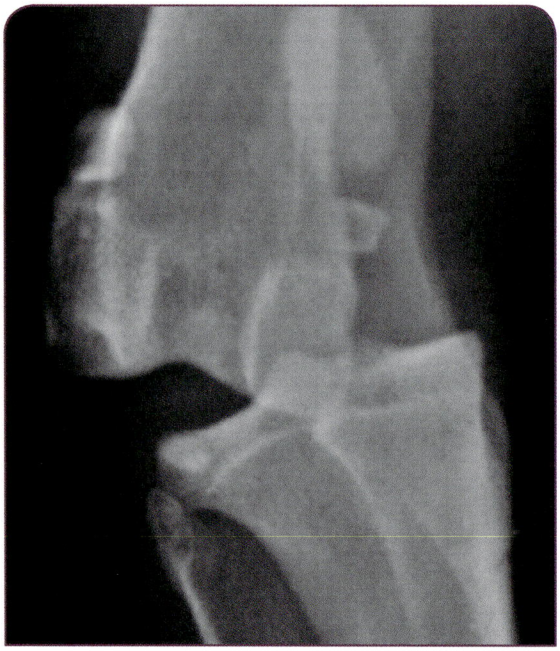

FIGURE 3. X-ray showing rupture of both collateral ligaments.

Rupture of the collateral ligaments

These injuries are more commonly observed in cats than in dogs. In many cases, rupture of the collateral ligament (especially the medial collateral ligament) is accompanied by rupture of the anterior cruciate ligament as well as the medial meniscus. Therefore, it is important to conduct a detailed clinical examination under anaesthesia. Rupture of the medial collateral ligament is much more common than rupture of the lateral collateral ligament (Figs. 2 and 3).

A swollen, very painful stifle joint is observed clinically. Stress X-rays are useful for diagnosis. Once the diagnosis is clear, it is advisable to perform surgery.

Surgical treatment

It is often possible to suture the ligament and then reinforce the suture area with a cerclage (Figs. 4 and 5). Although the wire generally wears out and breaks, it provides a restraint during the first four to six weeks. When implants are removed, care must be taken not to destroy the ligament scar tissue providing the new stability.

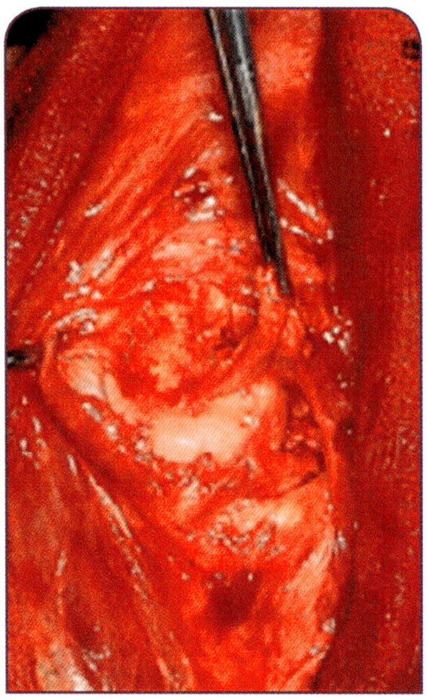

FIGURE 4. Rupture of the medial collateral ligament.

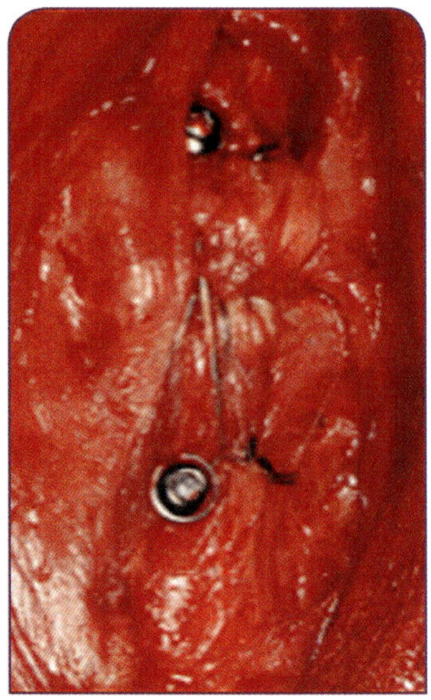

FIGURE 5. Surgical resolution with a prosthetic ligament fixed by screws.

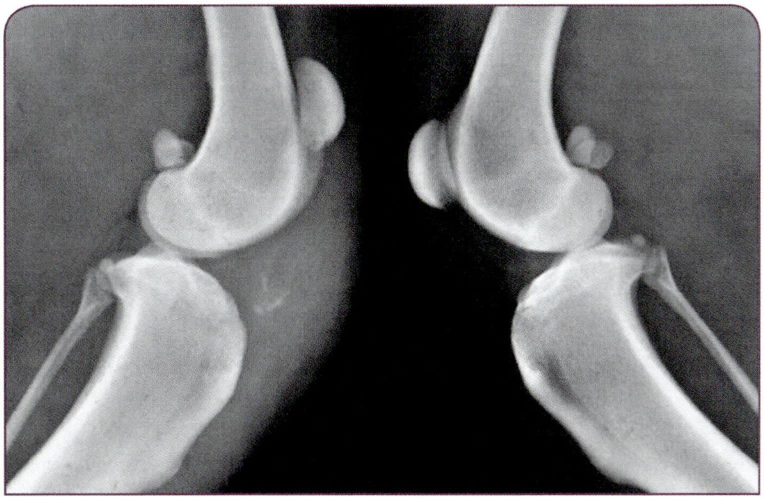

FIGURE 6. Rupture of the patellar ligament (left limb on the X-ray). Proximal displacement of the patella is observed.

Rupture of the patellar ligament

This is generally observed after penetrating trauma. The diagnosis is simple; patella alta and laxity of the patellar ligament are detected on palpation (Fig. 6). The patient is unable to extend the stifle joint.

Surgical treatment

Treatment involves suturing the ligament and then protecting tensile forces using fixation as described above for fractures of the patella (Figs. 7-11). It may also involve reinforcing the muscle fascia (Figs. 12 and 13).

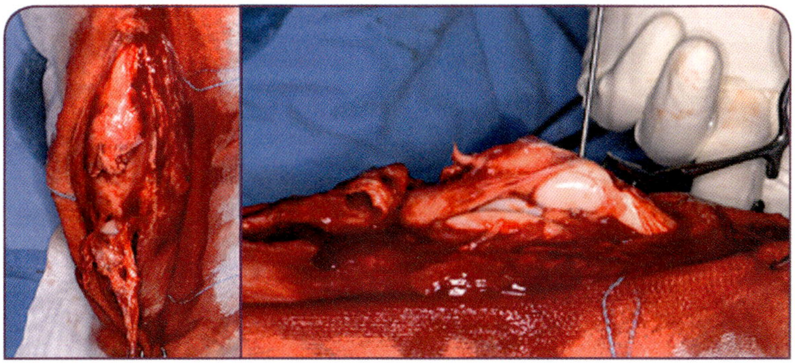

FIGURE 7. Surgical image of rupture of the patellar ligament.

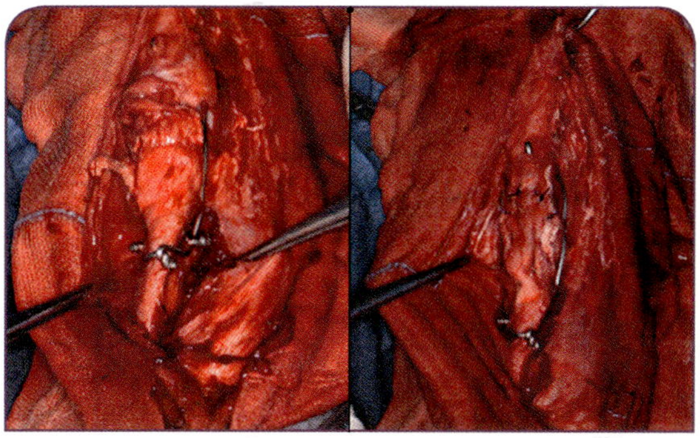

FIGURE 8. Surgical resolution of the ruptured patellar ligament by means of suture and additional fixation with cerclage.

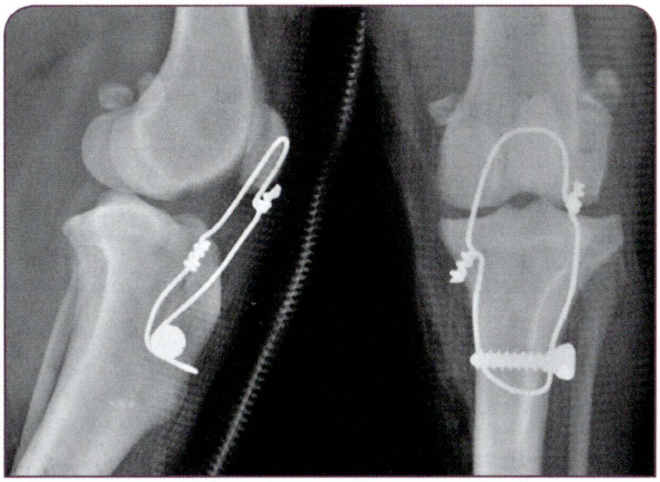

FIGURE 9. Postoperative X-ray.

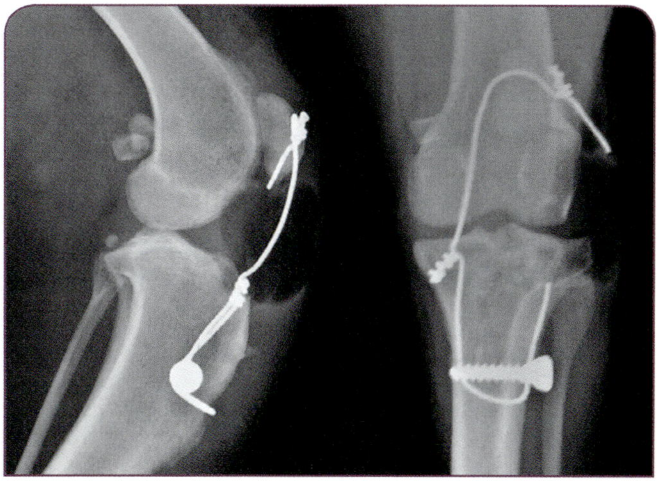

FIGURE 10. X-ray after eight weeks. The cerclage has broken but has fulfilled its function.

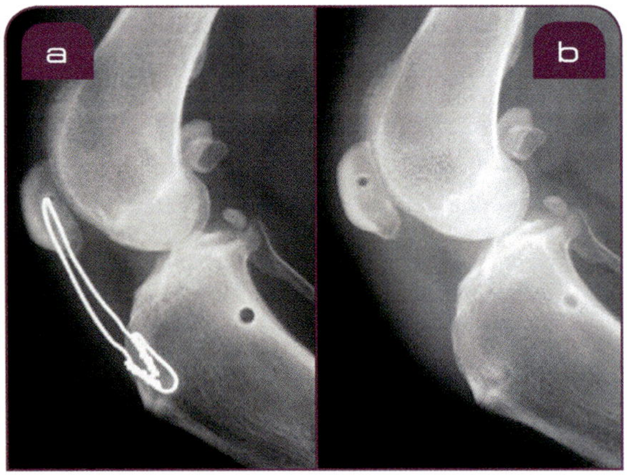

FIGURE 11. Surgical resolution with cerclage reinforcement of rupture of the patellar ligament six weeks after the operation (a) and 20 weeks after the operation (b).

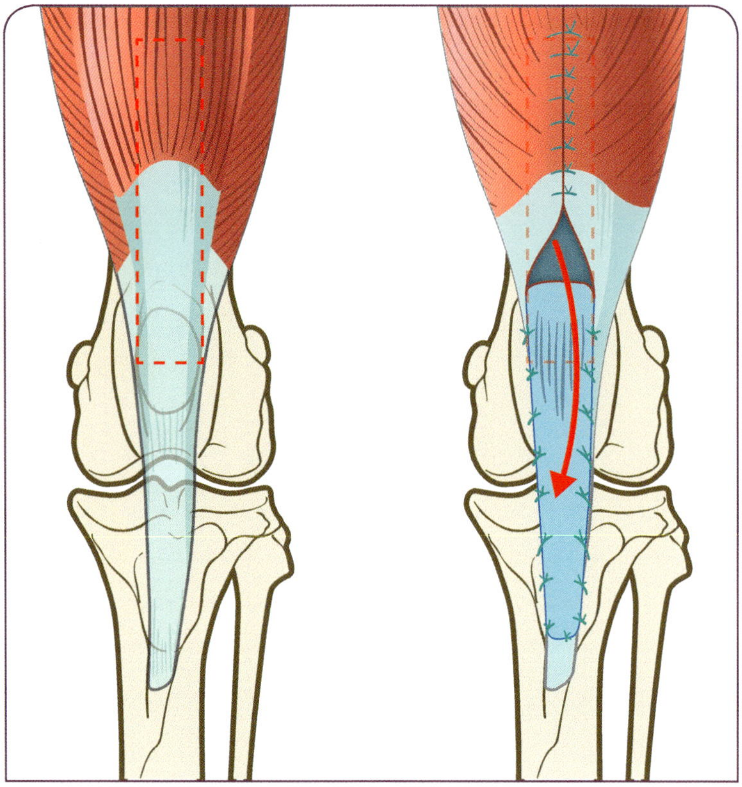

FIGURE 12. Technique of reinforcement using muscle fascia.

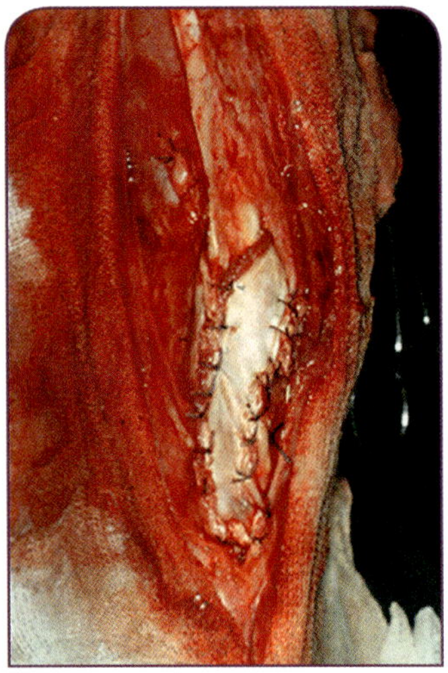

FIGURE 13. Reinforcement of suture of the patellar ligament using muscle fascia.

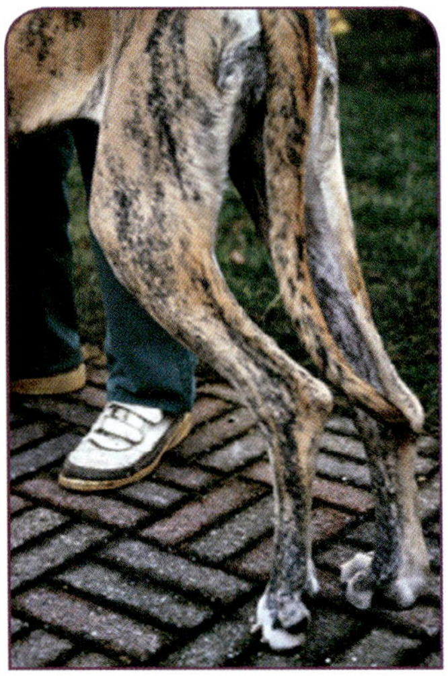

FIGURE 14. Clinical posture of an animal with tearing of the tendon of origin of the long digital extensor muscle.

Tearing and ossification of the tendon of origin of the long digital extensor muscle

This injury is particularly seen in young dogs (five to eight months old) belonging to giant breeds. The authors have particularly seen it in Great Danes (Fig. 14). After tearing occurs, lameness lasts around three to four weeks, disappears after this time and reappears after two to three months. The cause is hypertrophy of the residual bone fragment, which irritates the joint.

In the first phase, inflammation of the stifle joint is observed with occasional pain laterocranial to the patella. A lack of extension of the phalanges is generally not observed. In the second phase (hypertrophy) a hard swelling is palpated. This swelling may be clearly seen on X-ray.

Surgical treatment

Cases with hypertrophy and bone metaplasia of the end of the tendon (this is generally when the problem is diagnosed) require resection and conformation of the end of the tendon to the joint capsule (Figs. 15-17).

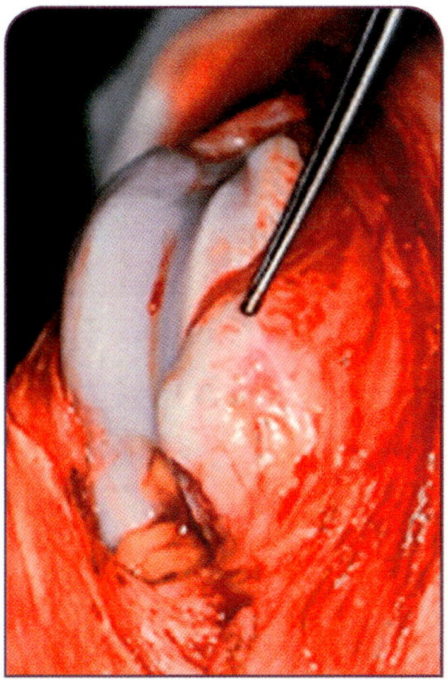

FIGURE 15. Tearing of the tendon of origin of the long digital extensor muscle.

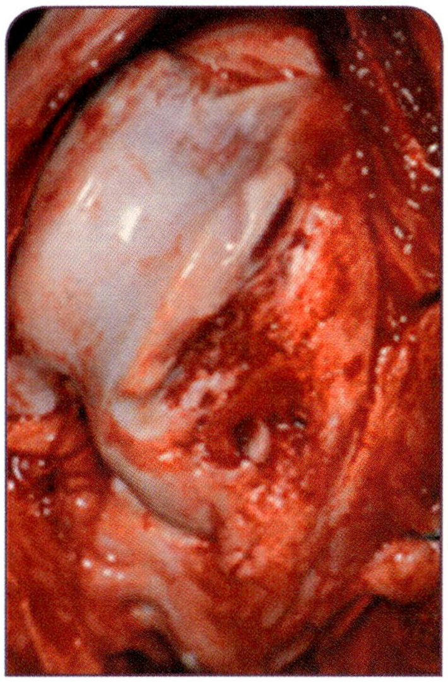

FIGURE 16. Surgical image following cleaning, debridement and resection of the tendon edges.

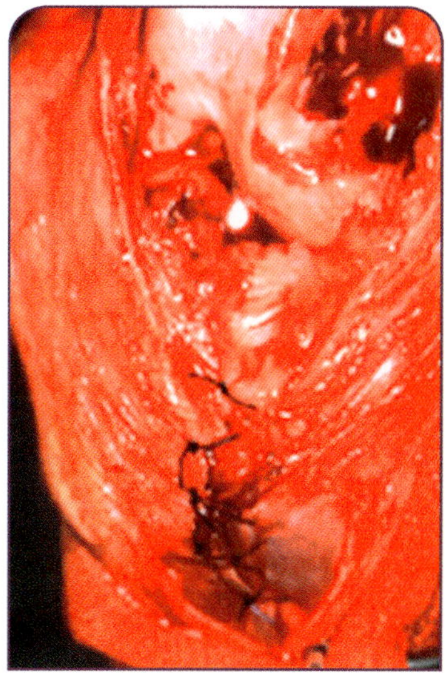

FIGURE 17. Surgical image following fixation.

Dislocation of the tendon of origin of the long digital extensor muscle

Clinical signs causing dislocation of the tendon of origin of the long digital extensor muscle (Figs. 18 and 19) are:

- Noise in the stifle joint when walking or during extension of the stifle joint with simultaneous internal rotation of the metatarsus (a "click" is detected that is similar to that heard when the meniscus is damaged).
- Local pain.
- Joint overload.

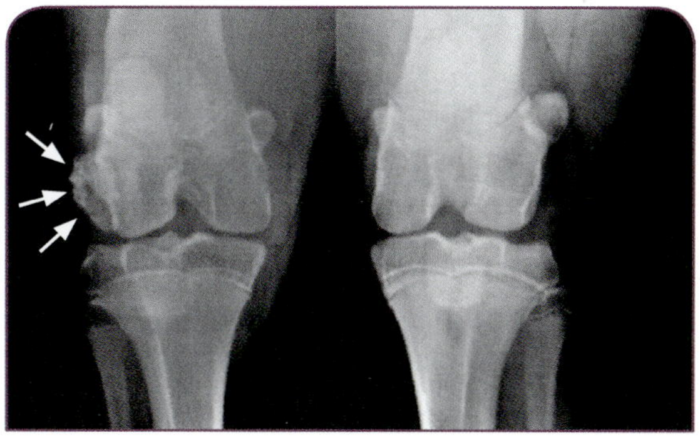

FIGURE 19. X ray of a dislocation of the tendon of origin of the long digital extensor muscle. The periosteal reaction to tendon friction can be seen.

Surgical treatment

Treatment involves repositioning the tendon and performing fixation with a flap of fascia lata (Fig. 20).

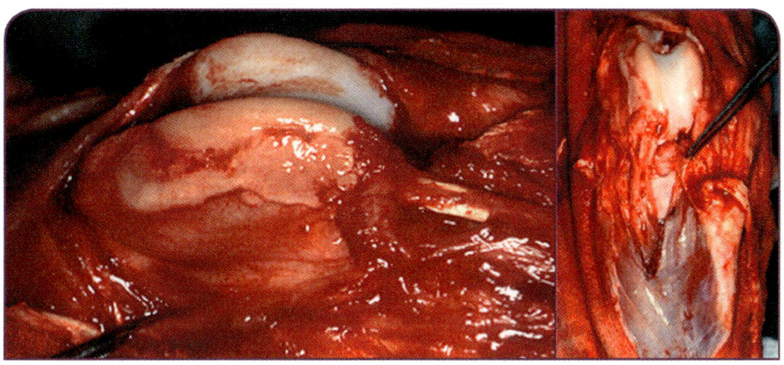

FIGURE 18. Dislocation of the tendon of origin of the long digital extensor muscle.

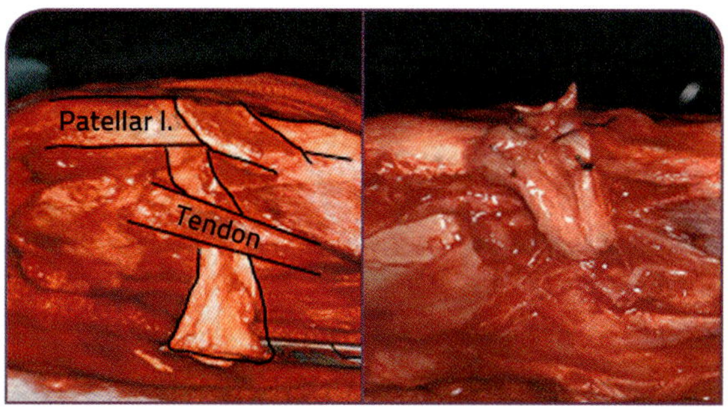

FIGURE 20. Surgical resolution of the dislocation. The tendon is replaced in its channel and prevented from dislocating again with a flap of fascia lata which runs along the patellar ligament and the tendon of the extensor muscle.

Osgood-Schlatter disease

This injury consists of avascular necrosis of the tibial tuberosity. The aetiology of these ossification abnormalities may be hereditary or traumatic. The authors particularly diagnose this condition in Bull Terriers and some very large breeds (e.g. Borzois).

Fairly pronounced lameness is observed with occasional pain at the level of the tibial tuberosity. An increase in synovial fluid volume does not tend to be observed as this is an extra-articular process.

Images of the injury on X-rays are characteristic (Fig. 21). It must not be mistaken for a fracture of the tibial tuberosity. In these cases a typical dislocation with elevation of the patella is always observed, while in Osgood-Schlatter disease there is no dislocation of the tibial tuberosity or proximal displacement of the patella; there is simply a radiotransparent area in the growth plate.

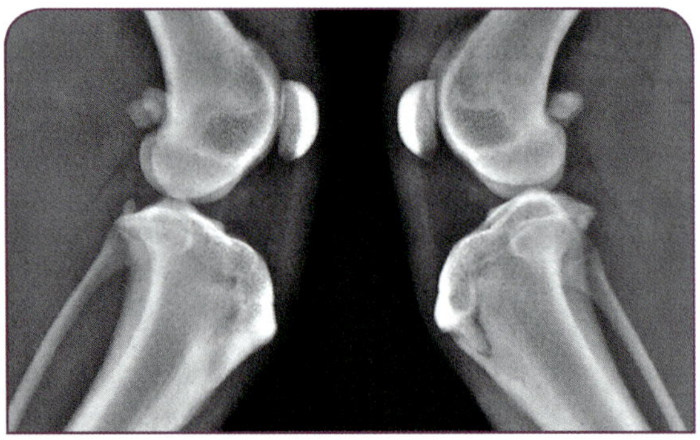

FIGURE 21. Osgood-Schlatter disease in the right limb. Both limbs must always undergo a radiological study as it aids in diagnosis.

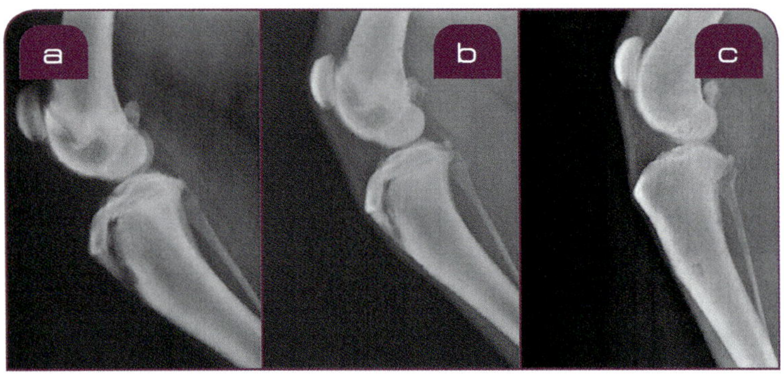

FIGURE 22. X-ray of a case of Osgood-Schlatter disease (a). Progress following the start of conservative treatment at rest (b and c).

Surgical treatment

Treatment is conservative (Fig. 22). Osgood-Schlatter disease may lead to a fracture if the patient is not kept at rest. Such fractures are treated as described in Chapter 3 in the section on proximal fractures of the tibia, specifically for fractures of the tibial crest, with a pin and a tension band.

Chondropathy or chondromalacia of the patella

This disease consists of necrotic softening in the patellar cartilage. It is caused by excessive pressure on the articular cartilage, especially if its weight-bearing capacity is decreased, as for example after prolonged immobilisation. It can also be attributed to metabolic disorders, joint lubrication abnormalities and so on (Box 1).

BOX 1

Aetiology of patellar chondropathy.

Lack of equilibrium between forces during weight-bearing and articular cartilage strength.

Increase in forces during weight-bearing:

- Dysplasia.
- Joint fractures.
- Errors in alignment.

Decrease in cartilage strength:

- Prolonged immobilisation.
- Metabolic disorders.
- Synovial disorders.
- Wear due to advanced age.

This injury is probably much more common than it is assumed to be. Therefore, the articular aspect of the patella must be carefully examined during an arthrotomy (Figs. 23 and 24).

Concerning clinical signs, the animal has trouble climbing stairs (bearing weight on the stifle joint in extension). Lameness of varying severity with pain in the stifle joint is observed, especially when attempting to dislocate the patella medially or laterally or striking the patella with a rubber hammer, as when examining the patellar reflex. Slight crepitation may be heard. Lameness is more severe in the morning when first getting up and resembles that observed in joint disease. Few changes are observed on X-ray. In bone scintigraphy hyperuptake is observed in the area (positive region of interest) (Fig. 25).

Surgical treatment

Optimal treatment involves surgically moving the tibial tuberosity cranially (Banti's operation* in human medicine) to decrease the pressure exerted on the articular surface of the patella (Figs. 26 and 27).

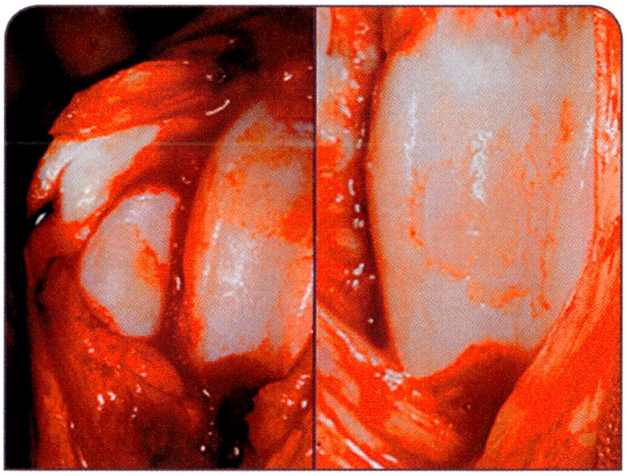

FIGURE 23. Patellar chondropathy.

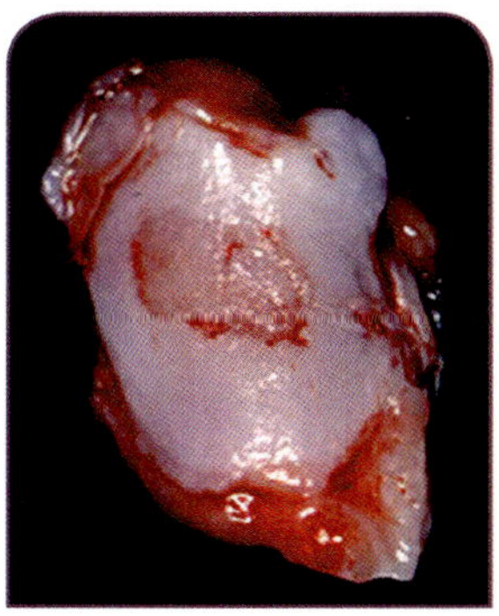

FIGURE 24. Patellar chondropathy.

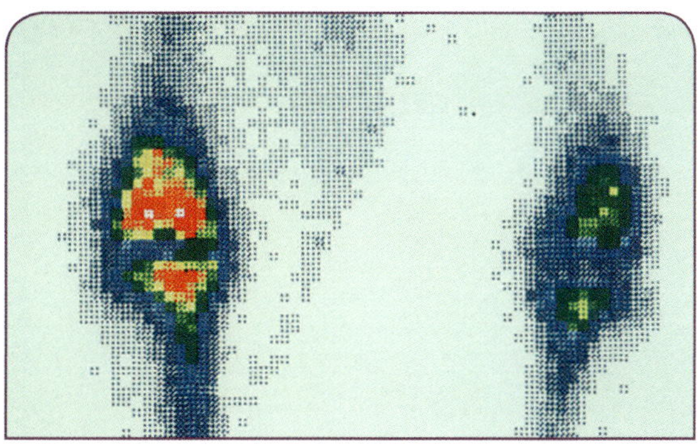

FIGURE 25. Bone scintigraphy of patellar chondropathy in the left limb.

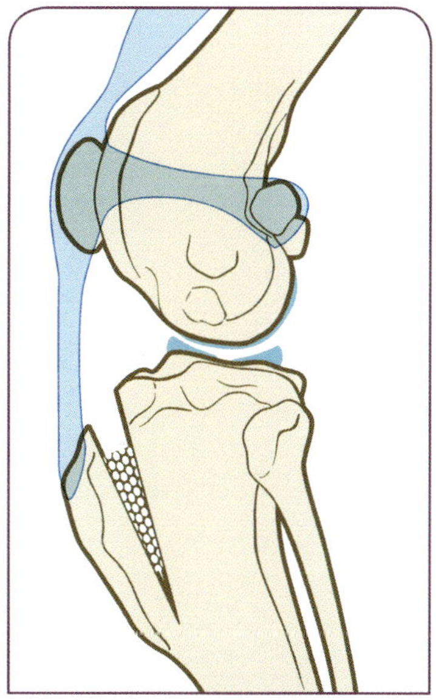

FIGURE 26. Technique of cranialisation of the patella (using a bone graft).

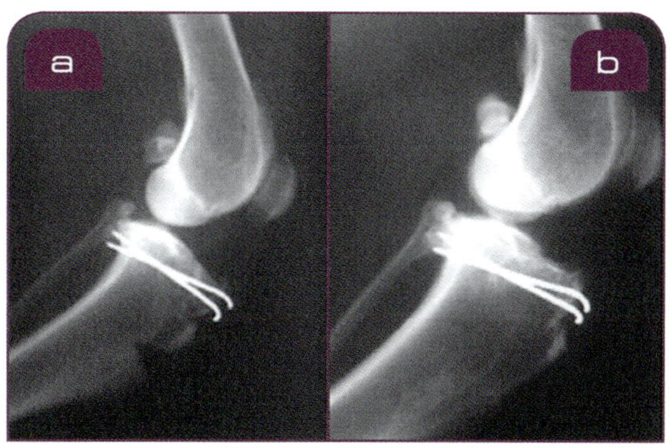

FIGURE 27. Technique of cranialisation of the patella. X-ray in the immediate postoperative period (a) and 15 months after the procedure (b).

*Surgical technique to treat patellar chondropathy, especially in athletes, which involved advancing the insertion of the patellar ligament. In human medicine it has lapsed into disuse as it has been replaced by more innovative techniques. However, in veterinary orthopaedics it is used with good results.

Dislocation of the stifle joint

This is an uncommon injury in general. It is seen more in cats, especially those with "high-rise syndrome". It is generally accompanied by rupture of several ligaments. Peripheral circulation must always be monitored, given that in these cases the popliteal artery may be compromised. This topic is discussed in greater detail in Chapter 5.

Surgical treatment

Treatment involves meticulously reconstructing the ruptured ligaments. It is advisable to start by replacing the anterior cruciate ligament (Westhues technique) and then focus on the collateral ligaments.

Fat pad abnormalities (Hoffa's disease)

Hypertrophy of the infrapatellar fat pad is considered to be not a disease in itself but a result of synovitis, which in turn derives from other orthopaedic problems. In general, once the primary problem has been treated the fat pad returns to normal. Even so, the authors have seen a Vizsla dog with a hypertrophic fat pad and no other injury. The abnormal fat pad was removed and the symptoms disappeared. The fat pad can be examined by means of ultrasound.

Tumours

Tumours are mainly observed in elderly dogs. Special attention must be paid to joint capsule tumours, given that the typical abnormalities on X-ray seen in cases of osteosarcoma are not seen in these cases.

If anything suspicious is observed during an arthrotomy, a biopsy and the corresponding histological examination must be performed without hesitation.

Surgical treatment

In this type of disease the histopathological diagnosis determines the surgical treatment of choice, which is either amputation or arthrodesis as a last resort (Figs. 28 and 29).

This chapter concludes with MRI scans of dog cadavers (Figs. 30-33).

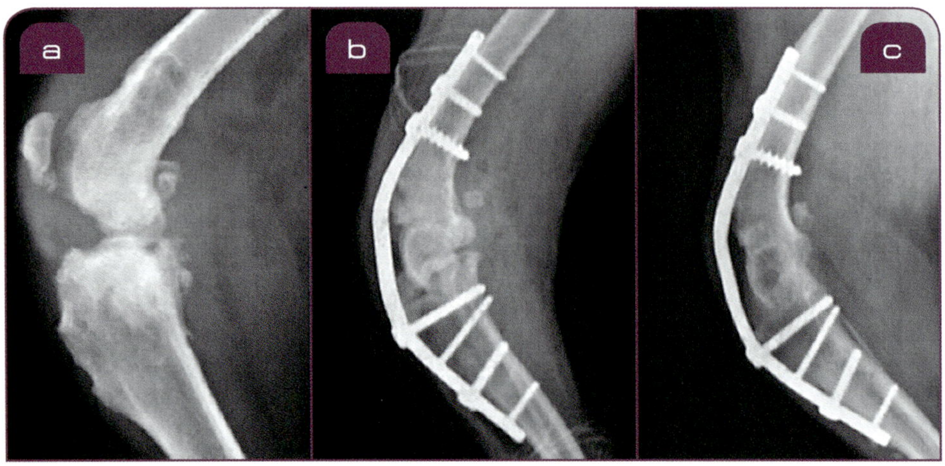

FIGURE 28. Arthrodesis of the stifle joint. X-rays in the preoperative period (a), in the postoperative period (b) and 12 weeks after surgery (c).

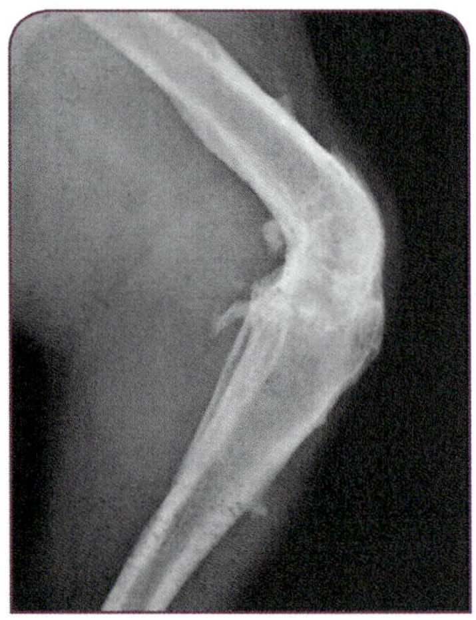

FIGURE 29. The ultimate goal of arthrodesis is ankylosis.

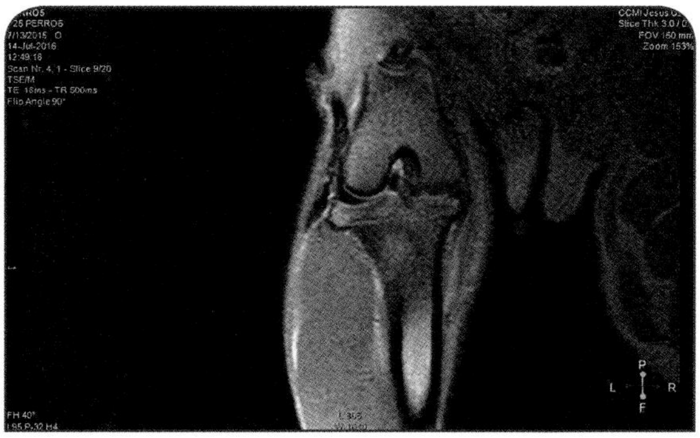

FIGURE 30. MRI scan. Rupture of the left collateral ligament. Sequence: T1 TSE.

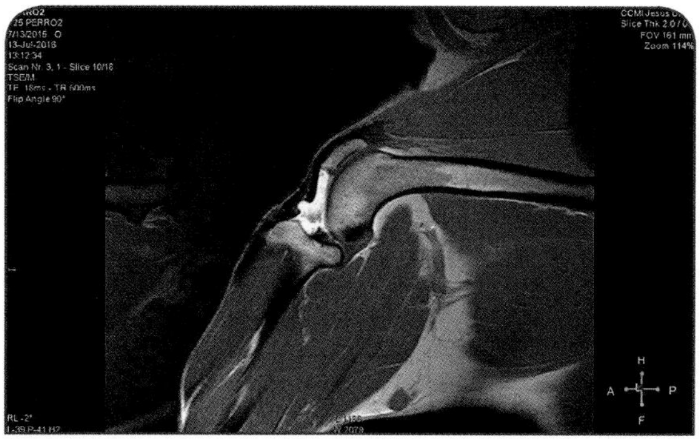

FIGURE 31. MRI scan. Rupture of the right patellar ligament. Sequence: T1 TSE.

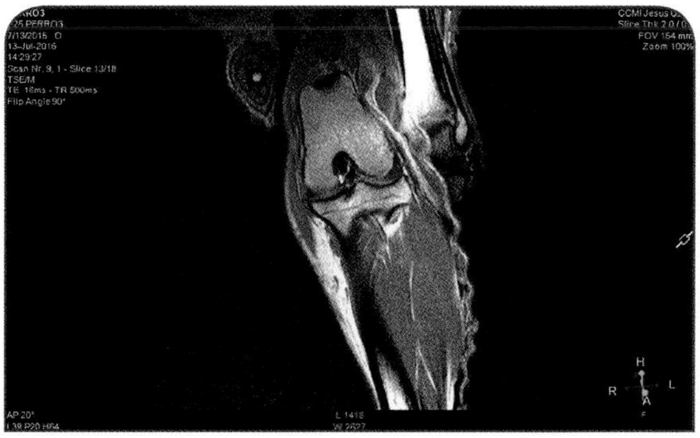

FIGURE 32. MRI scan. Left tearing of the long digital extensor muscle. Sequence: T1 TSE.

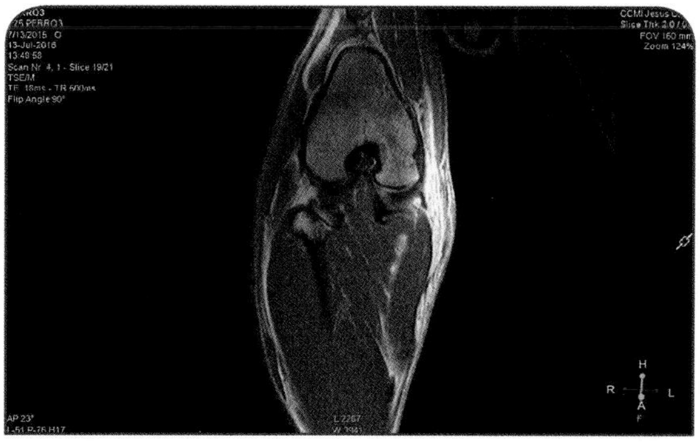

FIGURE 33. MRI scan. Right dislocation of the long digital extensor muscle. Sequence: T1 TSE.

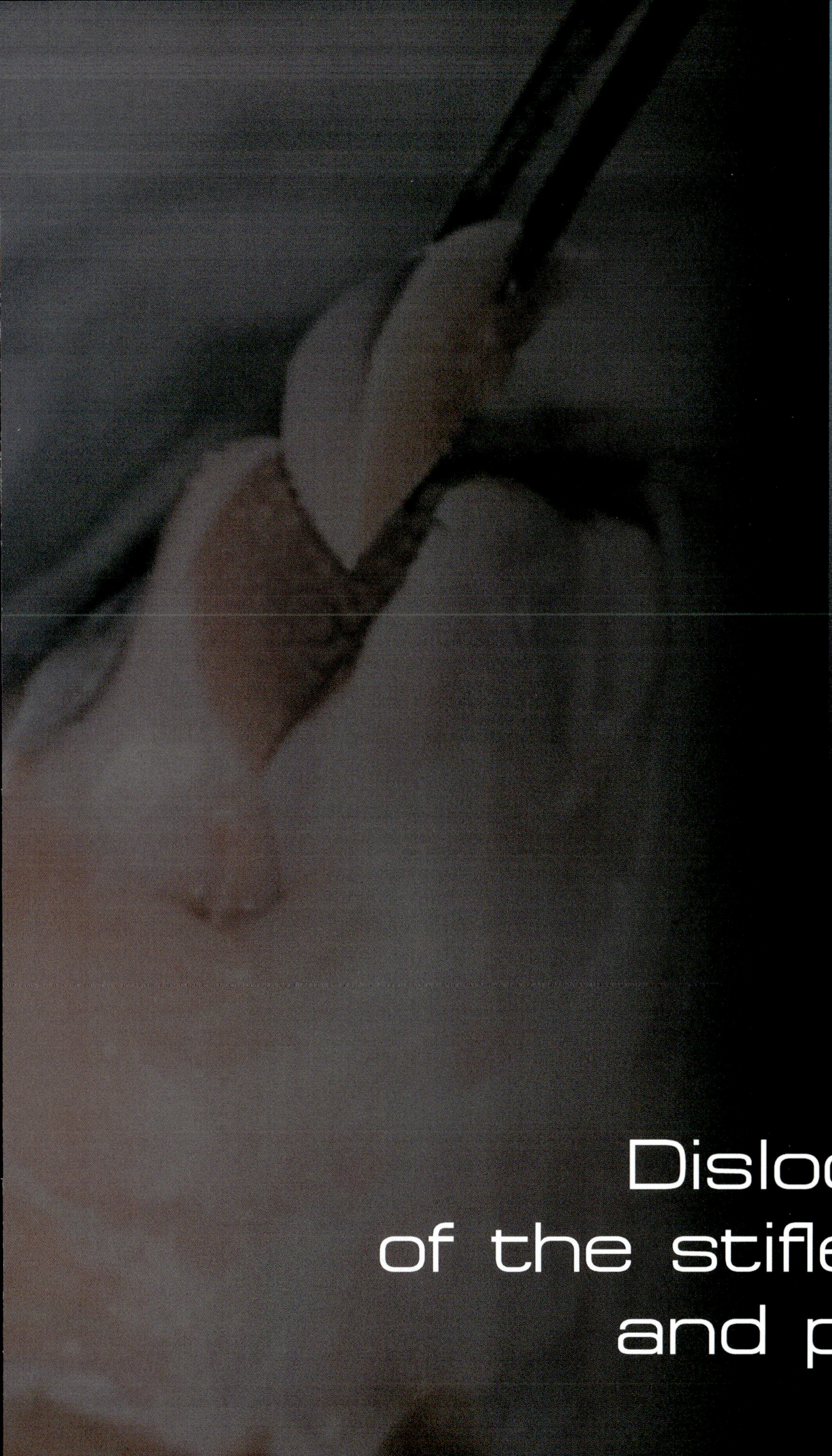

CHAPTER 5

Dislocation of the stifle joint and patella

Dislocation of the stifle joint

Displacement of structures comprising the stifle joint from their normal position has a traumatic origin. It is an uncommon injury, which is fortunate since it is usually associated with vascular and nerve injuries that are difficult to resolve.

Mechanism and classification

The classification is based on tibial movement:

- In **posterior dislocation** the tibia is caudal to the femur. It occurs due to an impact on the anterior aspect of the upper third of the tibia and requires trauma of substantial energy such as a traffic accident.
- In **anterior dislocation** the tibia moves cranially. This dislocation occurs due to hyperextension: at 10° the anterior cruciate ligament ruptures, at 30° the posterior cruciate ligament ruptures and at 50° the popliteal artery is injured.
- **Medial and lateral dislocations** result from varus or valgus trauma and involve rotation, as does rotatory dislocation.

Anterior and posterior dislocations represent 50 %–70 % of all dislocations of the stifle joint. One in five are open dislocations. Lateral dislocations account for barely 5 % of cases, while medial dislocations amount to nearly 20 % of cases. The former two are always traumatic. Lateral dislocations may be congenital but most are traumatic, while medial dislocations are always congenital in aetiology.

Associated injuries

The seriousness of dislocation of the stifle joint is due to the fact that it is commonly associated with vascular and nerve injuries (see vascular and nerve structures in Chapter 1).

Vascular injuries

The popliteal vessels are injured in 30 %–40 % of cases. They are attached proximally at the level of the adductor ring. This renders them more vulnerable in movement of the tibia. In addition, the collateral circulation of the stifle joint is insufficient to compensate for complete disruption of these vessels. Artery elongation is very common in such situations. This results in injury of the intima of the vessels, followed by thrombosis, which becomes more patent in cases in which the joint ends are not repositioned. Moreover, clinical signs and symptoms are not always sufficiently expressive since the presence of distal pulses does not rule out vascular injury. Therefore, in theory, artery injury must be assumed to be present until proven absent.

Nerve injuries

The incidence of injury of the common peroneal nerve is lower (15 %–30 %). It generally occurs in caudolateral dislocations. Injury ranges from neurapraxia to complete rupture. The prognosis tends to be poor and the potential for repair tends to be limited as these injuries are extensive due to traction.

Treatment

Following general and local clinical evaluation, in which special attention is paid to distal neurovascular status, treatment involves emergency reduction, even without X-rays, and if possible under anaesthesia. Particular care must be taken not to damage the popliteal fossa.

Caudolateral rotatory dislocation often requires surgical reduction due to capsular interposition.

It must be borne in mind that, given the extent of capsuloligamentous injuries, spontaneous reduction masking the true nature of the injury may occur at the site of the accident or in transit, especially in animals with multiple trauma. This should be suspected in significant varus or valgus instability, with the stifle joint in extension or hyperextension.

Following reduction, vascular status must be re-evaluated to make and implement a decision on eventual vascular repair (with or without an arteriogram) before six to eight hours have elapsed. Obviously, this is an option in large animals referred to hospital centres of reference with orthopaedic veterinary surgeons specialising in minimally invasive surgery and vascular and nerve surgery. If it is pursued, the joint should be stabilised using a Type II transarticular external fixator and any ligament interventions should be postponed. Vascular repair is generally performed with a contralateral saphenous vein graft. If limb ischaemia persists for more than six hours, a fasciotomy should be performed in the same surgical session as artery repair.

An algorithm of the clinical approach to dislocation of the stifle joint is shown in Chapter 2 (page 34).

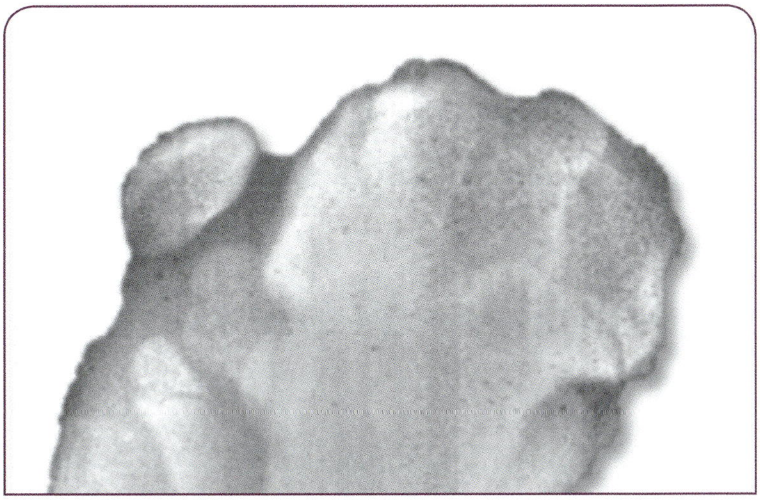

FIGURE 1. Lateral dislocation of the patella.

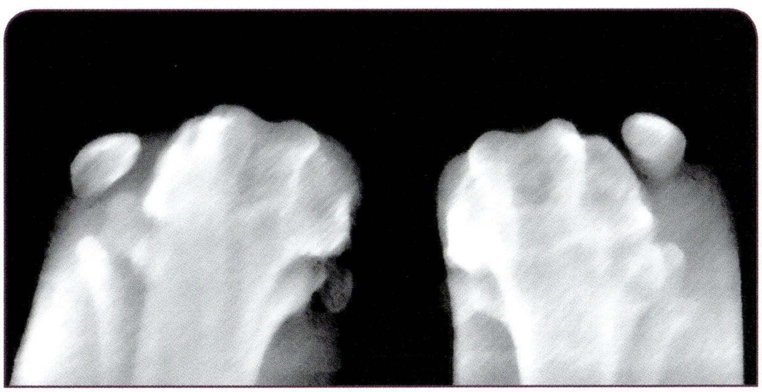

FIGURE 2. Bilateral dislocation of the patella.

In this surgical scenario, the trend is to wait for several weeks with the fixator in hopes of verifying vascular reperfusion and, only after two to three weeks, proceed to directly treat ligament injuries. The key element is the posterior cruciate ligament, which must be reinserted or reconstructed. The collateral ligaments and capsule must also be repaired. Anterior cruciate ligament reconstruction may be further delayed. Its indication depends on residual instability.

The reality is that such resources are not available to all clinicians. When a case cannot be referred to a private hospital specialising in orthopaedics and vascular surgery or a university hospital, complete arthrodesis of the stifle joint must be performed as an alternative.

Dislocation of the patella

This orthopaedic problem is very common. It is particularly seen in small breeds, but also occurs in large breeds (e.g. Samoyeds and Eurasiers) and cats.

Mechanism and classification

The classification depends on the direction of dislocation of the patella:

- Medial dislocation.
- Lateral dislocation (Figs. 1 and 2).
- Dislocation in both directions.

It also depends on the cause:

- Congenital dislocation.
- Traumatic dislocation.

Grades of medial dislocation in dogs belonging to toy breeds

- Grade I: the patella can easily be dislocated with the stifle joint extended. When it is released, the patella jumps back towards the lips of the trochlea. Normally this is a typical dislocation and lameness is intermittent. Rotation of the tibia is minimal and, when the stifle joint is flexed, it remains aligned without abducting the tarsal joint.
- Grade II: the patella is often outside of the articular groove of the lips of the trochlea. The limb bears weight with the stifle joint flexed. When the animal is examined under anaesthesia, the patella can be replaced by rotating the tibia laterally. When the tibia is released, the patella spontaneously dislocates again. The tibia can be rotated approximately 30° relative to the sagittal plane. Abduction of the tarsus is observed when the patella is dislocated medially.
- Grade III: the patella is permanently dislocated and the tibia can be rotated approximately 30°–60°. The limb can bear weight, but only with the stifle joint flexed.
- Grade IV: the tibial tuberosity can be rotated approximately 60°–90°. The patella is permanently dislocated. Generally the limb cannot bear weight and the patella is difficult to identify on palpation.

A tangential X-ray with the stifle joint flexed (skyline view) shows the depth of the trochlear groove of the femur (Figs. 3 and 4).

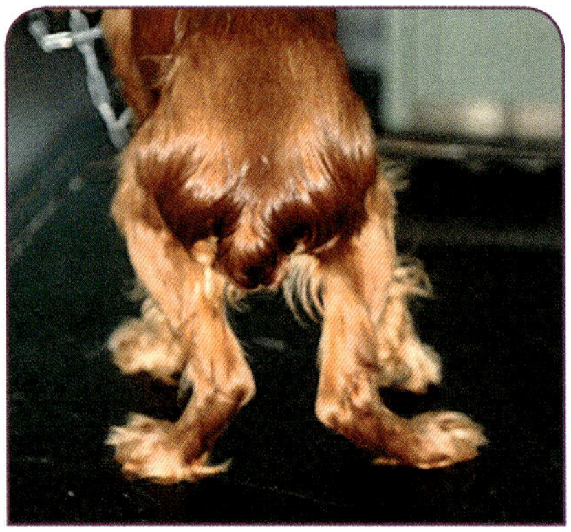

FIGURE 3. Clinical posture of the animal with bilateral dislocation of the patella.

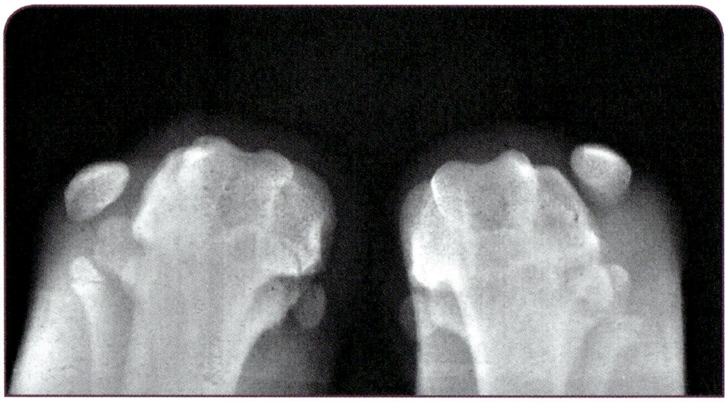

FIGURE 4. X-ray of the patient shown in the previous figure.

Images from the book *3D joint anatomy in dogs: main joint pathologies and surgical approaches* (Servet, 2014).

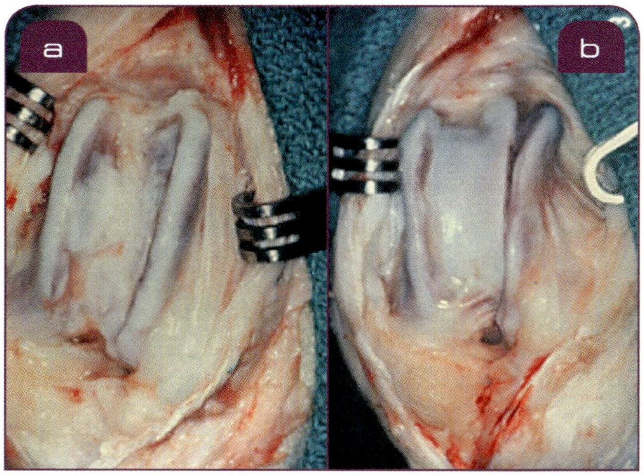

FIGURE 5. Trochlear reconstruction techniques. Sulcoplasty (a) and trochleoplasty (b).

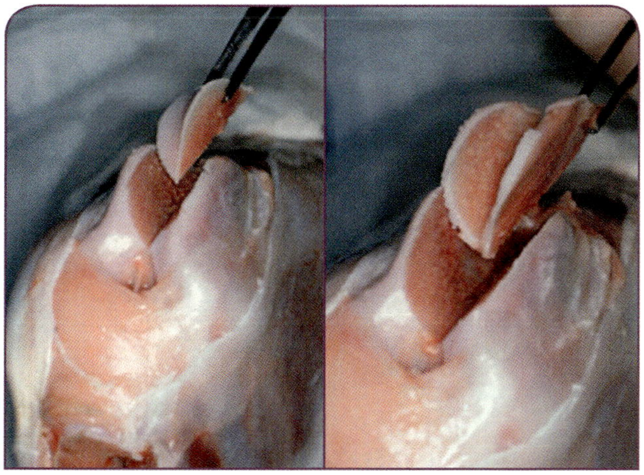

FIGURE 6. Wedge technique.

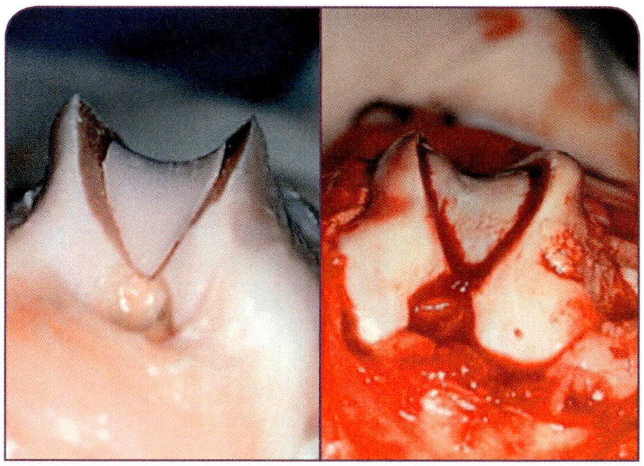

FIGURE 7. Wedge technique.

Images courtesy of Prof. Bruce Hohn.

Treatment

Although there is no strict protocol, the following diagram can guide treatment:

- **Grade I:**
  - Lateral/medial retinacular overlap, always on the side opposite the dislocation (often lateral).
  - Fixation of the tibial tuberosity to the sesamoid bone to prevent rotation of the tibia.
  - Lateral tibial tuberosity transposition, which prevents twisting of the fragment to be transposed and therefore also twisting of the patellar ligament and patella.
- **Grade II:**
  - Medial desmotomy to achieve repositioning.
  - Lateral tibial tuberosity transposition.
  - Trochleoplasty (Fig. 5).
  - Wedge technique (Figs. 6 and 7).
- **Grade III:**
  - Medial desmotomy to achieve repositioning.
  - Trochleoplasty.
  - Wedge technique.
  - Retinacular and lateral fascia overlap.
  - Fixation of the tibial tuberosity to the sesamoid bone to prevent rotation of the tibia.
- **Grade IV:**
  - Same procedures as in Grade III.
  - Osteotomies of the femur, tibia or both.
  - Arthrodesis.

In lateral dislocation, the techniques used are similar but performed towards the opposite side.

If the patient has a dislocation in both directions (lateral and medial) it is advisable to perform a trochleoplasty or wedge technique and retinacular overlap of both sides. In these cases the prognosis is guarded.

In traumatic dislocation, rupture of the joint capsule is generally observed. In this case it is sufficient to suture the joint capsule with loose stitches.

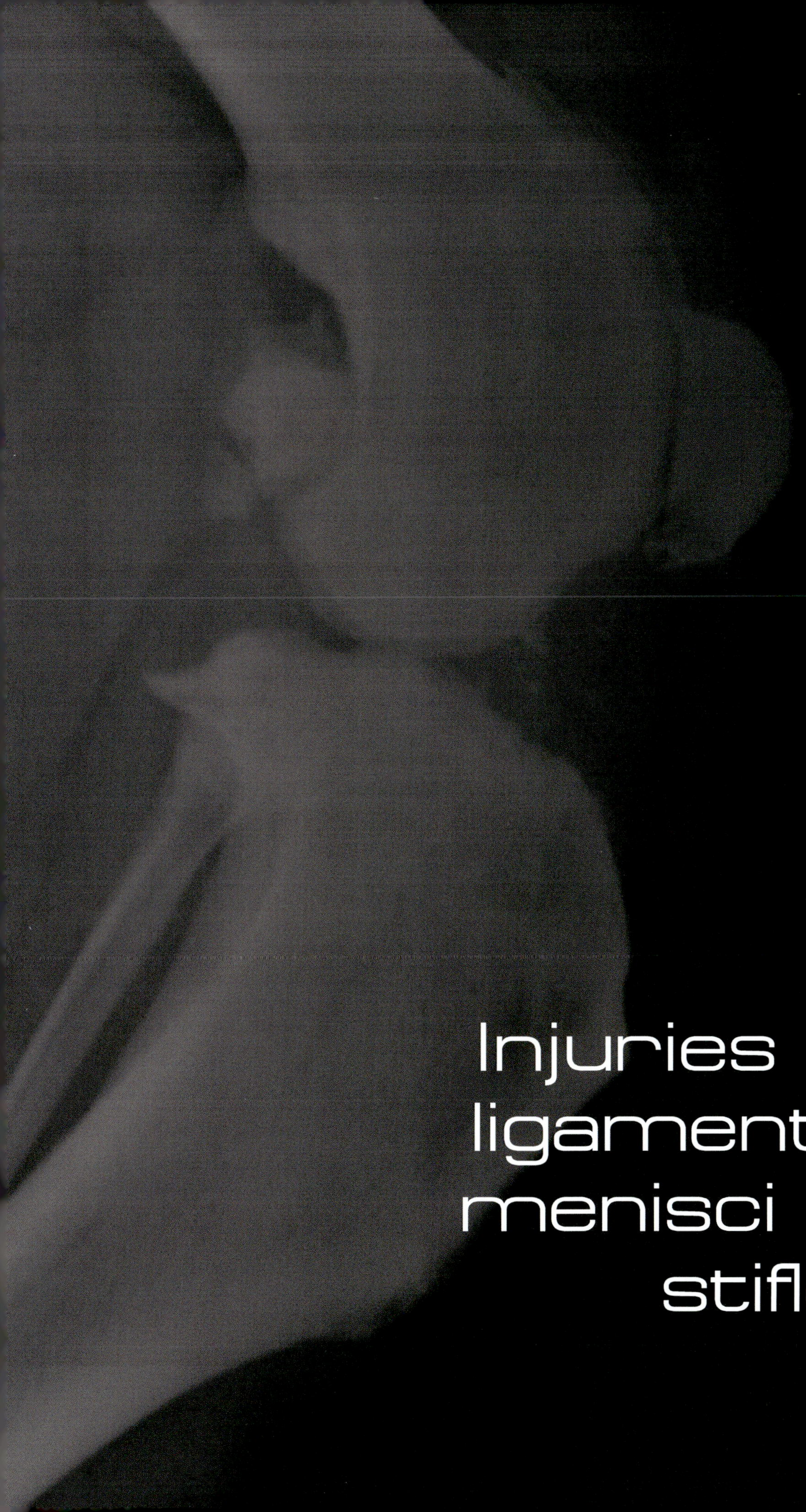

CHAPTER 6

Injuries of the ligaments and menisci of the stifle joint

Introduction

This is the most important, and therefore most extensive, chapter of this book, as the ligaments and menisci are the most widely injured structural elements of the stifle joint. It features a general review (not as comprehensive as desired) of all parts involved in injuries of the ligaments and menisci of the stifle joint, including anatomy, biomechanics and a broad overview of all techniques described to resolve the different ligament abnormalities of the stifle joint.

Knowledge of biomechanics has enabled the development of surgical techniques to offset ACL rupture. The technique of choice for this purpose is currently TPLO. Therefore, throughout this chapter, the biomechanical concepts of ACL rupture are linked to this technique, which is repeatedly referenced both directly and indirectly.

Injuries of the soft tissues of the stifle joint have taken on increasing importance given the current widespread popularity of recreational and competitive sporting practice. This is the most commonly injured joint in sporting activity, due in part to its characteristic biomechanical complexity. On the one hand, the joint is capable not only of flexion and extension (its most conspicuous movements), but also significant femorotibial rotation, which contributes to the mechanical efficacy of the extensors. On the other hand, the configuration of the articular surfaces offers limited stability, which must be strengthened in part by the menisci and in particular by a complex ligament system involving both extracapsular components (collateral ligaments and capsule reinforcements) and intracapsular components (cruciate ligaments). This system also acts as a coupling guide between the condyles of the tibia, the menisci and the femoral condyles during the different degrees of movement.

Biomechanics of the stifle joint

Capsule and ligaments

As stated, the functions of the capsule and ligaments are to supplement the stability conferred upon the stifle joint by the articular surfaces and menisci and to guide the combined movements of the stifle joint together with these elements. It has been confirmed that control of each movement depends on a specific ligament structure (primary stabiliser) whose action is supplemented by additional elements (secondary stabilisers), as shown in Table 1.

Both the strength of the tissue itself (relative to the density and thickness of the collagen bundles) and the morphology of the ligament influence the mechanical properties of the ligament. In vitro trials have confirmed that the resistance to rupture of the medial collateral ligament is similar to that of the ACL (340–390 N) and approximately 50 % of that of the PCL (780 N). The resistance of the patellar ligament is modestly higher than that of the first two ligaments, while the resistance of the individual tendons of the pes anserinus is distinctly lower.

Certain muscles help stabilise the stifle joint synergistically with some ligaments. The quadriceps muscle tends to move the tibia cranially (extension) at 0°–70° of flexion, thereby opposing the ACL and enhancing the action of the PCL. The flexors of the stifle joint (hamstring muscles) move it caudally. This has two important practical consequences. First, a lack of muscle relaxation (due to pain, fear, etc.) can "falsify" the results of the manoeuvres used to diagnose stifle joint ligament injuries. Second, proper muscle preparation can functionally offset to a certain extent the effects of ligament rupture.

TABLE 1. **Stabilising elements of the stifle joint.**

Movement	Primary stabiliser	Secondary stabiliser
Cranial tibial movement	ACL (85 %)	Medial collateral ligament and caudomedial capsule
Caudal tibial movement	PCL (95 %)	Lateral collateral ligament and caudolateral capsule
Varus	In flexion: lateral collateral ligament (70 %)	Caudolateral capsule
Valgus	Superficial and deep medial collateral ligament (80 %)	Cruciate ligaments, especially ACL
External tibial rotation	Superficial and deep medial collateral ligament	ACL
Internal tibial rotation	Lateral collateral ligament and caudolateral capsule	PCL

Menisci

The mechanical functions to which the menisci contribute can be summarised in the following points:

1. The differences in terms of both morphology and mobility between the medial and lateral menisci facilitate combined flexion–extension and rotation movements, during which it is often said that the fibrocartilage accompanies the tibial surface in its movements. Specifically, the final rotation movement in the last few degrees of flexion may be blocked if a fragment of meniscus is trapped between the articular surfaces.
2. Their wedge morphology helps distribute synovial fluid in a thin film, which facilitates cartilage lubrication and nutrition.
3. As they cover a great deal of the articular surface, they transmit 50 % (in extension) to 90 % (in flexion) of joint loads, as well as 20 % of stress waves on impact during walking, running and jumping. This explains why a total meniscectomy increases contact stress on cartilage to the point of causing degenerative phenomena in cartilage in the medium term.
4. Although their morphology may suggest that the menisci significantly contribute to the stability of the stifle joint, their absence has no clinical repercussions in this regard, except when associated with a concomitant ACL injury.

Their mechanical resistance is lower than that of articular cartilage and, as expected of an anisotropic material, greater in the main direction of their collagen bundles (longitudinal). This accounts for the frequency of longitudinal, vertical and horizontal tearing.

Rupture of the cruciate ligaments

The ACL is the main stabilising structure of the stifle joint in dogs. It may rupture by different mechanisms:

- Rupture by direct trauma.
- Partial rupture which continues little by little and ultimately becomes complete rupture.

Biomechanics in the failure of the anterior cruciate ligament mechanism

The anatomy of the stifle joint has been reviewed to supplement the traditional anatomical model (capsule, ligaments and menisci) with the function of the different muscle groups that act on and help stabilise this joint. The biomechanics of the entire stifle joint have also been very generally reviewed. Due to the extreme importance of ACL injury, this section takes a somewhat more detailed look at the evolution of stifle joint biomechanical models and their applications to the different surgical techniques developed to repair the ACL mechanism.

Development of the study of the cruciate ligaments

In 1952, Paatsama described the existence of various types of ligament ruptures that he called acute and chronic, determined the existence of partial and complete ligament ruptures and established the importance of the anterior drawer sign for diagnosis. He also identified the link between ACL rupture and injury of the caudal horn of the medial meniscus.

Moreover, he explained the pathogenesis of ACL rupture by two mechanisms:

- Internal rotation of the flexed stifle joint which causes the ACL to stretch and touch the PCL and/or the lateral edge of the intracondylar medial femoral groove.
- Hyperextension of the stifle joint in straight-legged breeds.

He described replacement of the ligament with a flap of fascia lata as treatment. His 1952 publication led to the establishment of a new school of thought and has guided most research on the ACL conducted to date.

Concerning repair technique, in 1967, Strande built upon the work of Paatsama by including other ACL repair materials. He reported that lameness after ACL replacement lasted three to six months, and that the onset of osteoarthritis decreased when the middle third of the patellar ligament was used, although postoperative lameness lasted longer still.

His study also found that bilateral ACL ruptures occurred in 28 % of cases and that the caudal horn of the medial meniscus was often damaged. He determined that partial ACL ruptures eventually progressed to complete ruptures in certain straight-legged dog breeds such as Chow Chows and Boxers.

Over time it became clear that intra-articular replacements yielded variable outcomes, and extracapsular techniques started to be used. Unfortunately, outcomes with extracapsular techniques also vary widely. As a result, there is a veritable arsenal of extracapsular techniques. Some of the most outstanding ones are as follows:

- De Angelis's lateral retinacular overlap (1970).
- Slocum's cranial fibular head transposition (1971).
- Hohn's posterior capsulorrhaphy (1973).
- Modified lateral overlap with suture of the sesamoid bone to the tibial crest or Flo's "three-in-one" technique (1975).
- Griffith's muscle sling (1976).
- Arnoczky's over-the-top technique (replacement of the ligament with aponeurosis and flap of the patellar ligament, with or without part of the patella) (1979).
- Milton's ACL prosthesis (1982).
- Smith's fibular head transposition (1985).

This plethora of procedures is a testament to the fact that their outcomes are highly variable. All that is generally agreed upon is that surgical treatment always yields better outcomes than conservative treatments, but in any case is abnormal if it does not confer normal function upon the joint in the postoperative period. Intra-articular procedures are intended to replace the ruptured ACL in order to remove the anterior drawer sign and maintain a full range of motion, as the ACL does in a normal stifle joint. Extra-articular procedures are also intended to remove the anterior drawer sign, although they sacrifice or remove some of the range of motion of the stifle joint. It is hypothesised that normal function is restored to the stifle joint once the anterior drawer sign is removed. The failing of these techniques is that they cannot restore the full function enjoyed prior to injury, regardless of breed, size or activity. Finally, it should be noted that in 1978 Henderson and Milton described the tibial compression test to demonstrate cranial movement of the tibia. This introduced a new biomechanical concept of the stifle joint.

The biomechanics of the stifle joint can be explained in two different ways: using a traditional passive model, as has been done to date, or using an active model introduced by Slocum (1993).

Traditional biomechanical model

The traditional model takes into account only the structures around the stifle joint; that is to say, those within the joint itself and in its environs. It is classically presented as a two-dimensional model with a single degree of freedom that moves on a single plane. This assumes:

- That it is a frictionless joint that can move on a single plane.
- That the ligaments go from bone to bone, thus limiting the longitudinal distance between its connections.
- That the union of four points produces movement of the stifle joint.

These four points correspond to the connections of both cruciate ligaments to the proximal tibia and distal femur.

With this model, the stifle joint completely depends on the ligaments, which passively limit any movement other than biplanar movement. This model would explain the cranial displacement of the tibia relative to the femur in ACL rupture, which is confirmed in routine clinical practice with the anterior drawer movement.

Arnoczky (1979) found that the ACL is the only structure that prevents cranial movement of the tibia. Therefore, this traditional model would explain ACL rupture following hyperextension of the stifle joint. The mechanism would be as follows: in hyperextension, the ACL stretches to the point of rupture, as the distance between its connection to the femur and the tibia exceeds its length. This was extensively documented by Paatsama (1952) and accounts for ACL rupture following hyperextension of the stifle joint, as commonly occurs in straight-legged breeds such as Chow Chows, Boxers and Bulldogs.

However, the traditional biomechanical model does not manage to account for serious discoveries such as partial or even complete ACL rupture with no prior hyperextension, serious trauma or degenerative disease.

In the last 40 years it has been demonstrated that some animals experience ACL rupture without prior trauma, or equivalently, with activities of daily living. The traditional biomechanical model is also contradictory in that it describes but does not explain rupture of the caudal horn of the medial meniscus. Finally, this model does not account for outcome disparities between the different intracapsular and extracapsular techniques, even in the hands of the most expert surgeons.

Active biomechanical model

Slocum developed an active biomechanical model of the stifle joint by expanding the traditional model to include the forces exerted by the muscles in the area and the weight borne.

This model is based on the premise that dogs use muscles to create forces that actively move or stabilise part of the body.

This system includes so-called active forces (muscles that go from bone to bone exerting a force) and so-called passive forces, which act when the stifle joint is in equilibrium (ligaments, bones and joint capsule). This biomechanical model takes into account the physical principles underlying the action of the muscles that form the different elements that create force. These include moment of force and point of equilibrium, which are not taken into account in the traditional model. This system establishes some two-dimensional simplifications which are explained below.

Two-dimensional simplifications

Slocum's system refers to the instant centre of the stifle joint. For purposes of simplification, the stifle joint is considered to be a single point. This means that an instant centre always remains perpendicular to a fixed plane, which tends to be the sagittal plane by default (Fig. 1).

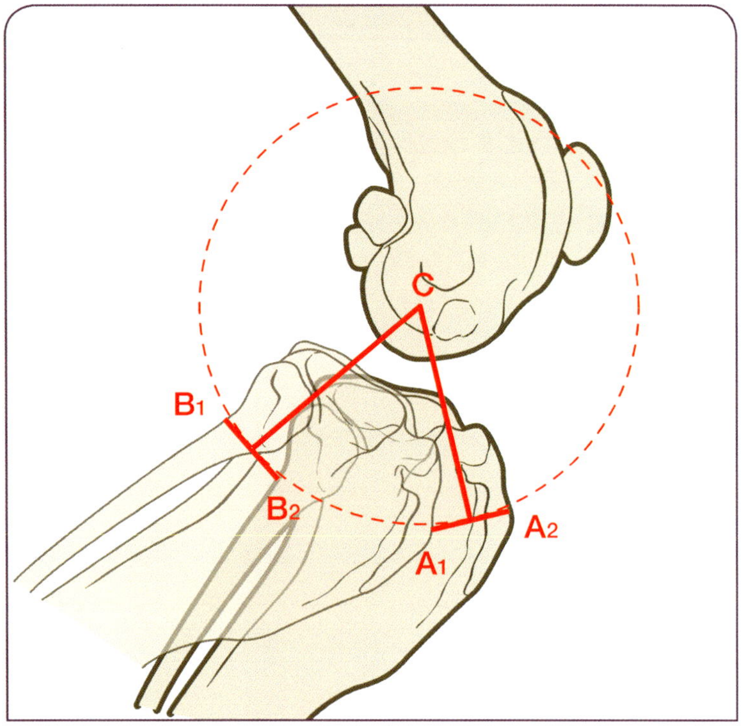

FIGURE 1. How to find the instant centre of the stifle joint considering the mobile tibia relative to the immobile femur, thus assuming that movement only occurs on the A–B plane in the diagram, and taking into account the positions at the start and the end of a movement which are A_1–B_1 and A_2–B_2. Therefore, the instant centre is C, which is found by tracing the bisectors and looking for their points of intersection with A_1, A_2, B_1 and B_2.

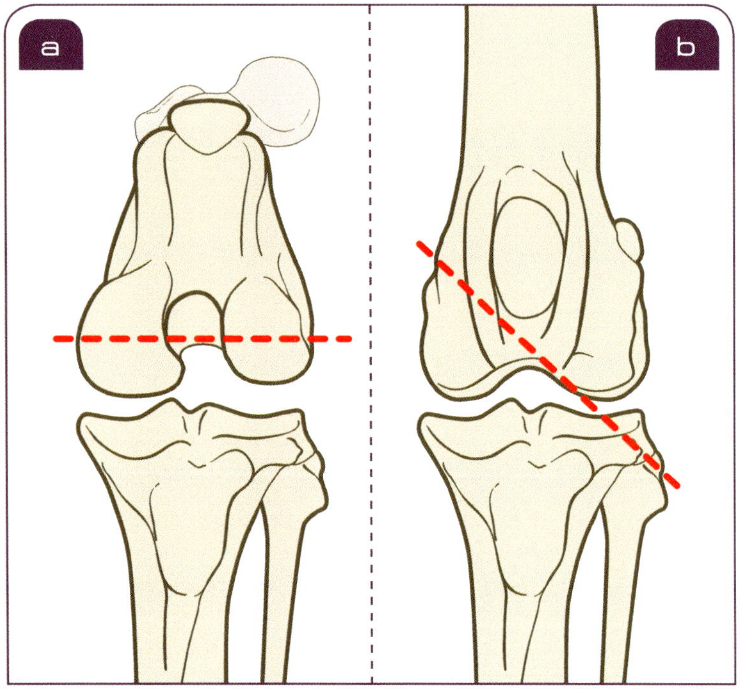

FIGURE 2. Positions of the instant centres of flexion–extension with the stifle joints in flexion (a) and extension (b).

If this is so, the points at which the consecutive positions of the instant centre intersect with a selected plane are known as instant centres, and the curve that connects the consecutive positions of the instant centre characterises movement. Since the two bodies, the femur and the tibia, move in relation to one another, the path of the instant centre relative to the femur will not be the same as that relative to the tibia, and it is important to specify the one in question. In 1971, Frankel et al. applied the simplification to humans. These researchers took profile X-rays of knees not bearing weight at intervals of 10°–20° from full extension to 90° of flexion. They discarded X-rays obviously showing significant rotation around the longitudinal axis of the tibia, thus attempting to remain within the constraints imposed by the hypothesis that the instant centre does not move. They found that it does move (Fig. 2).

They determined that while in normal knees the instant centre was always located such that relative movement at the articular surfaces was tangential, in abnormal knees there was a perpendicular movement component at the articular surfaces. This may be of little importance with respect to the bulk of movement of one segment of the limb relative to another.

In 1978, Denham and Bishop found in their experiments with cadaver knees that a point several centimetres along the tibial diaphysis traced a circular path relative to the femur. They reached this conclusion with a great deal of accuracy by attaching a pencil to the tibia and placing a sheet of paper relative to the femur.

Control of movement

As the articular surfaces are highly incongruous and the menisci that reduce their incongruity are flexible and mobile, these surfaces cannot control joint movement; therefore, the ligaments and musculature must play a role. The collateral ligaments help limit nearly all possible movements through elastic forces, but acting alone they would not be able to control craniocaudal sliding with any precision. Therefore, the cruciate ligaments and the muscles of flexion and extension of the stifle joint make a significant contribution.

The system consisting of the femur, the tibia and the cruciate ligaments, which of course appear to intersect when viewed laterally, has been described in kinematics as a four-bar linkage. In that linkage, the instant centre is always at the intersection of two bars. Therefore, in a two-dimensional system with rigid connections, the positions of the instant centre along the entire trajectory of motion are well demarcated. Figure 3 shows the path of the instant centre of a four-bar linkage with connections arranged much as in a representative stifle joint. The stifle joint differs from this model in three regards:

- Its motion is not two-dimensional.
- The cruciate ligaments may stretch under the influence of a load.
- Its ligaments may be lax.

With the simplified model (wherein a single point is taken as an instant centre of movement of the stifle joint), if the moments of force around the instant centre of movement are evaluated, the opposing forces that act on the stifle joint, essentially those of flexion and extension, are seen to equilibrate.

Cranial tibial thrust arises from the action of an active force created by weight-bearing plus the compression exerted by the tibial plateau against the femoral condyles through the muscles (Fig. 4). Equilibrium is achieved by the action of the flexor muscles of the leg (active components) as well as the ACL and the caudal horn of the medial meniscus (passive components).

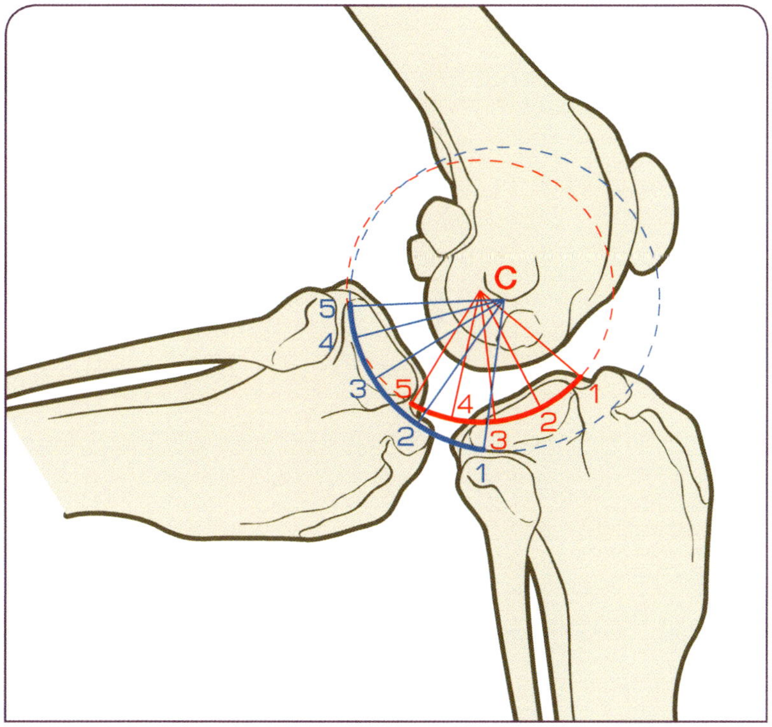

FIGURE 3. Potential trajectory of the instant centre of the tibia relative to the immobile femur, where it is assumed that movement only occurs on a single plane and also that the ligaments are connections comprising a four-bar linkage, kinematically speaking. Five consecutive positions of the instant centre are numbered.

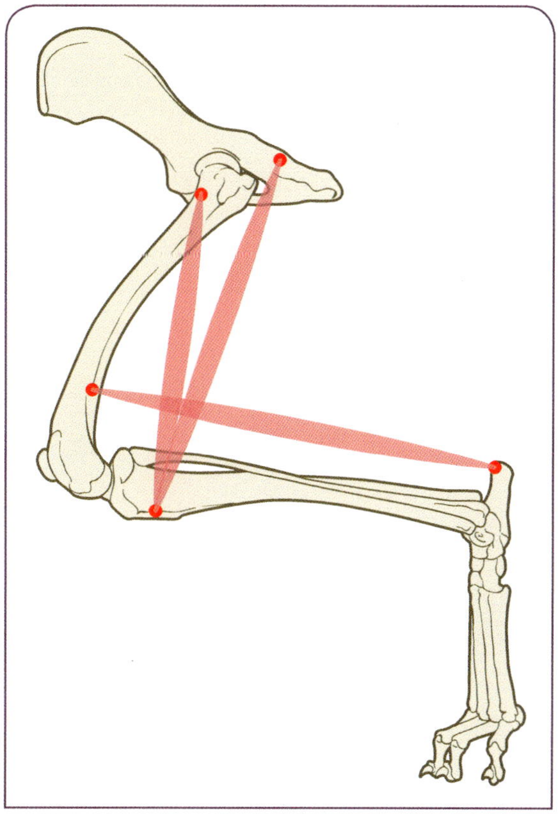

FIGURE 4. Muscle action which creates tibial compression.

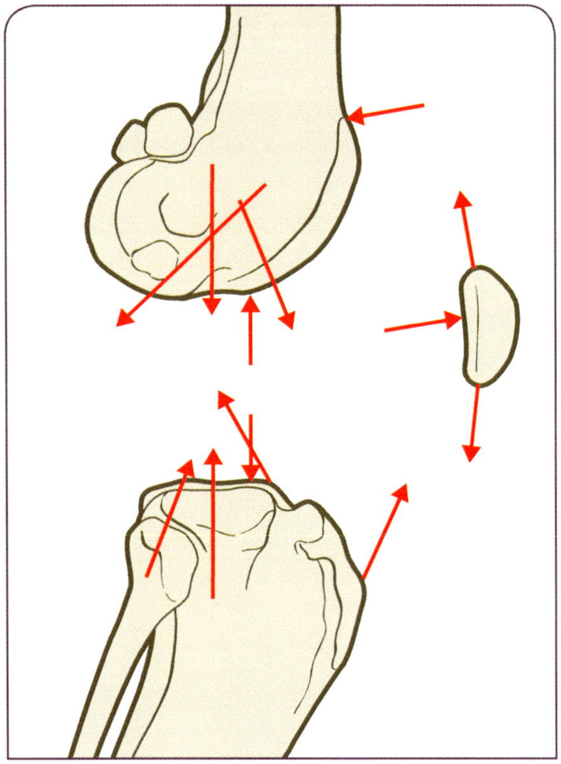

FIGURE 5. Results of force showing the approximate direction of action of the different forces applied between the femur, patella and tibia.

From a physical perspective, for the stifle joint to maintain a nearly constant angle in flexion during the weight-bearing phase, the moments of force of flexion and extension around the centre of movement of the stifle joint must add up to zero (Fig. 5).

Given the above, one may wonder why the cruciate ligaments exist, if the geometry of the condyles is consistent with joint rotation movement and the articular surfaces cannot control movement by themselves. The answer may be in large part that incongruous articular surfaces with very low friction can control movement if the forces applied always remain perpendicular to the surfaces at the point of contact. In the absence of this particular requirement, the articular surfaces would slide and the joint would tend to destabilise. The cruciate ligaments can exert forces with some significant components parallel to the articular surfaces. Since the capsule and the collateral ligaments cannot do this, the cruciate ligaments allow the joint to remain stable even on a trajectory under weight-bearing conditions.

The tangential tibiofemoral forces calculated by Denham and Bishop (1978) and the forces of the cruciate ligaments measured by Trent et al. (1976), which are the forces referred to herein, suggest that these ligaments play an important role in some activities such as climbing stairs.

This question can be explained on the basis of the two-dimensional simplification described above. In fact, the two articular surfaces of the tibia are not exactly the same shape, the lateral and medial femoral condyles are not exactly the same shape either and the cruciate ligaments do not remain on one plane. These things point to the three-dimensional nature of the actual motion of the stifle joint.

Muscle moment of force

Muscle moment of force is defined as the perpendicular distance from the line of muscle rotation to the centre of joint movement times the magnitude of force. Therefore, the stifle joint is neither flexed nor extended when the sum of the moments of force in flexion equals the sum of the moments of force in extension. Here the stifle joint is said to be in muscle equilibrium.

Origin of the forces of the stifle joint

This being said, the forces transmitted through a normal stifle joint, specifically their origin, will now be examined. The stifle joint, like other joints of the pelvic limb, transmits force due in part to the weight that it bears and in part to the muscles that act through it to perform ambulatory movements. Occasional accessory forces also occur when at least one segment of the body has been accelerated.

It must be borne in mind that, if there were no muscle action, each femorotibial joint would in theory transmit half the weight of the part of the body above the stifle joints. For example, if an animal were missing a pelvic limb, one stifle joint would transmit all the weight of the body minus the weight of the segment of the leg below that stifle joint. In fact, some muscles are always acting, and any tensile force between two segments of the body increases compression force through the joint in question.

The length of the lever arms of the muscles around the stifle joint (or any other joint) is less than the distances to the centres of gravity of the body segments and in general less than the muscle and joint forces. Consequently, in other activities, said forces acting on the stifle joint mechanism will exceed the weight of the relevant body segments.

These forces thus explained are applied to the system of articular surfaces, capsules and ligaments. The forces in the latter two are tensile and tend to increase compression force through the articular surfaces. However, as the forces in the capsule and the ligaments vary when a trajectory is inferior to that of the muscle forces, their effect on the forces transmitted to the articular surface is lower.

Having explained this theoretical aspect of the origin of the forces, it must be borne in mind that, during the weight-bearing phase, the extensor muscles of the stifle joint and tarsal joint, as well as the tarsal tendon, prevent the collapse of the limb and the caudal muscles of the thigh stabilise the stifle joint, but mainly act as extensors of the hip to propel the dog forwards. Therefore, tibial compression is created by the extensors of the limb and weight-bearing forces.

Provided that the compression elements are in line between the centres of the tarsal joint and stifle joint, the compressed components are in equilibrium. From a biomechanical perspective, active and/or passive forces are needed to provide equilibrium and prevent the tibia from protruding cranially, as the point of contact between the femur and the tibia is cranial to this line.

The biceps femoris muscle and the semitendinosus muscle provide active force which stretches the proximal tibia caudally. When the force exerted is insufficient to prevent cranial movement of the tibia, passive resistance (the ACL and the caudal horn of the medial meniscus) counteracts this cranial displacement.

It is important to bear in mind that cranial tibial thrust is created by compression exerted between the femur and the tibia. The magnitude of tibial thrust depends not only on the amount of compression exerted, but also on the slope of the tibial plateau relative to the line between the centres of movement of the stifle joint and the tarsus.

Compression varies because the amount of force that the dog produces on the ground varies with activity.

Therefore, cranial tibial thrust can be controlled by changing the slope of the tibial plateau, with the help of muscle control and, as mentioned, bearing in mind that the articular surfaces, which are incongruous, can control movement if the forces applied always remain perpendicular to the surfaces at the point of contact. Tibial plateau levelling contributes to this.

This chapter concludes with a reminder that the forces involved in cranial tibial thrust are active and passive:

- The active forces are caudal forces provided by the tendons of the pes anserinus and the caudal muscles of the leg. They are responsible for the activity of the dog and cannot be controlled.
- The primary passive force of the ACL can be controlled by modifying its properties through surgical repair. The secondary passive force of the caudal horn of the medial meniscus can potentially be controlled through meniscal repair.

As main conclusions accounting for failures in the ACL mechanism and the general ideas that have led authors such as Slocum and Montavon to propose new techniques for repair of this defective mechanism, it can be affirmed that the functions of the capsule and ligaments are, as stated, passive stabilisation of the stifle joint, with which they supplement the stability conferred upon the stifle joint by the articular surfaces and menisci. All these elements guide the combined movements of this joint.

> It has been confirmed that control of each movement depends on a specific ligament structure (primary passive stabiliser), whose action is supplemented by additional elements (secondary passive stabiliser) and active stabilisers (musculature of the area).

As mentioned above, both the strength of the tissue itself relative to the density and thickness of the collagen bundles and the morphology of the ligament influence the mechanical properties of the ligament. The action of active stabilisers (muscles) has also been highlighted as fundamentally important in the conceptual development of TPLO, which is based on the fact that certain muscles cited help stabilise the stifle joint synergistically with some ligaments.

All this has essential practical consequences (essential point of the technique), as proper muscle action, once the tibial plateau has been levelled, functionally compensates for the effects of cranial tibial movement following complete or partial ACL rupture.

To summarise these biomechanical concepts, it can be affirmed that the TPLO technique best resolves ACL mechanism failure and fundamentally differs from all other techniques to date. The purpose of this surgery, according to Slocum, its developer, is to neutralise cranial tibial thrust, not to remove the anterior drawer sign. Ultimately, the stifle joint is redesigned so that the ACL is not needed to stabilise the joint; instead, stabilisation is achieved under active muscle force, and the outcomes alone speak to the efficacy of this concept. Given the importance of this technique, it is discussed in depth in a separate chapter.

However, there may be two causes for concern in the use of this technique:

- First, when there is no ACL (complete rupture) there is no mechanism to support muscle action controlling cranial tibial thrust. This predisposes the tibia to move cranially relative to the femur under compression, and this is a determining factor in whether or not osteoarthritis subsequently develops. Any lack of equilibrium between cranial tibial thrust and active muscle force leads to compression by cranial movement of the tibia, and this predisposes the caudal horn of the medial meniscus to be crushed by the femoral condyle. Therefore, it is best to excise the medial meniscus in surgery for complete ruptures; otherwise, it will likely need to be removed within a year of surgery. In partial ACL ruptures, normally the joint is relaxed and osteoarthritis changes are minimal. The caudal horn of the medial meniscus usually remains intact. The protection conferred upon the caudal horn of the medial meniscus by the remaining ACL shows that meniscal damage occurs following rupture of this ligament. It has been demonstrated that not all ACL ruptures are due to hyperextension. This is especially true of partial ACL ruptures. Physical examination of the affected joint or joints (often both) will reveal increased ACL laxity. A TPLO without a medial meniscectomy is known to restore the normal function of the animal (once the ACL ruptures a meniscectomy is needed).
- The second cause for concern around the TPLO technique is that it may lead to iatrogenic over-rotation of the tibial plateau. This may create extra pressure on the partially ruptured ACL and cause it to stretch. If this happens, proper walking function is not restored, and the integrity of the ACL must be properly evaluated, especially in trauma cases. A TPLO must never be performed on animals with an intact ACL.

This chapter concludes with Slocum's description of this technique as a pleasure for him and a blessing for his patients, since they go home the same day of surgery and recover in a reasonable time. It is safe to say that this technique has definitively replaced the plethora of techniques that came before it and has undoubtedly set the standard for a new understanding of treatment of a defective stifle joint mechanism. Other ideas such as the surgical technique for tibial tuberosity advancement (TTA) have arisen from this initial idea.

Clinical signs

Clinical signs that can be seen in affected animals are:

- Acute or chronic lameness.
- Joint inflammation.
- Pain on palpation of the area, especially during hyperextension.
- Positive drawer sign.
- Positive Finochietto's jump sign when there is an injury of the meniscus.
- In chronic cases, hypertrophy of the joint capsule and increase in synovial fluid.
- Muscle atrophy.
- Osteoarthritis changes along the edge of the trochlea.

There are two types of candidates for ACL rupture. One type consists of purebred animals and animals no more than five years old which are overweight and subjected to a sedentary lifestyle. The other type consists of particularly predisposed animals belonging to various breeds including Rottweilers, Chow Chows, Boxers, Bulldogs, Neapolitan Mastiffs, etc.; these are all straight-legged breeds (Fig. 6).

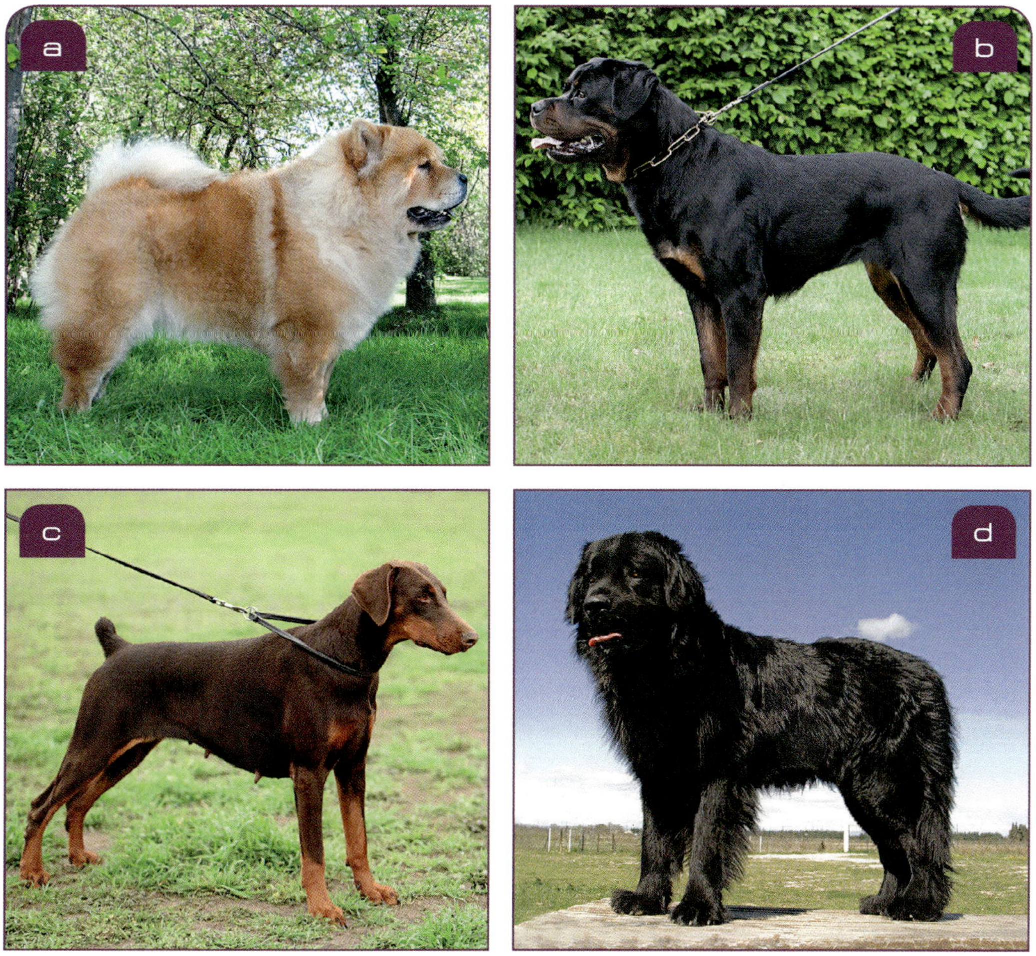

FIGURE 6. Examples of dogs belonging to the Chow Chow (a), Rottweiler (b), Doberman Pinscher (c) and Newfoundland (d) breeds.
Images from tandemich (a), wims-eye-d (b), Stieber (c) and cynoclub (d), Shutterstock.com.

Diagnosis

The diagnosis is based on:

- Medical history data.
- Clinical examination (Fig. 7).
- Drawer sign under local or general anaesthesia.
- Radiological examination.

Rupture of the cruciate ligaments is easy to diagnose using the drawer sign test. This test may be difficult to perform in some animals belonging to large breeds with a great deal of muscle contraction. The tibial tuberosity compression test may be easier in these cases (Fig. 8). It must be borne in mind that this test carries less diagnostic certainty than the drawer sign test (Fig. 9). Often it is essential to evaluate the joint with complete muscle relaxation.

The drawer sign test is performed with the stifle joint in extension to diagnose ACL rupture and with the stifle joint in flexion to diagnose PCL rupture. The clinician must be very careful to bear this in mind as PCL rupture does not require surgery. In these cases muscle compensation is complete and deforming joint disease virtually does not develop.

It is always advisable to examine both limbs, since the problem may be bilateral. Recent ACL rupture with aseptic arthritis or with an injury of the medial meniscus may be observed in one limb. In this case, the patient exhibits lameness in that limb, even though it may have experienced ACL rupture on the opposite side several weeks ago.

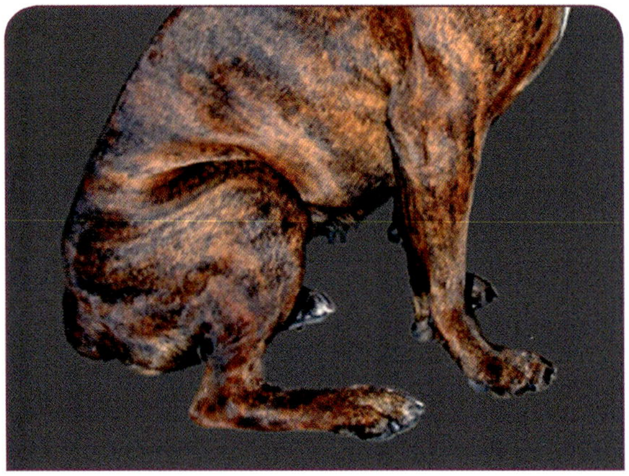

FIGURE 7. Sitting test. Typical posture adopted by patients with an ACL mechanism injury as they are unable to perform full flexion of the limb with abduction.

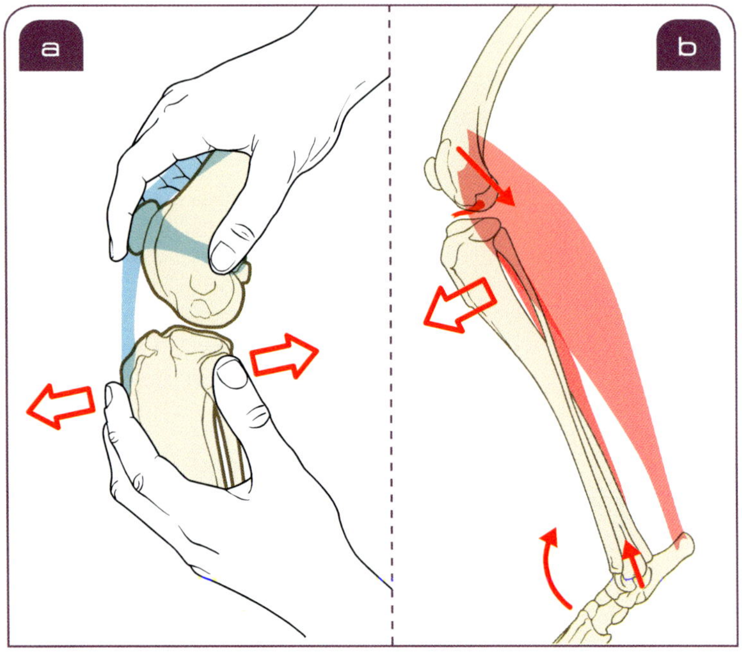

FIGURE 8. Diagnosis of ACL rupture. Position of the hands and movement in the anterior drawer sign test (a). Cranial displacement of the tibia with the tibial compression test (tibial thrust) (b). The reader can supplement both images by reading Chapter 2.

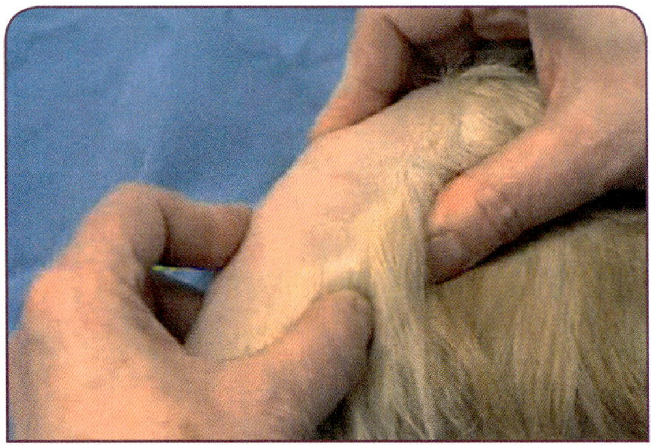

FIGURE 9. Positive anterior drawer test result.

It is advisable to take an X-ray of the stifle joint and pelvis (Figs. 10 and 11). Very often there is serious coxarthrosis of the hip joint opposite the affected stifle joint. It is important to diagnose this to make a proper prognosis. It is also best to view the deforming joint disease before performing surgery. This spares the owner some disappointment if the lameness does not completely disappear after surgery.

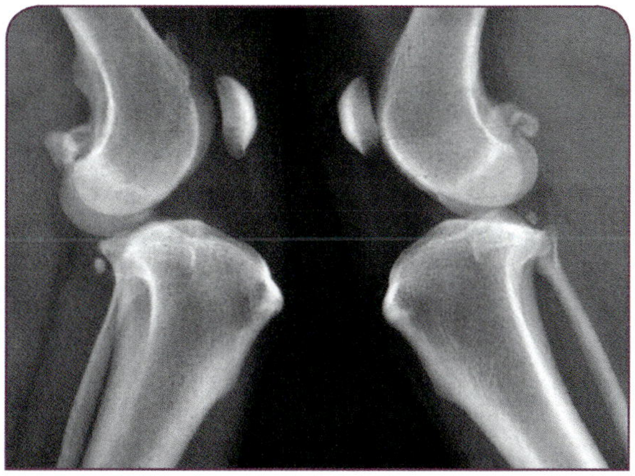

FIGURE 10. X-ray showing a stifle joint with ACL rupture (left) compared to a healthy contralateral stifle joint (right).

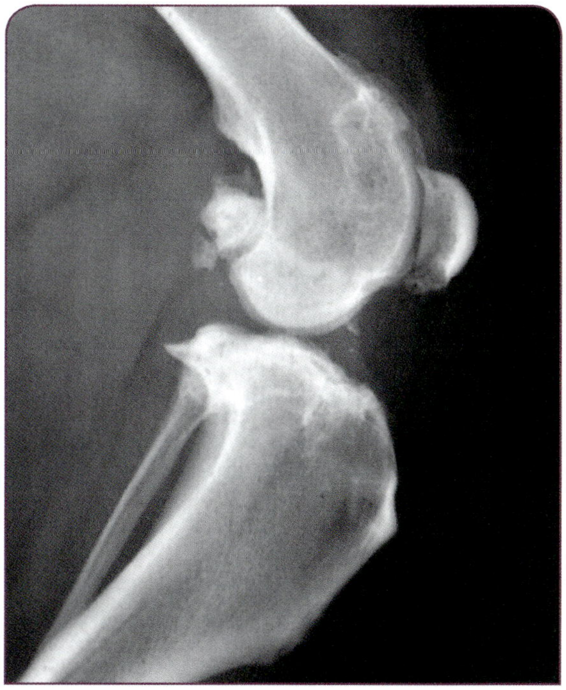

FIGURE 11. Serious joint osteoarthritis which betrays ligament and/or meniscal injury.

Treatment of rupture of the cruciate ligaments

In reality there is no optimal technique and new methods are constantly being developed. Accredited intracapsular and extracapsular techniques are as follows:

- Cranial fibular head transposition.
- Replacement of the ligament with a prosthesis (non-resorbable thread).
- Arthrotomy and surgical debridement of the stumps of the ruptured ligament as well as partial resection of the meniscus (cleaning up) without replacement of the ligament.
- Replacement of the ligament with an aponeurotic flap of the fascia lata.
- Lateral retinacular overlap and modified retinacular overlap technique.
- Replacement of the ligament with aponeurosis and flap of the patellar ligament, with or without part of the patella (over-the-top technique).
- TPLO.
- Surgical technique for TTA.

Regardless of the technique to be used, the patient is positioned in supine decubitus and the affected limb is placed on a stand so that the joint can be flexed and extended during surgery.

Cranial fibular head transposition

Fibular head transposition (Fig. 12):

- Is an extracapsular technique.
- Uses the lateral collateral ligament.
- Prevents internal rotation and cranial displacement of the tibia.

This method is very suitable for dogs belonging to large breeds. A lateral surgical approach is used and the parapatellar fascia lata is cut. First the fibular head is mobilised together with the distal attachment of the lateral collateral ligament. To do this, the tibiofibular joint must be released by cutting the ligaments that cover it while of course keeping from injuring the peroneal nerve.

The full length of the joint capsule must be cut so that all structures may be inspected. It is preferable not to injure the fat pad. To prevent postoperative seromas, it is advisable to aspirate the synovial fluid and not let it reach extracapsular tissue from the surgical approach. The patella is dislocated medially; flexing the stifle joint achieves good exposure for examination.

Finally, with the limb in extension, pointed forceps are used to move the fibular head cranially and separate it from the fibular articular aspect until craniocaudal instability disappears. The head of the fibula can be fixed to the tibia with a traction screw or a threaded Steinmann pin. Once the pin has been inserted, the tip is cut and bent (Fig. 13).

Next the joint capsule is closed. It is advisable to use loose stitches for the capsule. The aponeurotic edges are closed with a continuous suture, like the subcutaneous aponeurosis. Polyglactin is exclusively advised as a suture material in deep planes. The skin is closed with loose stitches. It is not necessary to apply a postoperative bandage. Exercise is of course limited for the next four weeks and gradually increased starting from the fifth week. Generally it is not necessary to administer antibiotics following the operation (Fig. 14).

One disadvantage that must be mentioned is that sometimes the limb rotates slightly outwards from the tarsal joint. The technique requires meticulous preparation.

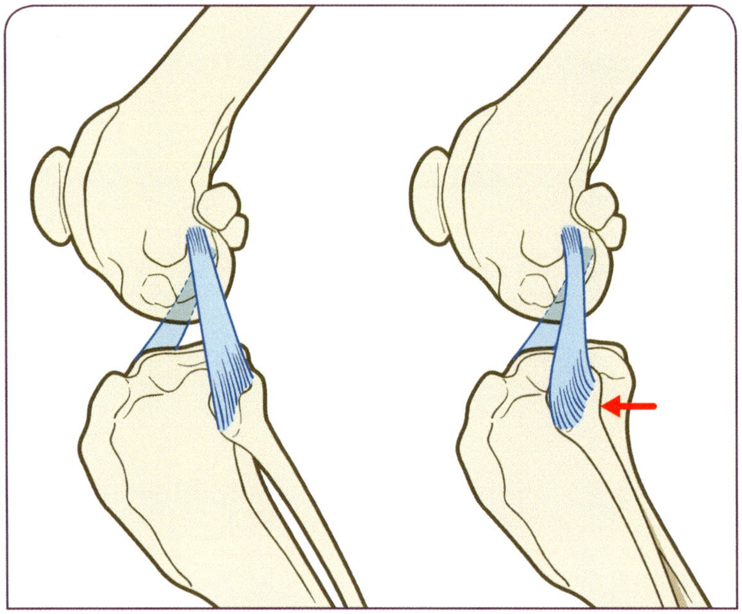

FIGURE 12. Representation of the change that occurs with fibular head transposition.

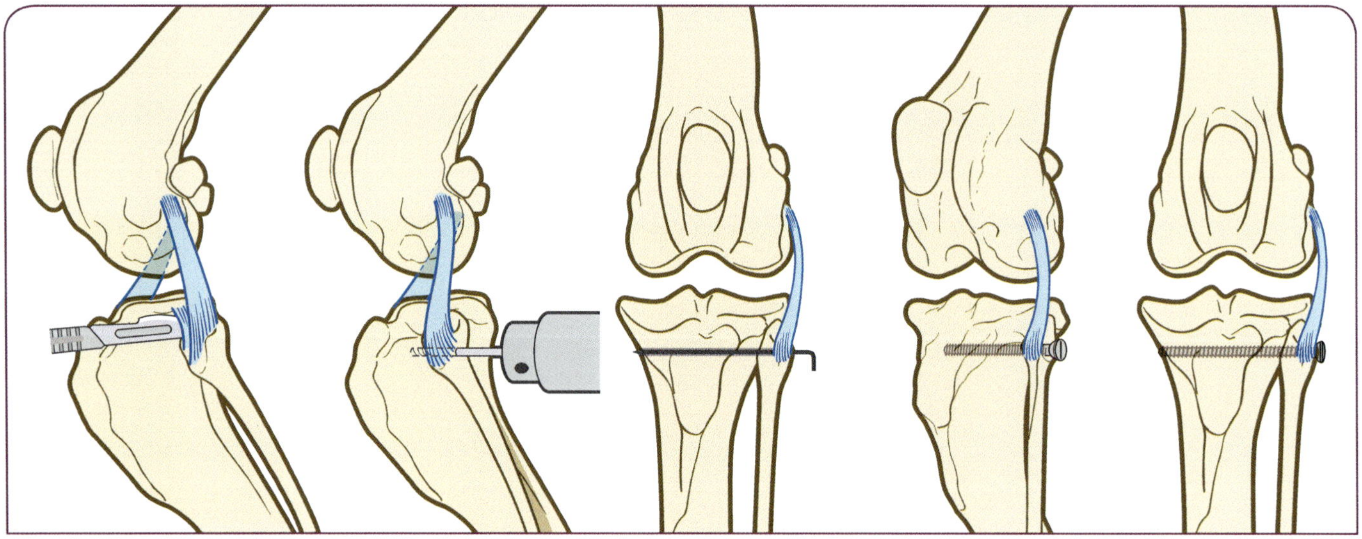

FIGURE 13. Representation of the different steps of the technique.

Replacement of the ligament with a prosthesis (non-resorbable thread): Westhues technique

This technique is mainly used in cats, in which both ACL rupture and PCL rupture are generally diagnosed. This rupture is often accompanied by injury of one or both menisci or one of the collateral ligaments. In other words, it often occurs in a stifle joint with multiple trauma.

For this technique four perforations must be made: two in the femur and two in the tibia.

After the usual arthrotomy is performed from the lateral side, a first perforation is made from the lateral condyle of the femur towards the point of origin of the ACL. Next a second perforation is made from the point of insertion of the ACL into the cranial part of the tibial plateau to the base of the medial margin of the tibia. Next, the tibialis cranialis muscle is separated and with a smaller bit a perforation is made through the tibial tuberosity. The fourth perforation is made through the femur, from the lateral distal area towards the medial proximal area. These smaller perforations must be made at an angle of around 90° relative to the larger perforations. Next the threads are passed through the perforations starting from the distal part. Once the threads are in place, they must be selected so that the corresponding ends may be knotted. The knots must be outside of the articular recess. It is advisable to flex the stifle joint a little and place it at a normal angle with slight outward rotation of the tibia before knotting the threads. The threads are at optimal tension if joint instability disappears after they are knotted (negative drawer sign). It is better to use a number of thin threads rather than a few thick threads (the principle underlying rope) (Figs. 15-19).

The joint and other planes are closed as described above.

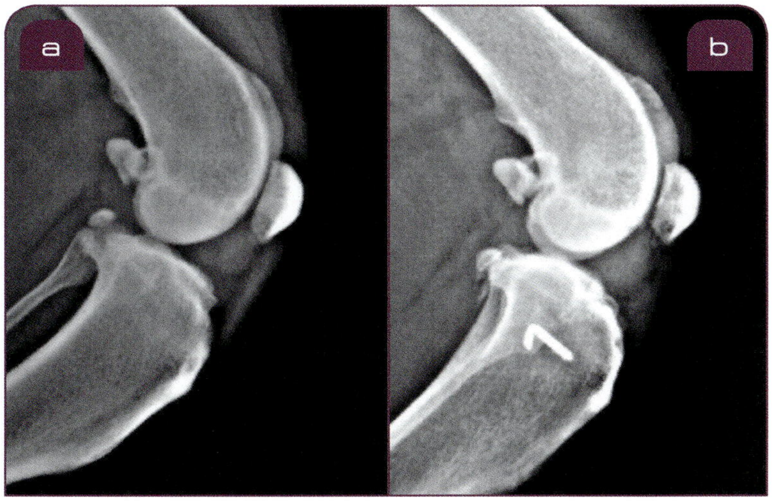

FIGURE 14. Preoperative X-ray of a candidate for fibular head transposition surgery (a). X-ray after the fibula has been advanced and secured with a pin (b).

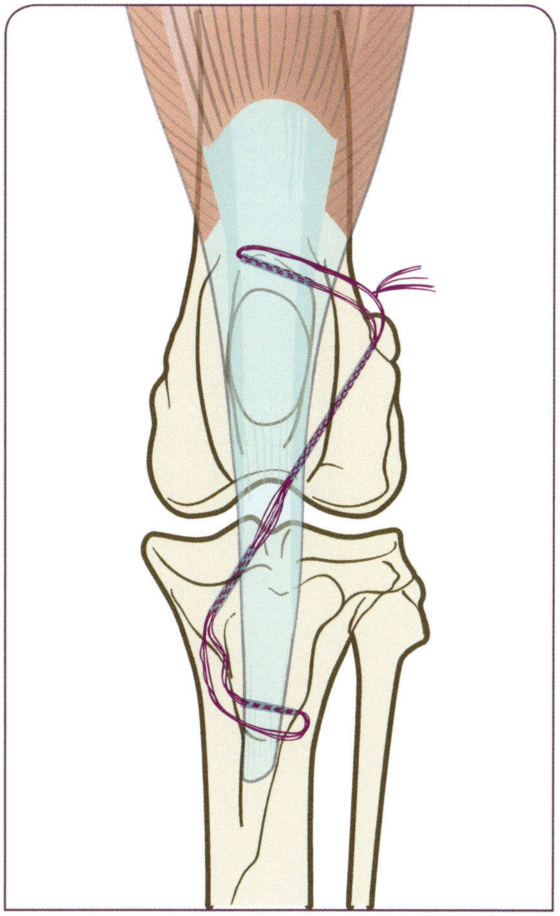

FIGURE 15. Replacement with non-resorbable threads: Westhues technique.

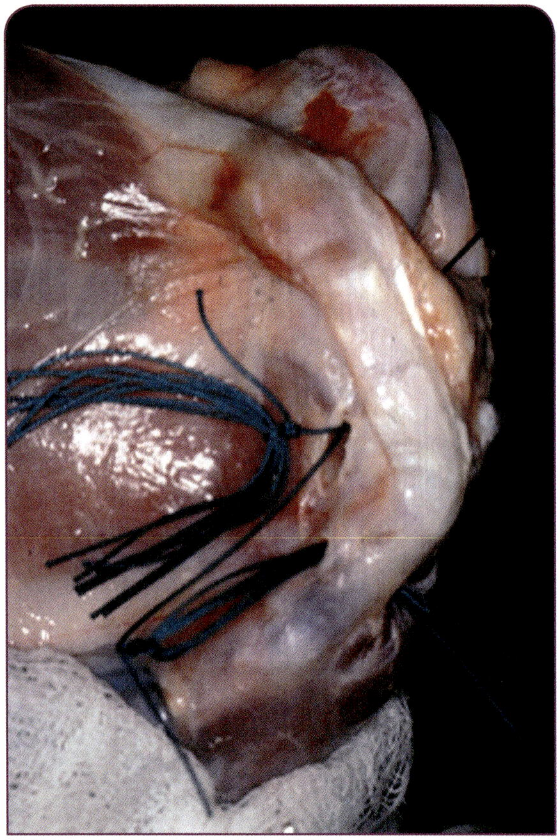

FIGURE 16. Placement of the threads prior to their knotting.

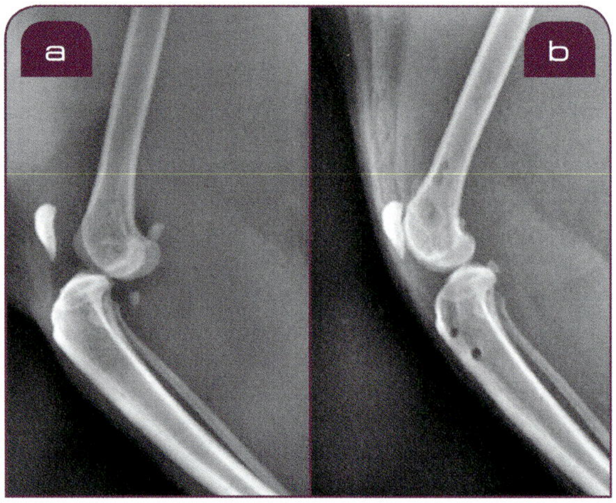

FIGURE 17. Technique of cruciate ligament replacement in a cat before (a) and after (b) surgery.

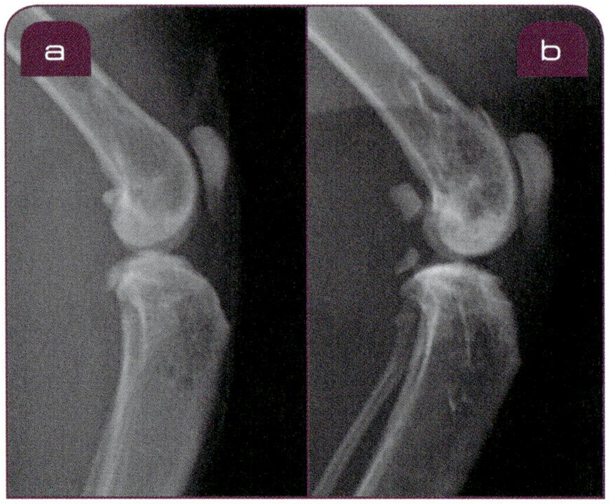

FIGURE 18. Westhues technique. Preoperative X-ray of a cat that is 12 years old (a). Appearance two years after surgery (b).

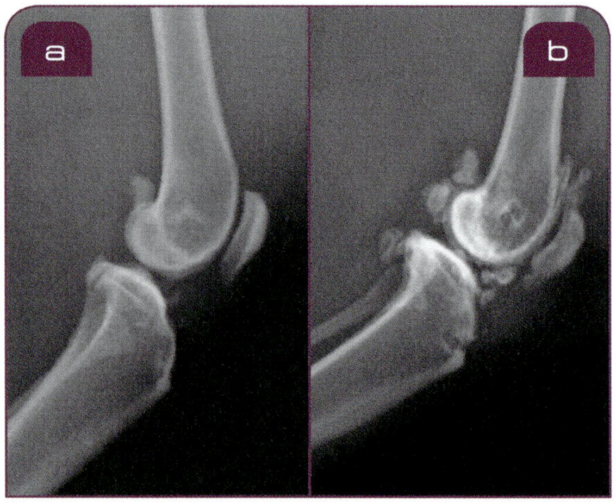

FIGURE 19. Westhues technique. Preoperative X-ray of a cat that is 17 years old (a). Appearance four years after surgery (b).

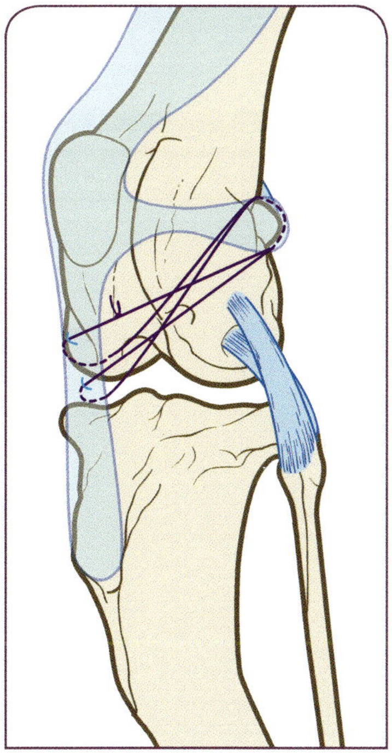

FIGURE 20. Lateral retinacular overlap. Suture between the sesamoid bone and the patellar ligament.

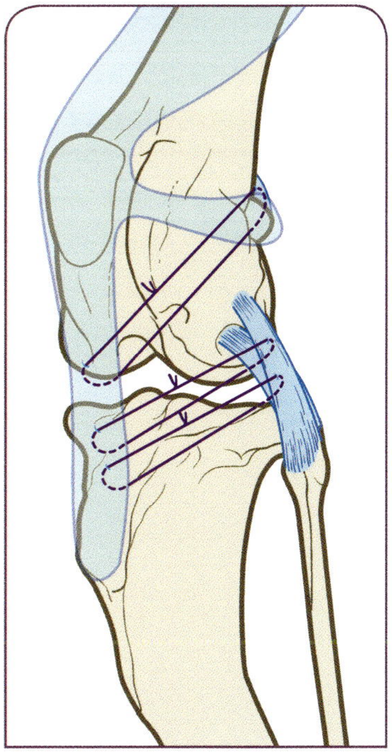

FIGURE 22. Modified lateral suture technique (three-in-one technique).

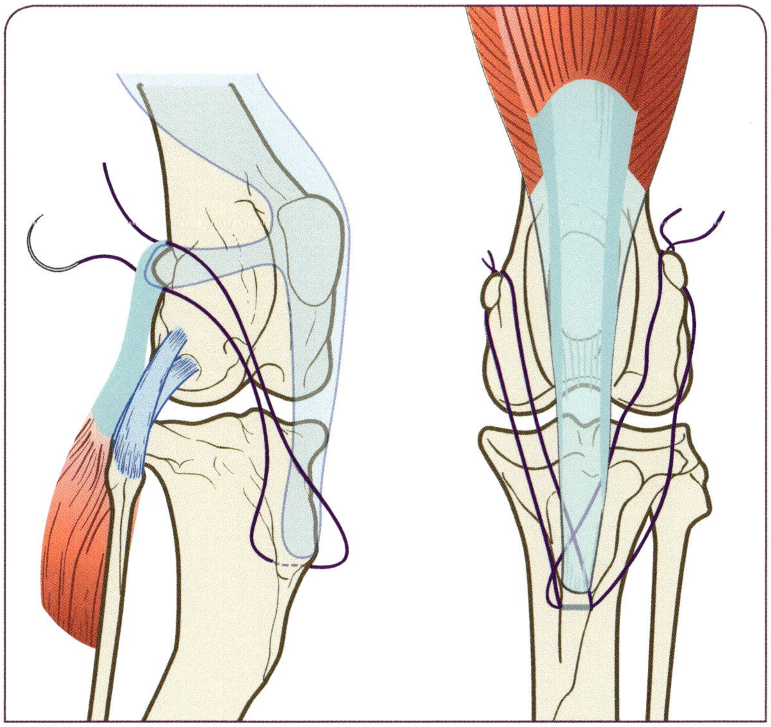

FIGURE 21. Modified lateral retinacular overlap. Sutures are placed on both the lateral and medial side through a bone tunnel in the tibial tuberosity.

Arthrotomy and surgical debridement without replacement of the ligament

To perform the technique of arthrotomy and surgical debridement of the stumps of the ruptured ligament, with partial resection of the meniscus (cleaning up) and without replacement of the ligament, a lateral approach is used as described above. Examination of the different structures is similar. The stumps of the ruptured cruciate ligament are meticulously resected. The meniscus is partially resected if it is injured. This technique is considered to be suitable for breeds that produce strong scar tissue (e.g. Boxers).

Replacement of the ligament with an aponeurotic flap of the fascia lata

Fascia lata overlap can be performed with a Lembert suture pattern with polydioxanone or polyglactin thread.

Lateral retinacular overlap technique

This involves placing a suture between the sesamoid bone and the patellar ligament. This technique is used in small dogs (weighing less than 10 kg) and cats (Fig. 20).

In modified lateral retinacular overlap a bone tunnel is made in the tibial tuberosity and sutures are placed on both the medial and lateral side (Fig. 21 and 22).

The disadvantage of retinacular overlap sutures is that they are not very reliable. They loosen or break over time, so joint stability depends exclusively on any pericapsular fibrosis that has occurred before this happens. Variants of reinforcement have been developed for this purpose (Figs. 23-25). Olmstead's lateral suture with wire has been a very popular technique, as it causes a great deal of extracapsular fibrosis, although it does not stop osteoarthritis.

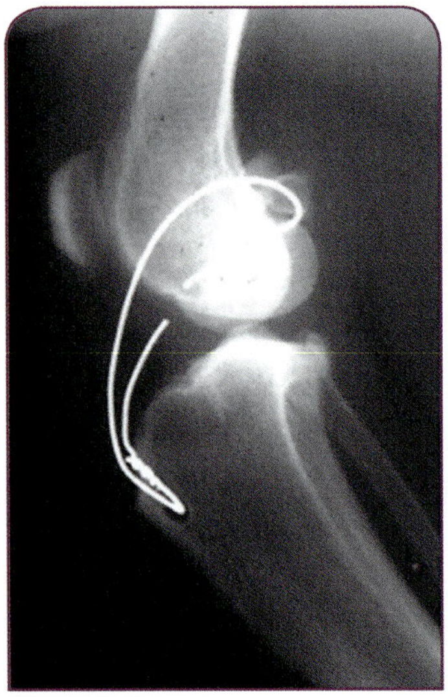

FIGURE 23. Monitoring X-ray of a retinacular suture with wire. Olmstead's technique.

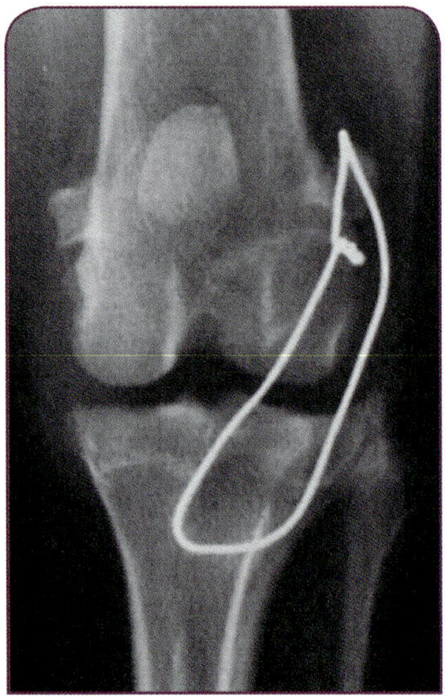

FIGURE 24. Olmstead's technique. Lateral overlap with cerclage.

Replacement of the ligament with aponeurosis and flap of the patellar ligament, with or without part of the patella (over-the-top technique)

One of the first intracapsular techniques was developed by Saki Paatsama in the 1950s. It remains a popular cruciate ligament surgery technique among clinicians. This method involves dissecting a strip of patellar ligament with fascia lata with a width of 1–2 cm from the thigh and leaving it connected distally. The femur and tibia are perforated to create holes at the anatomical origin and insertion of the ruptured cranial cruciate ligament. Care must be taken to keep from injuring the caudal cruciate ligament. The end of the strip of fascia lata is passed through each hole with a knotted wire. Then the graft is firmly pulled and secured with sutures along the patellar ligament.

There are different variants of this initial technique taken from human medicine. This method, developed by Arnoczky et al. and called the over-the-top technique,

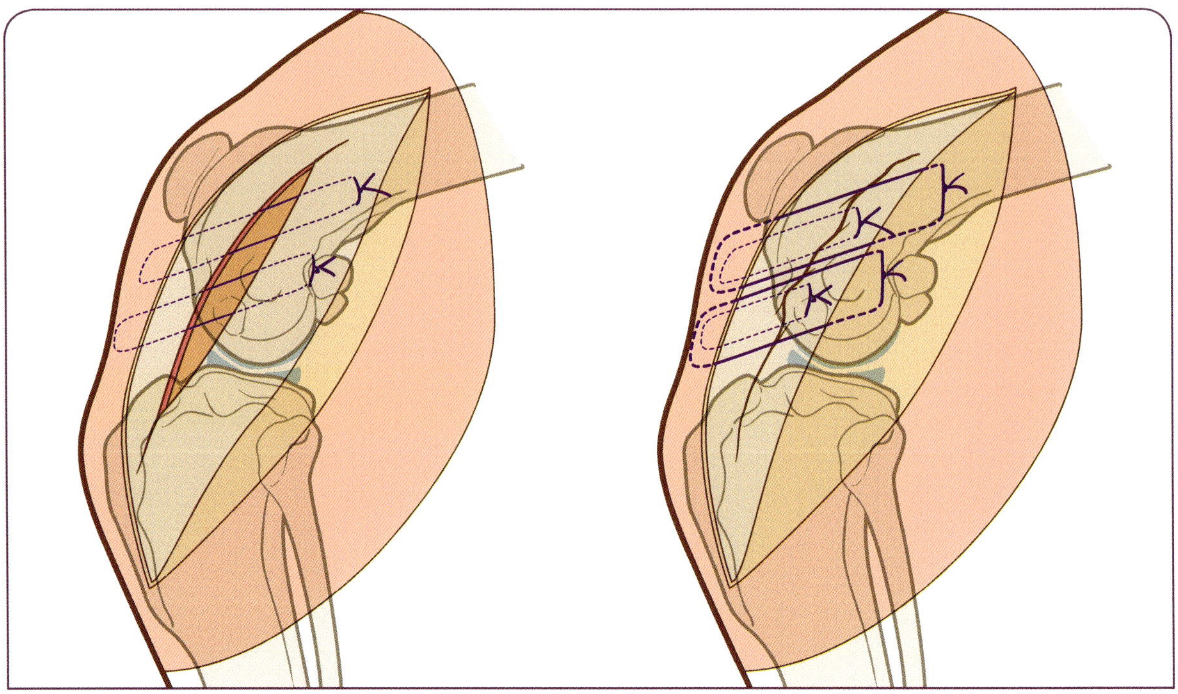

FIGURE 25. Meutstege's lateral overlap technique.

involves replacing the cruciate ligament starting from the medial third of the patellar ligament, part of the patella and the tendon of the quadriceps muscle (Fig. 26). It must be considered only in athletic dogs weighing 25–30 kg. The process of obtaining this graft is very technically difficult and entails a risk of severe injury of the patella. The graft is passed through the joint above the lateral condyle and sutured. This prevents the need to pass it through a bone tunnel, which in turn prevents the graft from potentially fraying at the bone edges, as occurs in the Paatsama technique.

After a medial arthrotomy has been performed, the medial third of the patellar ligament is separated from the rest of the ligament but left connected to the tibia and patella. The incisions in the patellar tendon and fascia lata are continued proximally. Part of the medial edge of the patella is divided with a small osteotome. Care must be taken not to penetrate the articular cartilage of the patella. The proximal and distal connections of the patellar ligament must be preserved. When the bone fragment is cut, the dissection is continued proximally in the fascia lata, where the strip is prepared as described below in the four-in-one technique. The strip, consisting of fascia, bone and ligament, must be only twice the distance from the tibial tuberosity to the patella. The incision in the medial capsule is continued as far as possible and as needed proximally to allow lateral dislocation, retraction of the patella and exposure of the lateral condyle. Forceps are used to pull the strip of the fascia through the joint from inside of the capsule. After the strip has been fixed to the periosteum, fascia and lateral collateral ligament, the joint is closed.

Another method or variation on the above is the under-and-over technique, which uses a strip of fascia lata as in the Paatsama technique. However, the strip extends as far as the tibia. A tunnel is made under the intermeniscal ligament and the graft is passed under this ligament as far as the inside of the joint. Next the strip is pulled through the joint and passed through the upper part of the region of the lateral condyle/sesamoid bone. The graft is pulled quite firmly to eliminate the drawer movement and then fixed to the lateral condyle of the femur with a screw and washer.

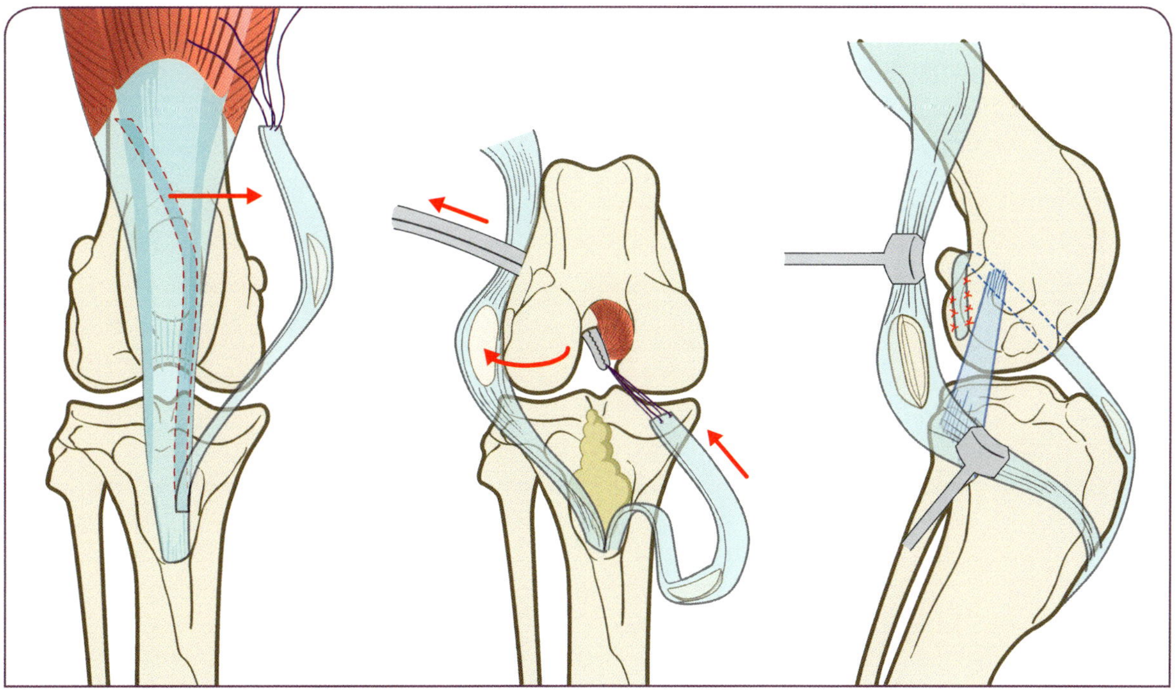

FIGURE 26. Diagram of the classic over-the-top technique.

Slocum's technique for tibial plateau levelling osteotomy

This technique is described at length in Chapter 7 by Dr Juan M. Martí of Veterinary Surgical Specialists in Chesapeake, Virginia (United States).

Surgical technique for tibial tuberosity advancement

This technique is described at length in Chapter 8 by Dr Tomás G. Guerrero of the University of Zurich (Switzerland).

Injuries of the meniscus

In examination of the stifle joint it is important to review the following structures:

- Joint capsule.
- ACL.
- PCL.
- Joint cartilage of the patella and condyles of the femur.
- Menisci (especially the medial meniscus).

The proximal end of the tibia must be moved cranially to view the medial meniscus. This is easily achieved by slightly extending the stifle joint and using a Hohmann retractor as a lever to keep from injuring the articular cartilage (Figs. 27 and 28).

In small animals, injury of the menisci is generally secondary; in approximately 55 % of cases with ACL rupture there is an injury of the medial meniscus. The lateral meniscus is more commonly injured in cats following multiple joint trauma. Injury of the meniscus can occur during trauma or movement with an unstable stifle joint. After the meniscus has ruptured, the medial portion may dislocate cranially and caudally between the femoral and tibial condyles. This dislocation causes an audible, palpable popping called Finochietto's sign or Finochietto's jump sign.

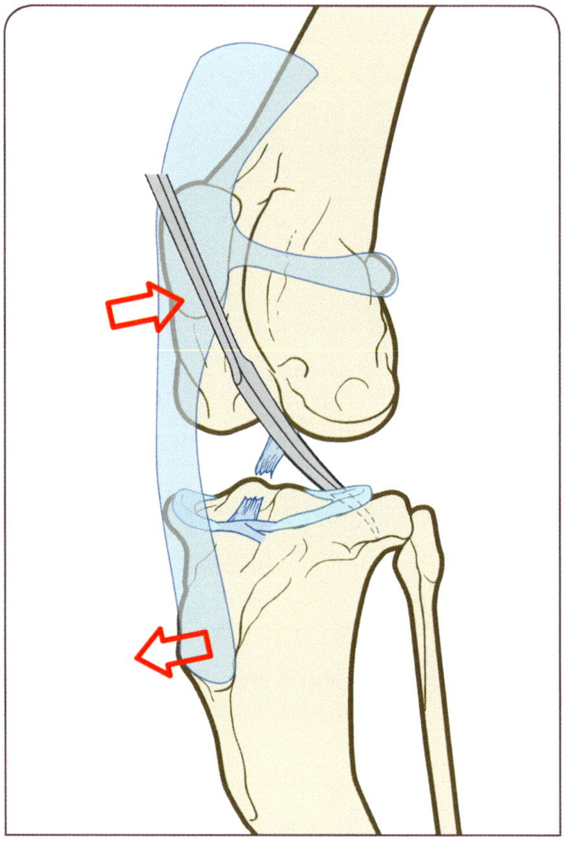

FIGURE 27. Position of the Hohmann retractor to visualise the caudal horn of the medial meniscus.

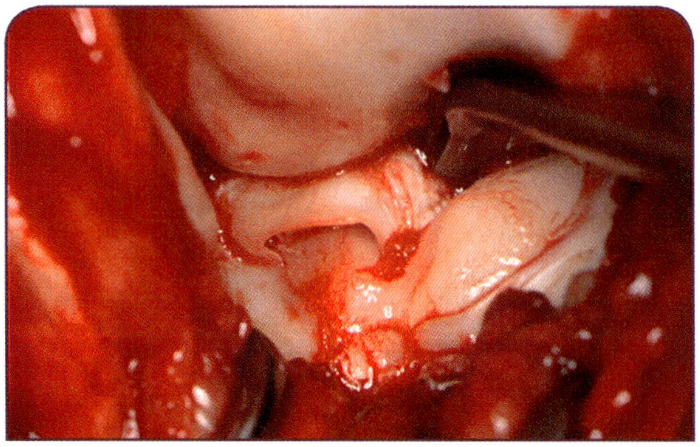

FIGURE 28. Intraoperative image of the medial meniscus with the Hohmann retractor in position and the stifle joint fully flexed.

Three types of complications must be prevented during a meniscectomy:

1. Laceration of the articular cartilage.
2. Excision of the cranial portion of the meniscus (generally undamaged) which leaves the caudal portion injured.
3. Laceration of the medial collateral ligament in an overly extensive excision.

If tearing of the meniscus (in most cases in the medial meniscus) is observed then a partial meniscectomy is performed. It is better to remove too much damaged meniscus than to perform an insufficient resection. The meniscus regenerates by means of connective tissue, and in most cases turns into a fibrocartilaginous disc. Moreover, it is necessary to prevent joint destabilisation, which would lead to secondary osteoarthritis. The articular cartilage must not be damaged during the meniscectomy.

Concerning osteophyte removal, the authors consulted hold completely contradictory opinions. In practice osteophytes stopped being removed around two years ago.

In summary, generally the medial meniscus is affected. Concerning diagnosis:

- The menisci cannot be visualised on X-ray (Fig. 29) and are somewhat difficult to visualise on arthroscopy.
- MRI scans allow for less invasive visualisation, although it is also necessary to have experience to diagnose meniscal injuries (Figs. 30-32).
- Arthroscopy is highly advantageous in that it not only confirms the diagnosis but also can be performed in the same session as a total or partial meniscectomy. It requires extensive experience.

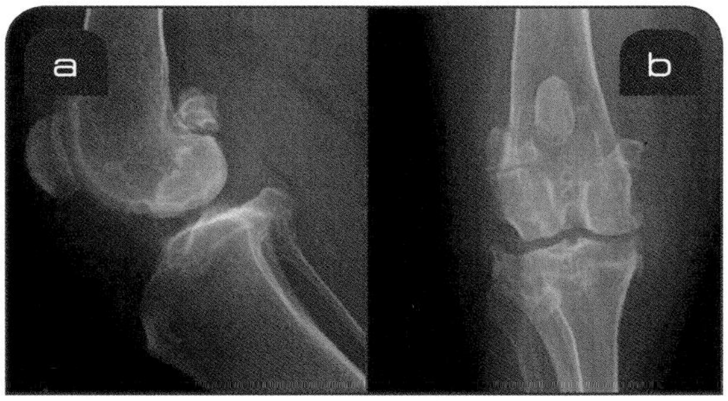

FIGURE 29. The patient suffers from a meniscal injury that does not appear on X-ray. Lateral projection (a) and craniocaudal projection (b).

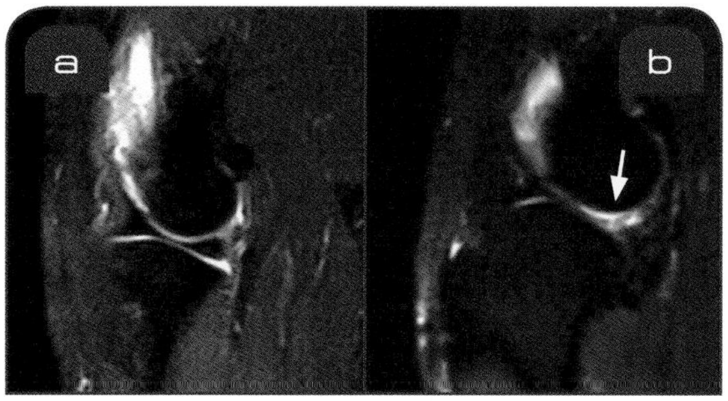

FIGURE 30. MRI scans of an intact meniscus (a) and an injured meniscus (b).

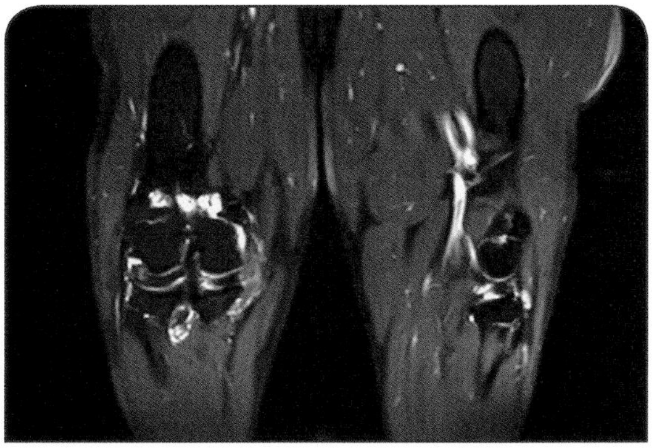

FIGURE 31. MRI scans of a healthy meniscus.

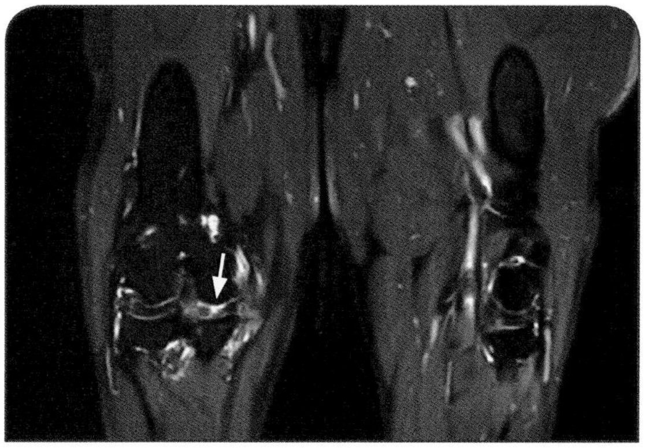

FIGURE 32. MRI scan of an injured medial meniscus (arrow).

Postoperative care

After surgery, animals must remain at rest with supervised exercise until radiological evidence of ossification is obtained. Normally, animals that have undergone surgery are capable of toe-touch weight-bearing 10 days after surgery; however, this figure can range from three days to three weeks.

After four weeks, a radiological study is performed. At this point, the owner usually mentions that it is difficult to keep the patient at rest, and this is a good sign. It may even be necessary to prescribe sedatives to keep the patient at rest. After eight weeks, another radiological examination is performed. After 12 weeks, the patient walks normally, and it is difficult or impossible to tell which limb has undergone surgery. Starting from this time, the animal is allowed to exercise freely, although it is best to establish a rehabilitation period which can consist of four phases:

- The first phase aims to stretch the scar tissue in the stifle joint.
- The second phase aims to develop the caudal muscles of the leg, in particular the biceps femoris muscle.
- The third phase includes swimming. The animal cannot dive into the water but can otherwise swim without restrictions.
- The fourth and final phase involves a return to normal function when the biceps femoris muscle has acquired normal tone and consistency.

This chapter concludes with MRI scans taken in dog cadavers showing some of the injuries described (Figs. 33-38).

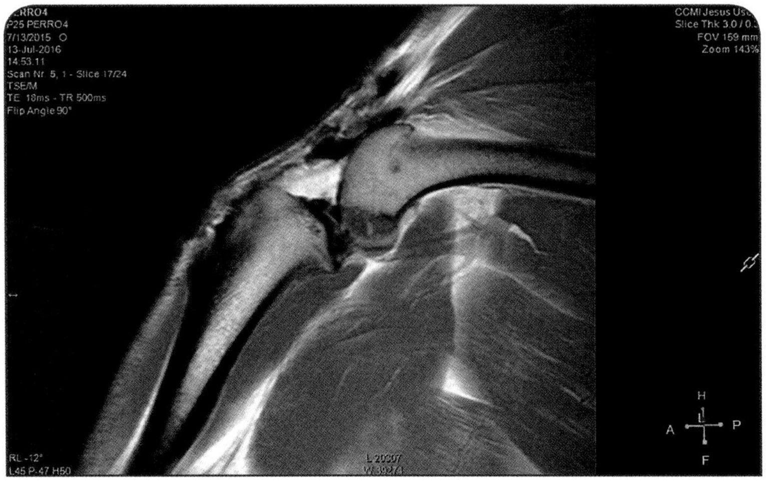

FIGURE 33. MRI scan. Partial tearing of the anterior cruciate ligament of the left stifle joint.

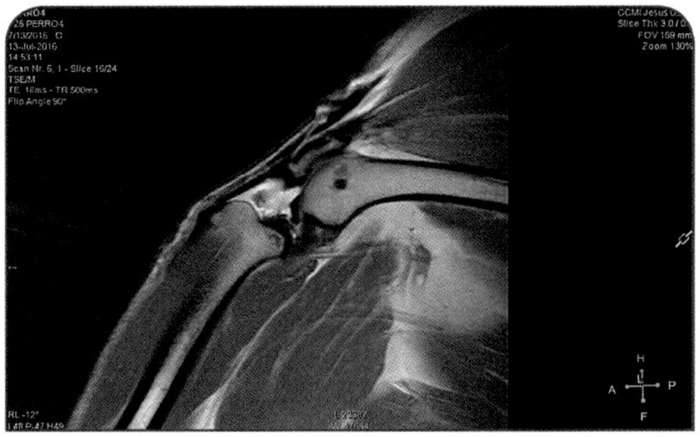

FIGURE 34. MRI scan. Complete tearing of the PCL of the left stifle joint.

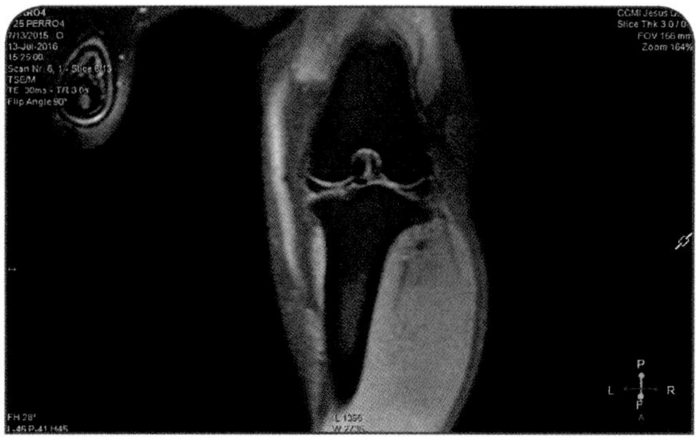

FIGURE 35. MRI scan. Injury of the lateral meniscus of the right stifle joint.

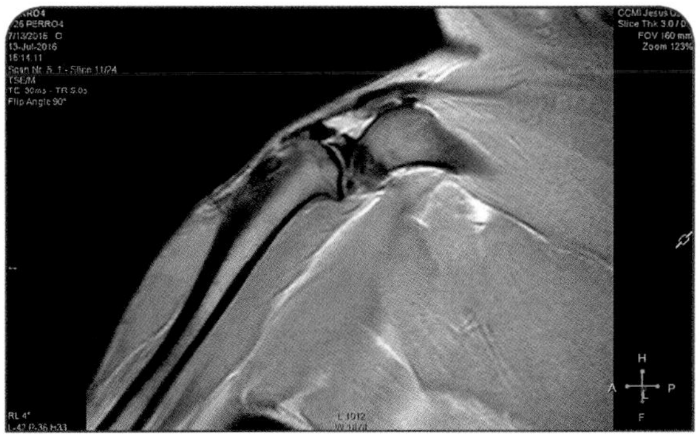

FIGURE 36. MRI scan. Injury of the lateral meniscus of the right stifle joint.

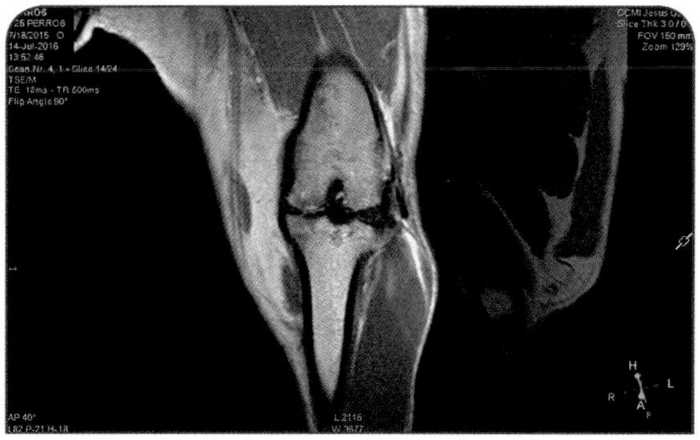

FIGURE 37. MRI scan. Injury of the medial meniscus of the left stifle joint.

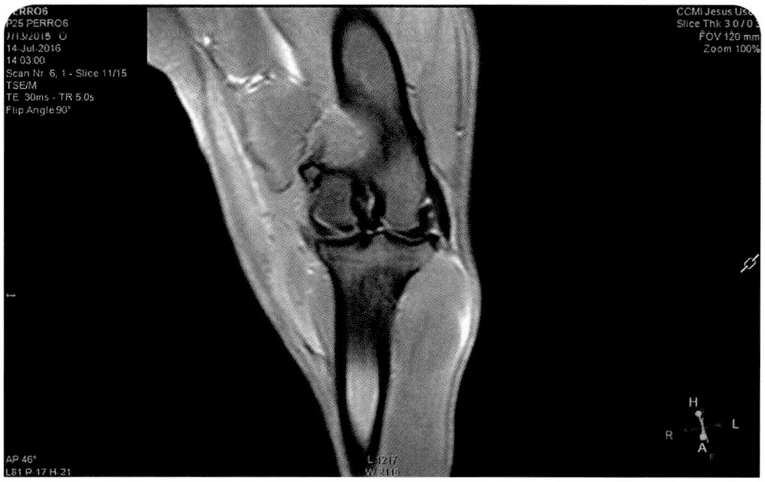

FIGURE 38. MRI scan. Injury of the medial meniscus of the right stifle joint.

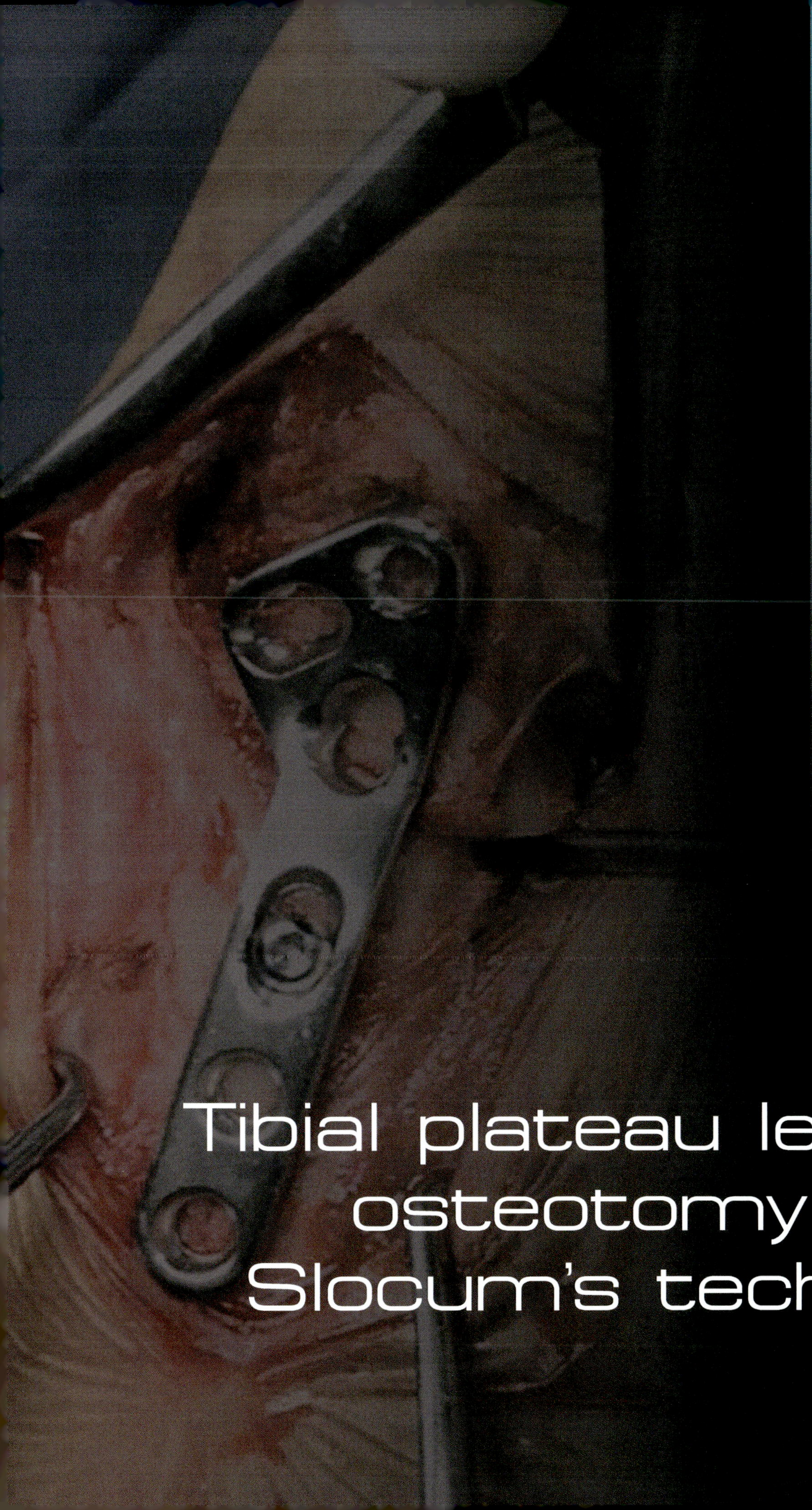

CHAPTER

7

Tibial plateau levelling osteotomy using Slocum's technique

Juan M. Martí

Introduction

TPLO is a technique described and patented by Slocum (1993) with licence available for Slocum Enterprise (Eugene [Oregon], United States) to restore the function of the stifle joint with a deficient ACL.

The end goal of the surgery is to neutralise the effects of uncontrolled cranial tibial thrust. It does not attempt to repair injuries of passive joint elements (ACL and caudal horn of the medial meniscus). It does attempt to control cranial displacement of the tibia by levelling the tibial plateau, which increases the efficacy of control of the so-called active forces created by the flexor muscles of the leg. First the extent to which the tibial plateau is to be rotated must be determined based on X-ray. A medial approach is used. To properly rotate the tibial plateau a curved osteotomy of the tibia must be performed and the fragments must then be fixed with a special plate. This technique is highly advantageous in that different limb alignment errors such as genu valgum and genu varum can be corrected.

It is of course a complicated technique. For this reason a prior course should be taken to master it.

This is probably the best surgical technique; however, long-term postoperative monitoring and proper comparison to other techniques must be done before a definitive opinion may be issued.

Basic biomechanics and history of the technique

The first mention of a surgical technique to modify the angle of the tibial plateau in order to treat instability caused by cranial cruciate ligament rupture in dogs was published by Slocum in 1984. In this surgery, the tibial plateau becomes perpendicular to the longitudinal axis of the tibia through resection of a bone wedge. This neutralises cranial tibial movement, which in turn reduces mechanical stress in the additional technique that the surgeon has selected to stabilise the stifle joint with ACL rupture (generally, the use of a patellotibial suture).

Later, in 1993, Slocum published his first description of what is known today as TPLO. This technique turns cranial tibial movement in weight-bearing into minimal caudal movement of the tibia, limited by the caudal cruciate ligament, and into tibial compression towards the femoral condyles, through rotation of the proximal tibial fragment following a radial osteotomy in the proximal metaphysis of the tibia. The proximal fragment is rotated so that the slope of the tibial plateau is nearly perpendicular to the longitudinal axis of the tibia (the ideal angle of the tibial plateau has been determined to be around 5° over the axis perpendicular to the longitudinal axis of the tibia) (Figs. 1 and 2). The osteotomy is fixed with an osteosynthesis plate and screws, which are available in different sizes and models and are specially designed for this surgery.

The need to surgically examine the stifle joint, especially with respect to inspecting the menisci, remains a controversial topic. Options range from performing a complete arthrotomy, with articular lavage, debridement of remnants of the ligament and superficial osteophytes, and meniscal inspection, to not opening the joint cavity. Intermediate options include performing an arthroscopic examination of the joint and using a limited approach exclusively to inspect the caudal horn of the medial meniscus.

> The most widely accepted recommendation to treat rupture of the medial meniscus, which is affected in a large proportion of chronically unstable stifle joints, especially in dogs belonging to large breeds, is to remove the injured portion.

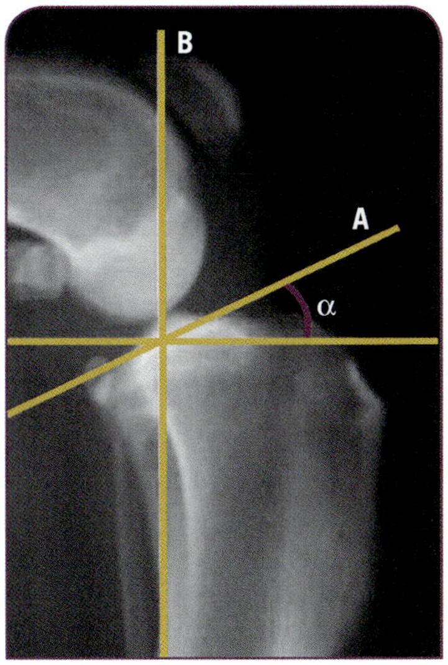

FIGURE 1. The ideal angle of the tibial plateau is 5° over the axis perpendicular to the longitudinal axis of the tibia.

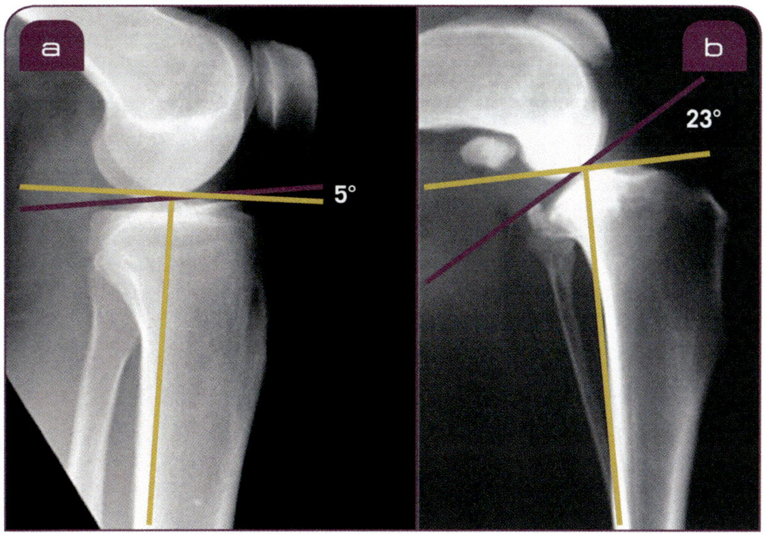

FIGURE 2. Comparison of the physiological slope of the tibial plateau of a human (a) and of a dog (b).

The risk of a postoperative meniscus injury, with its potential for an associated second surgery, has led some authors to recommend prophylactic "meniscal release". This involves radially transecting the full thickness of the meniscus to separate the caudal horn from the two cranial thirds. This allows this caudal horn to move with the medial femoral condyle and thus in theory decreases its potential for being pinched and crushed (Fig. 3). Although meniscal release was very popular for a few years after it was described, subsequent mechanical studies have demonstrated deleterious effects due to overload on the articular cartilage, and it no longer enjoys the popularity it once did.

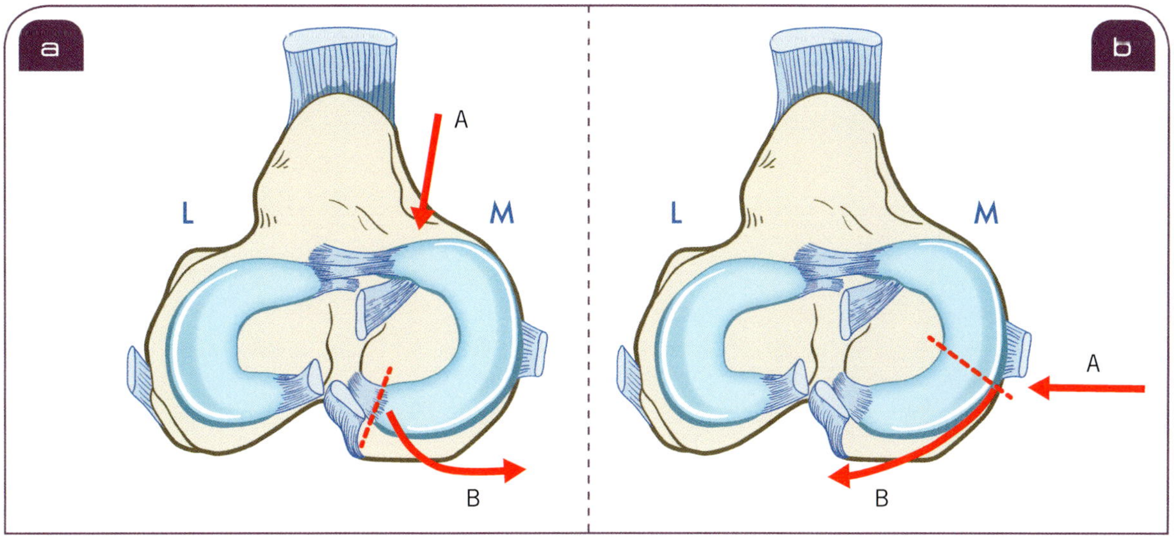

FIGURE 3. Two ways to perform the meniscus release technique: using a craniomedial approach (a), where the letter A indicates the direction of the approach and the letter B indicates the direction in which the caudal horn proceeds after the meniscus is released; and using a caudomedial approach (b), where the letter A shows the caudal approach to the medial collateral ligament and the letter B shows the direction in which the medial horn proceeds (caudal) after the meniscus is released.

Clinical efficacy studies of the TPLO technique generally show very favourable outcomes compared to other more traditional techniques, particularly in the long term and in medium and large dogs. The outcomes are less development of degenerative osteoarthritis, greater functional stability and better preservation of joint flexibility and muscle mass. At this time, there are still no definitive studies comparing the clinical outcomes of a TPLO to other popular tibial osteotomy techniques such as a TTA, wedge ostectomy and so on (Figs. 4-12).

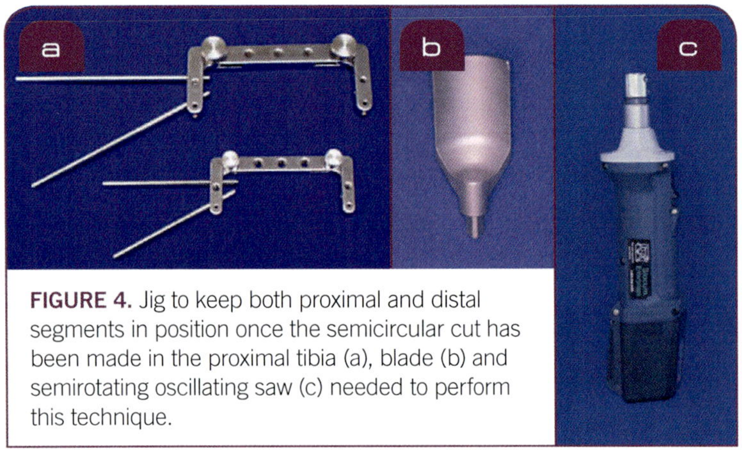

FIGURE 4. Jig to keep both proximal and distal segments in position once the semicircular cut has been made in the proximal tibia (a), blade (b) and semirotating oscillating saw (c) needed to perform this technique.

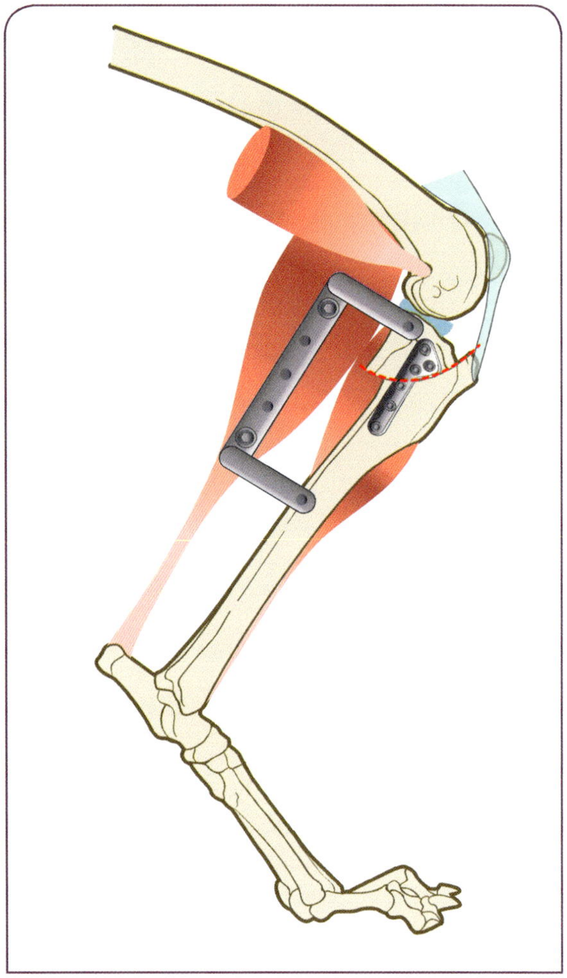

FIGURE 5. Diagram of how the external fixator is used to keep both segments stable and aligned following the cut.

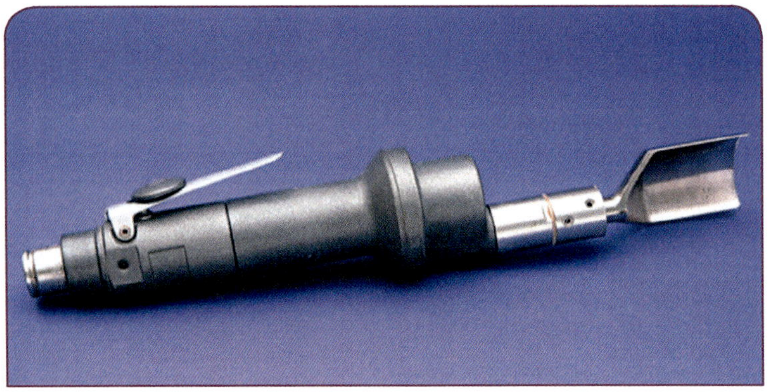

FIGURE 6. Another image of a saw, this one with the blade inserted, which works in a semirotating fashion.

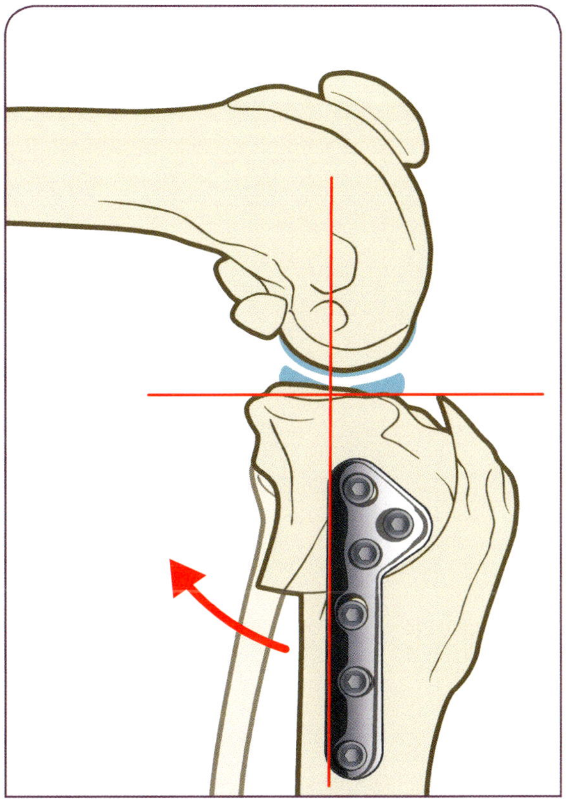

FIGURE 7. Diagram of how the proximal segment of the tibia must be moved caudally a number of millimetres determined based on the initial degrees of slope of the tibial plateau. Once this technique has been properly performed, the tibial plateau is seen to be perpendicular to the longitudinal axis of the tibia.

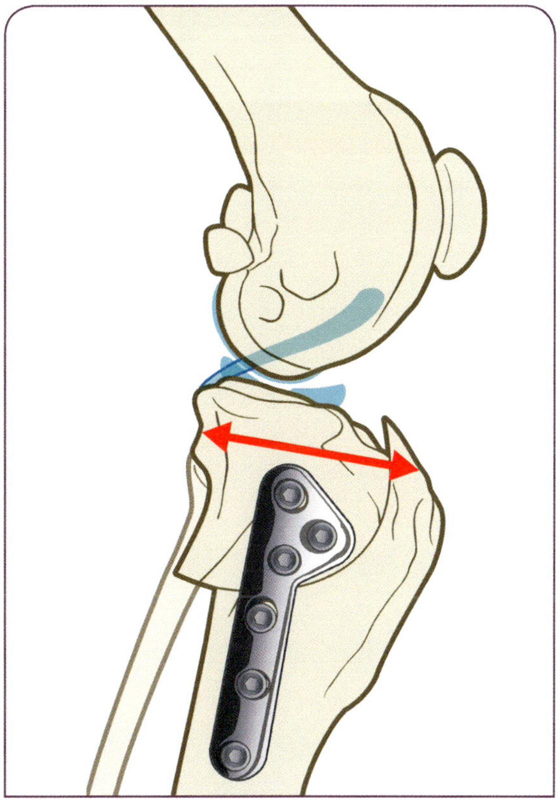

FIGURE 8. Diagram of the position of the posterior cruciate ligament following surgery. Plateau levelling causes it to lose its laxity and properly perform its function.

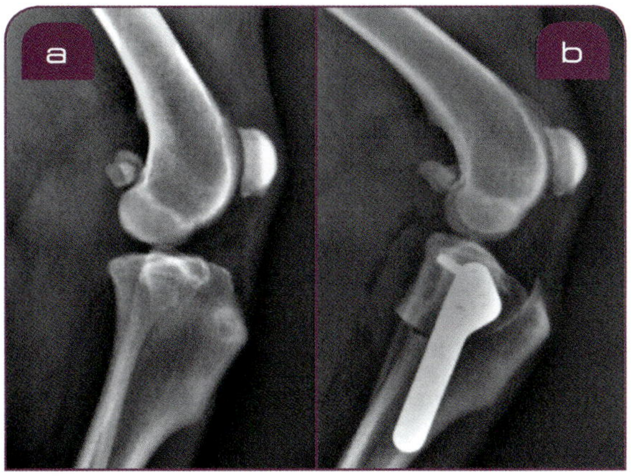

FIGURE 9. Case study of TPLO surgery using Slocum's technique. Preoperative image (a) and postoperative image (b).

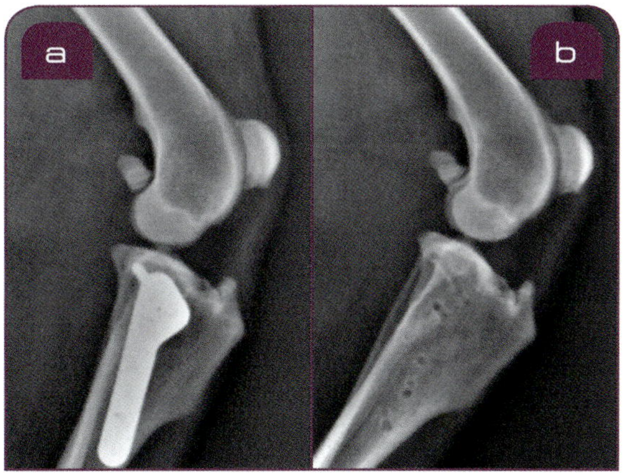

FIGURE 10. Follow-up of the previous case 20 weeks after the operation (a) and one week after the implant has been removed (b).

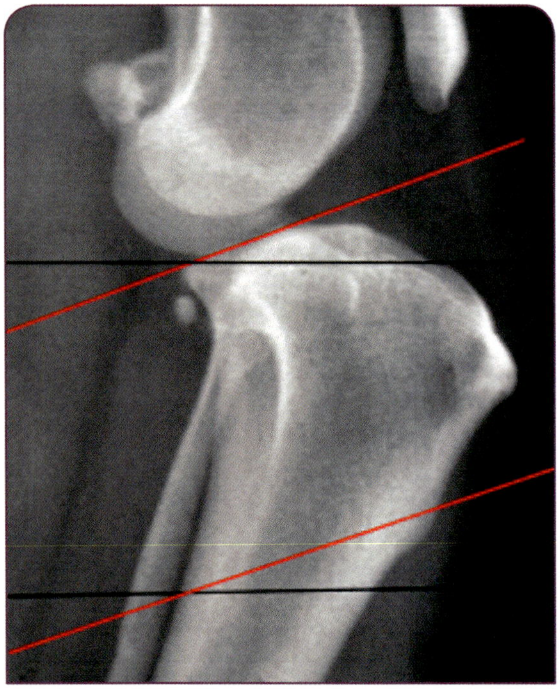

FIGURE 11. The wedge technique was first described by Slocum, who abandoned it in favour of the TPLO technique. The red line indicates the initial angle of the stifle joint, and the black line indicates the final angle following wedge resection.

A patent was granted for the TPLO technique itself, and other patents were granted for the instruments needed to perform the technique. This created an unprecedented situation in the field of veterinary surgery in which a company completely controlled the teaching of training courses in the technique and the sale of the surgical instruments. This ensured accuracy among surgeons in the chain of learning and sought to minimise deviations from the original technique. However, due to the growing popularity of TPLO and the limitations on access to the training courses, the veterinary surgical community (especially in Europe) started to develop analogous tibial plateau levelling techniques to free itself of patent restrictions. Today, although alternative techniques have been successfully developed, the TPLO technique still enjoys great popularity all over the world, especially in the United States, where it was developed and still dominates the tibial osteotomy market.

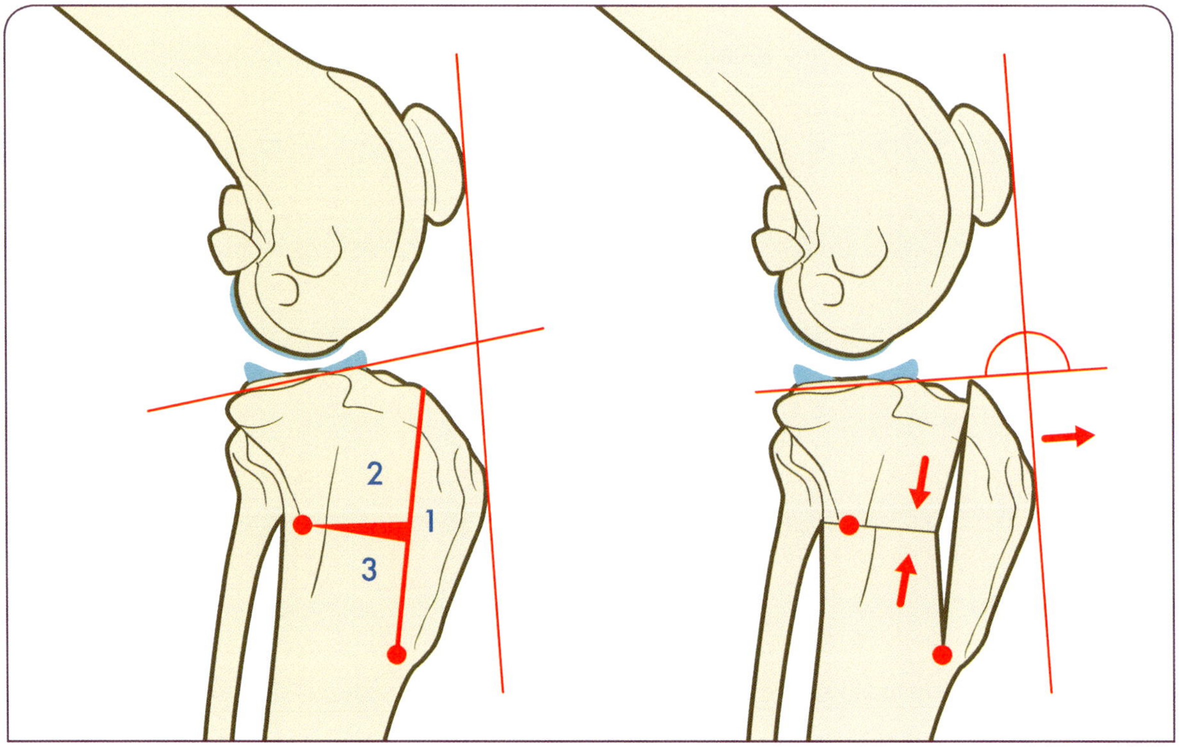

FIGURE 12. Wedge technique. Biomechanical justification for the wedge resection technique.

Surgical technique

The technique is described in general terms below to offer an appreciation of the biomechanical solution developed to control the deficient action of the ACL mechanism.

First, in the diagnosis phase special emphasis must be placed on thoroughly evaluating the ACL using the drawer test and the tibial compression test. It is known that muscle action can falsify this test in excessively nervous animals. Therefore, prior calming or even general anaesthesia might be needed to allow the surgeon to neutralise these active forces which are so decisive in this diagnosis phase.

A meticulous medical history can provide a very high percentage of the information needed to diagnose partial ruptures. This abnormality must be suspected in animals with subtle lameness of the pelvic limb that does not completely prevent the activity of the limb but does always appear after exercise and disappear with rest. It must always be checked by means of an arthrotomy or arthroscopy prior to a TPLO.

Cases in which continuous lameness in weight-bearing is observed but the dog remains just as active tend to involve an ACL rupture without rupture of the caudal horn of the medial meniscus. Cases in which this lameness progresses to an antalgic gait without any sort of weight-bearing probably involve a prior ACL rupture with rupture of the caudal horn of the medial meniscus.

The technique itself consists of an approach to the proximal end of the tibia through the medial side (see annex of surgical approaches). The skin incision extends from the distal end of the femur to the proximal end of the tibia and passes over the medial epicondyle of the femur. The first structures thus revealed are the descending artery of the stifle joint and the caudal belly of the sartorius muscle. The fascia that covers the artery must be cut parallel to this artery and reflected caudally, while the remaining medial fascia is brought cranially. This incision is extended distally, immediately cranial to the medial meniscus, at the caudal boundary of the fat pad. The patella is dislocated laterally and all branches of the genicular artery are ligated around the vastus medialis muscle.

Following an arthrotomy the preoperative diagnosis is verified, although the trend is to separate the meniscus without performing an arthrotomy. If the rupture is partial it should be evaluated, and if the ligament that remains unruptured is strong enough to continue functioning as a passive element (it is said that at least a third of the original ACL must be maintained), the meniscus is not touched. If the meniscus is completely ruptured, it is ideal to perform TPLO and a medial meniscectomy.

It is important to reflect the insertions of the gracilis and semitendinosus muscles and the caudal belly of the sartorius muscle at the middle proximal part of the tibia while taking care to leave the medial collateral ligament intact.

The steps involved in a TPLO are as follows:

1. A special fixator (registered by Slocum Enterprise) is applied to the sagittal plane of the medial and proximal tibia and care is taken to leave the medial collateral ligament intact (Figs. 13-17).
2. Next a cylindrical cut is made in the proximal tibia with a special oscillating saw (registered by Slocum Enterprise). It is important for the surface of the bone cut and the saw to have the same radius to match the TPLO (Figs. 18-21).
3. The fragment is rotated to the degree previously planned following the corresponding study and X-ray measurement of the degrees of levelling needed (Figs. 22-26).
4. A plate (registered by Slocum Enterprise) is conformed to keep both fragments in the new position with the tibial plateau in its corrected position (Figs. 27-31).

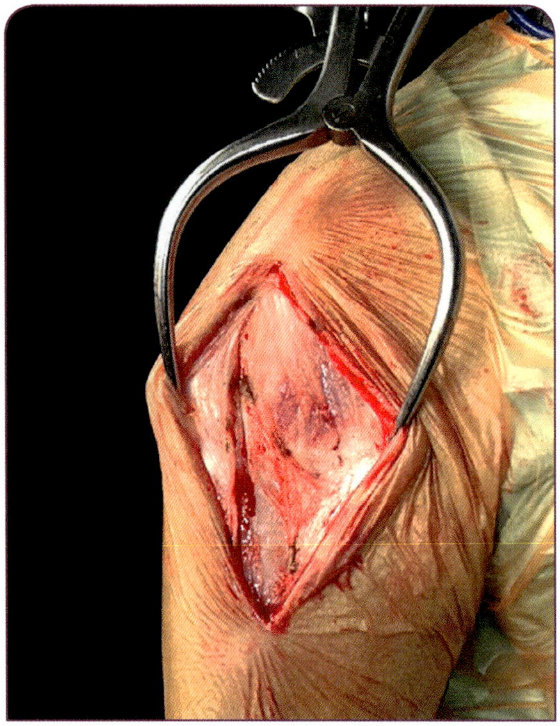

FIGURE 13. Preparation of the area through a medial approach to the proximal region of the tibia.

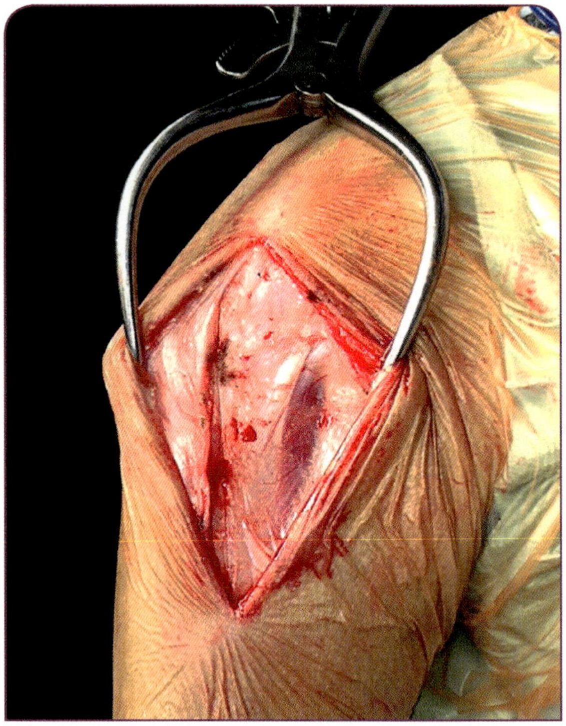

FIGURE 14. The tendons of the pes anserinus are reflected caudally and the medial collateral ligament is shown.

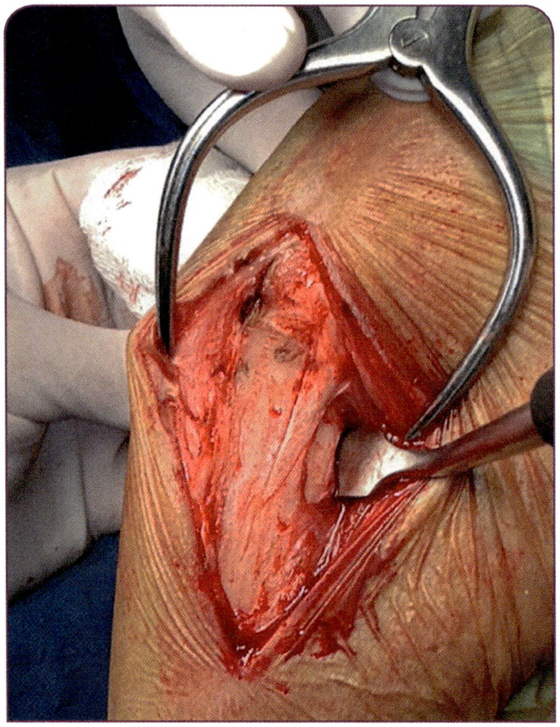

FIGURE 15. The insertion of the popliteus muscle is partially released on the caudal cortex of the tibia, caudal to the collateral ligament.

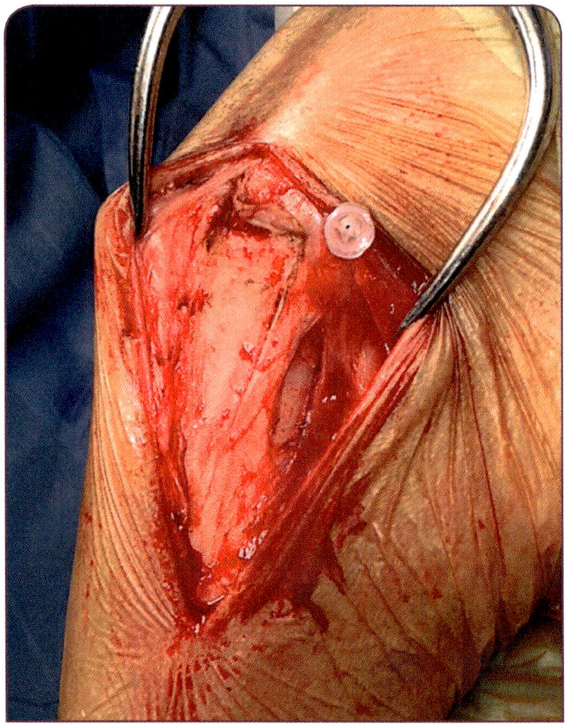

FIGURE 16. A hypodermic needle is inserted into the joint to delimit the edge of the medial condyle of the tibia.

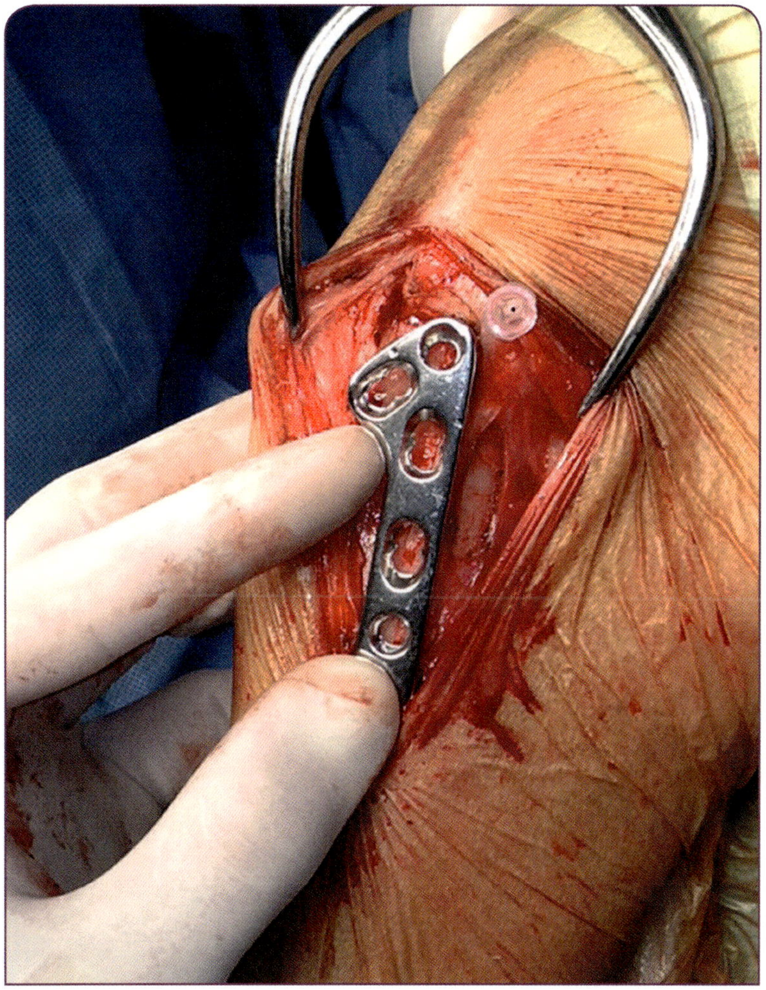

FIGURE 17. At this time the size of the plate to be used can be decided upon, based on the space available and the weight of the patient.

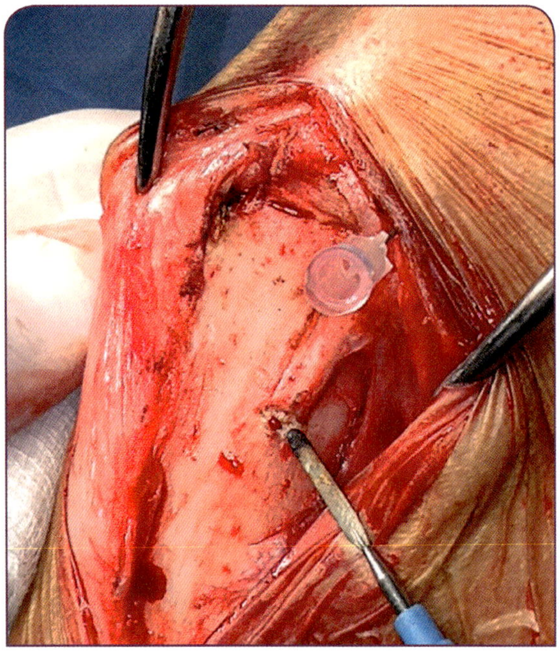

FIGURE 18. Cautery marks the two points, cranial/proximal (over the area of the fat pad) and caudal/distal (generally at the level of the distal fibres of the collateral ligament), where the saw will be supported to start the radial osteotomy.

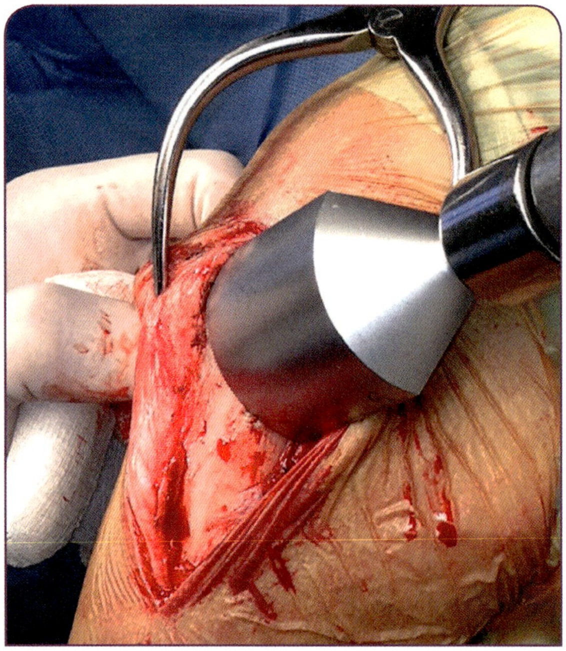

FIGURE 19. Start of the osteotomy with the radial saw.

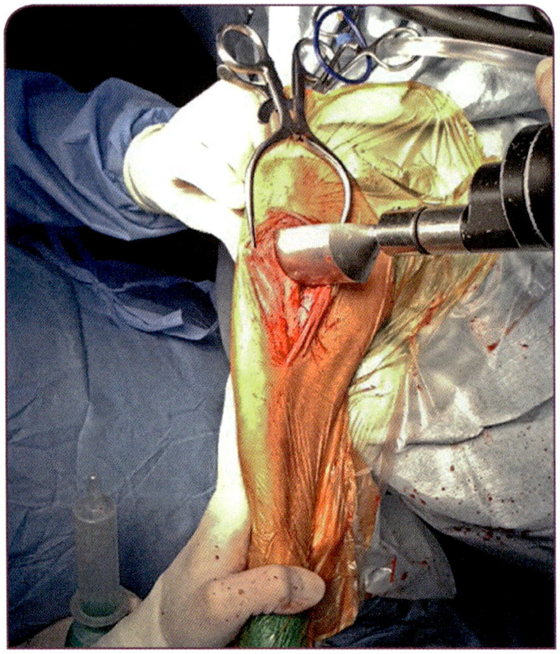

FIGURE 20. The saw must be perpendicular to the longitudinal axis of the tibia and perpendicular to the medial cortex.

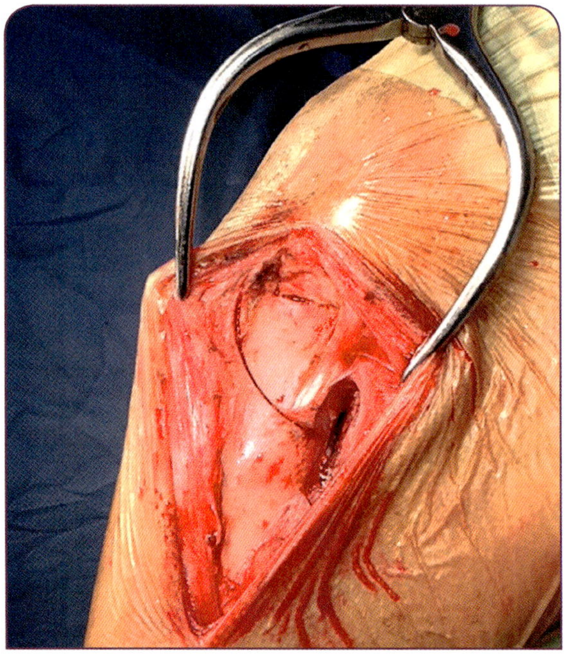

FIGURE 21. Partial-thickness osteotomy.

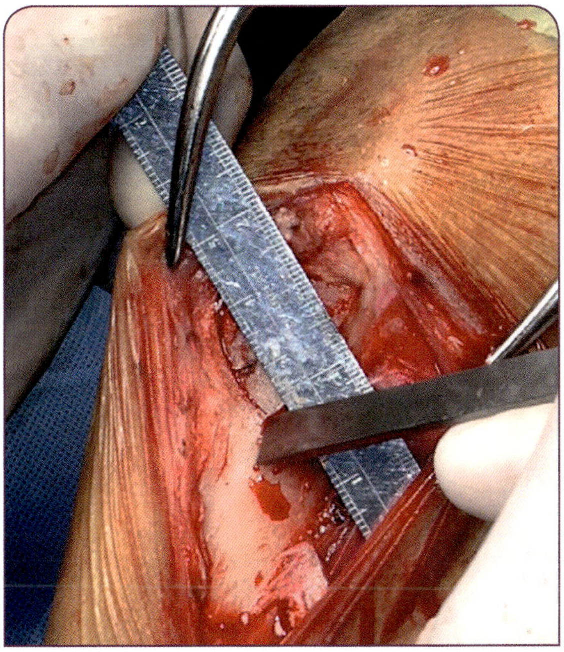

FIGURE 22. Depending on the preoperative lateral X-ray, the angle of the tibial plateau is measured and correction tables are used to decide upon the distance of rotation of the TPLO fragment to achieve the desired degree of rotation of the tibial plateau in the postoperative period. At this time the cortices on both sides of the osteotomy are marked with two stitches that distance apart.

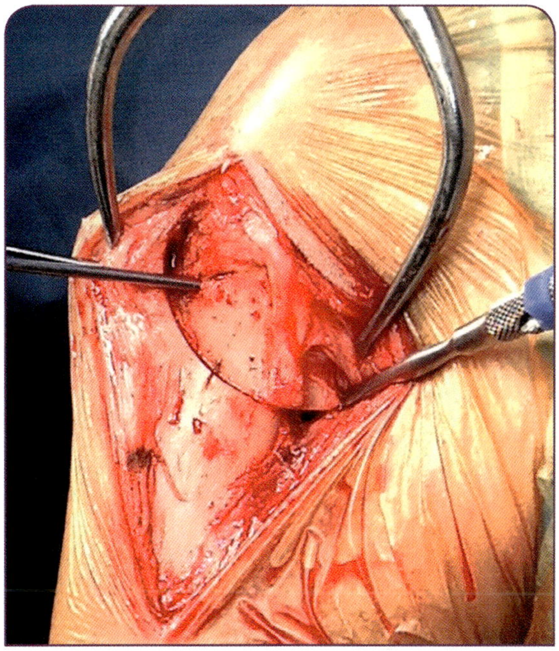

FIGURE 23. The partial-thickness osteotomy is continued, a pin is inserted and the fragment is rotated until the two marks are aligned.

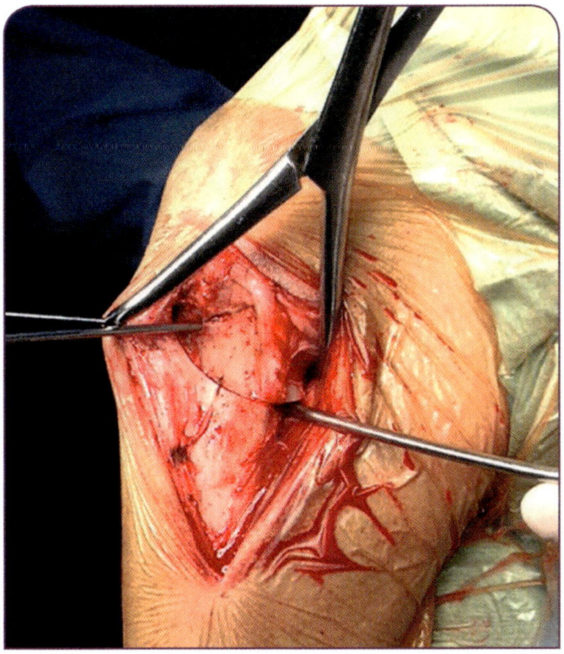

FIGURE 24. A small Kirschner wire inserted from the tibial tuberosity is used to ensure this position. Reduction forceps may also be used as the image indicates.

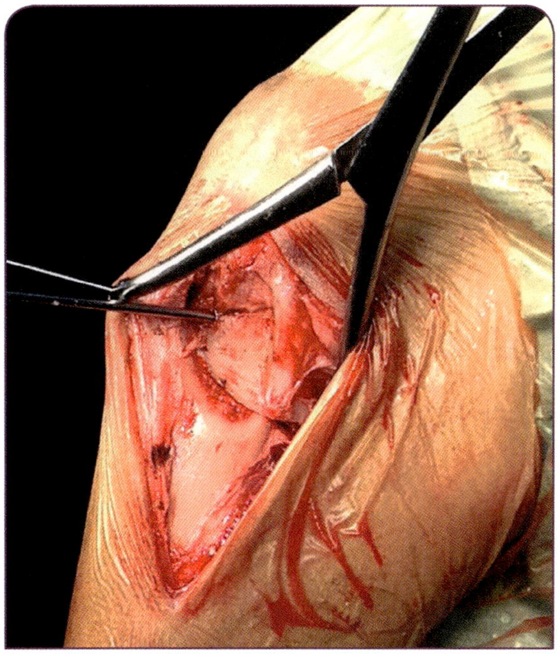

FIGURE 25. The raised element formed in the osteotomy can be lowered with the same radial saw to help the plate perfectly conform to the bone (this is less necessary if locking plates are used).

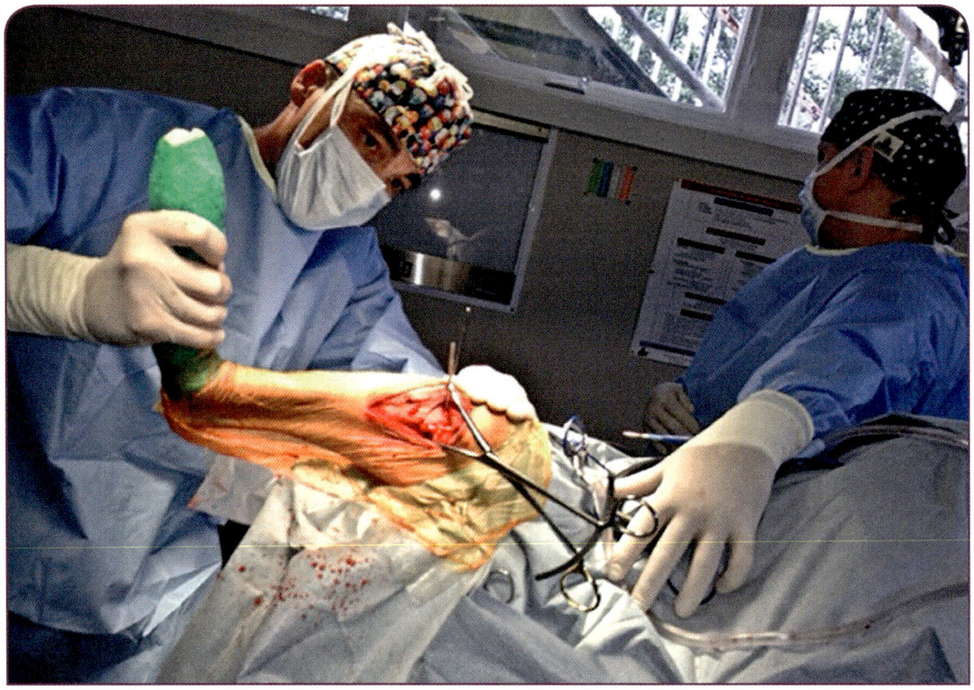

FIGURE 26. At this time the alignment of the limb and the disappearance of cranial tibial thrust can be confirmed before definitive fixation is performed.

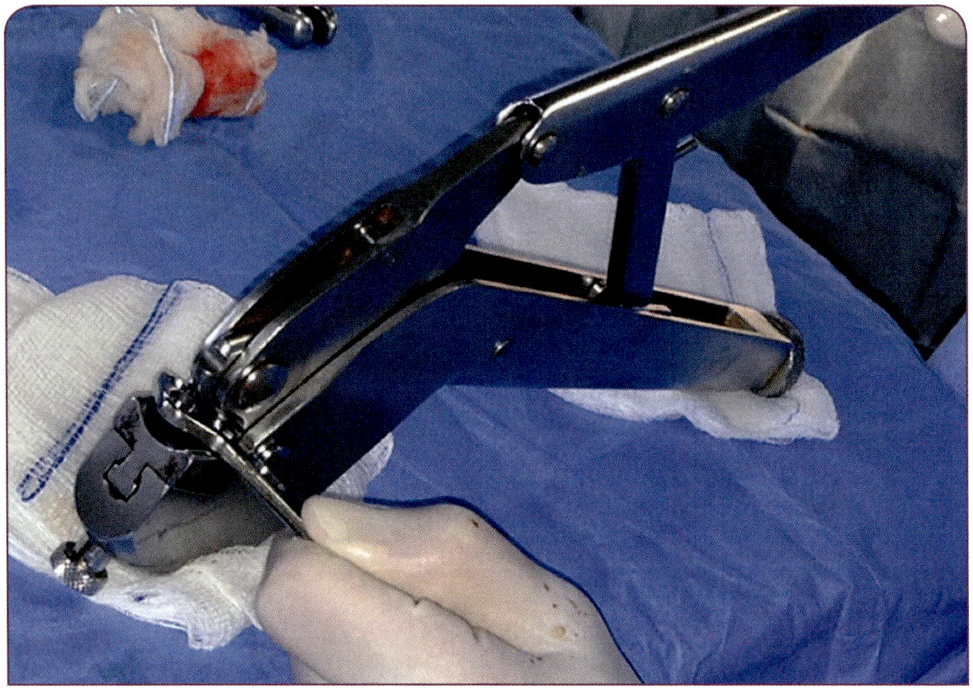

FIGURE 27. Moulding of the plate is achieved with implant benders and must be as complete as possible when traditional (nonlocking) plates are used.

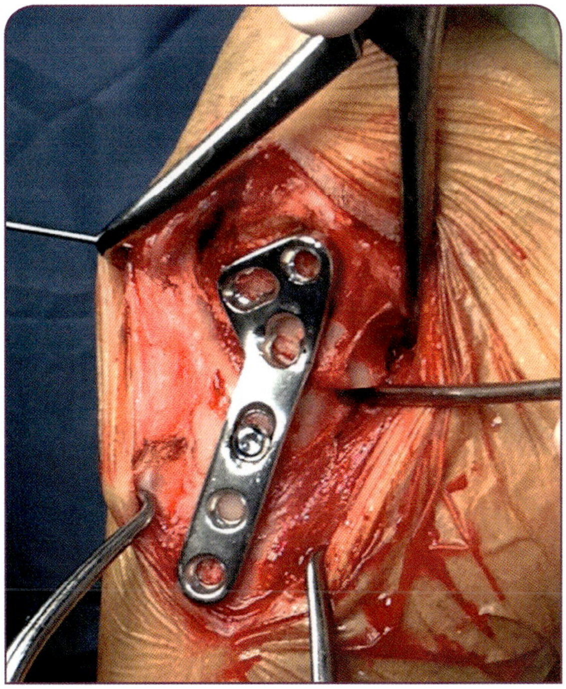

FIGURE 28. TPLO plate in position with a distal screw.

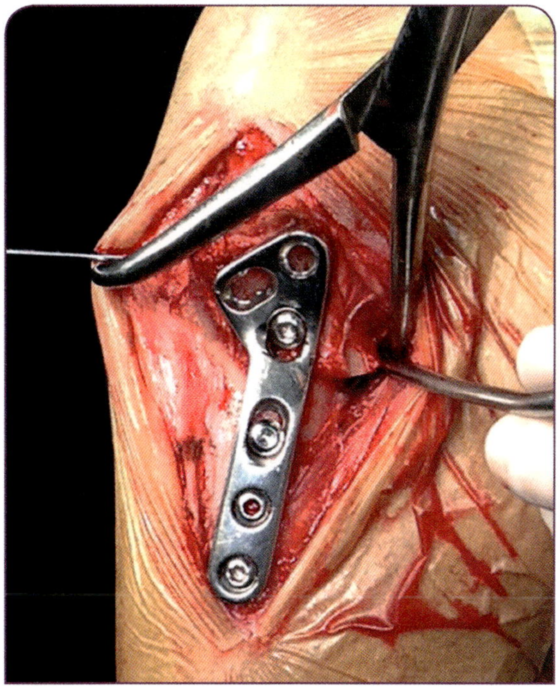

FIGURE 29. Three distal screws and one proximal screw are placed.

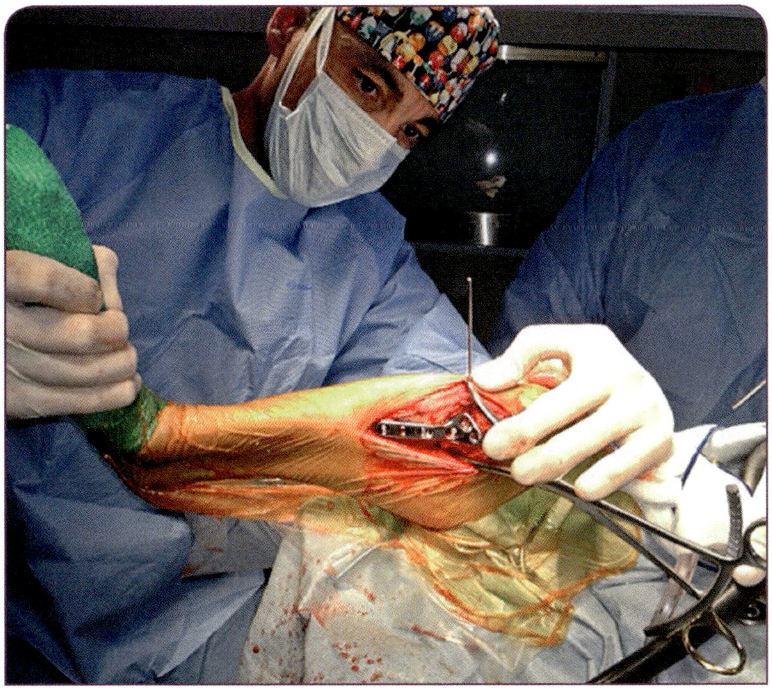

FIGURE 30. At this point the alignment and stability of the stifle joint are checked to ensure that they have not changed before the rest of the screws are placed.

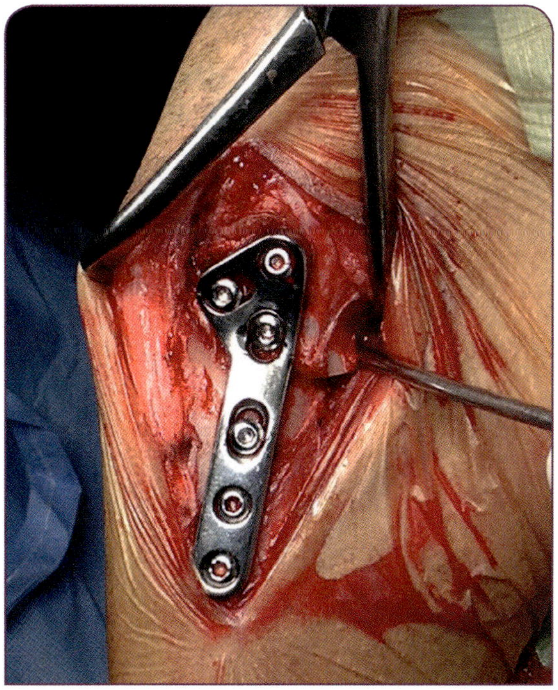

FIGURE 31. View of the finished surgery. The wound is closed in layers: periosteum, pes anserinus, subcutaneous tissue and skin.

Postoperative care

Following surgery, animals must remain at rest with supervised exercise until X-ray evidence of ossification is obtained.

Normally, animals are already toe-touch weight-bearing 10 days after surgery; however, this figure ranges from three days to three weeks.

After four weeks, the patient undergoes another radiological examination. At this time, the owner tends to report that it is difficult to keep the animal at rest, and this is a favourable sign. It may even be necessary to prescribe sedatives to keep the animal at rest. After eight weeks, another radiological examination is performed. After 12 weeks, the animal walks normally and it is difficult to tell which limb has undergone surgery. Starting from 12 weeks, the animal is allowed to move freely, although it is best to establish a rehabilitation period which may consist of three or four phases:

- The first phase aims to stretch the scar tissue in the stifle joint.
- The second phase aims to develop the caudal muscles of the thigh and leg, in particular the biceps femoris muscle.
- The third phase includes swimming. The animal cannot dive into the water but can otherwise swim without restrictions.
- The fourth and final phase consists of a return to normal function when the biceps femoris muscle has acquired normal tone and consistency.

Postoperative evaluation of the stifle joint

There are five main criteria to evaluate the success of a TPLO:

1. The animal must be fully capable of flexing the stifle joint. This may be calculated by examining the capacity of the animal to sit on its haunches with its weight over the region of the tarsus. This must happen within 12 weeks of surgery. This period may be slightly longer in the most chronic cases.
2. Complete muscle development of the affected limb occurs simultaneously with normal use of this limb. This should happen within 12 to 16 weeks of surgery. It is recognised by measuring the circumference of the affected limb and the circumference of the unaffected limb with a tape measure and comparing the measurements.
3. Absence of inflammation in the stifle joint, which should completely resolve within three months of the operation. It is easily observed by palpating and noting the soft, spongy structure of the joint capsule which becomes firm when the tissues are no longer inflamed.
4. Cessation of osteoarthritis progress, which must be evaluated on X-ray.
5. Complete return to normal activity 12 to 16 weeks after surgery. This is an especially important point in working and athletic animals. The traditional anterior drawer criterion lacks value, since a TPLO does not eliminate it; this movement constitutes a passive force created by the surgeon. A TPLO does eliminate cranial displacement of the tibia with the functional load of the animal itself.

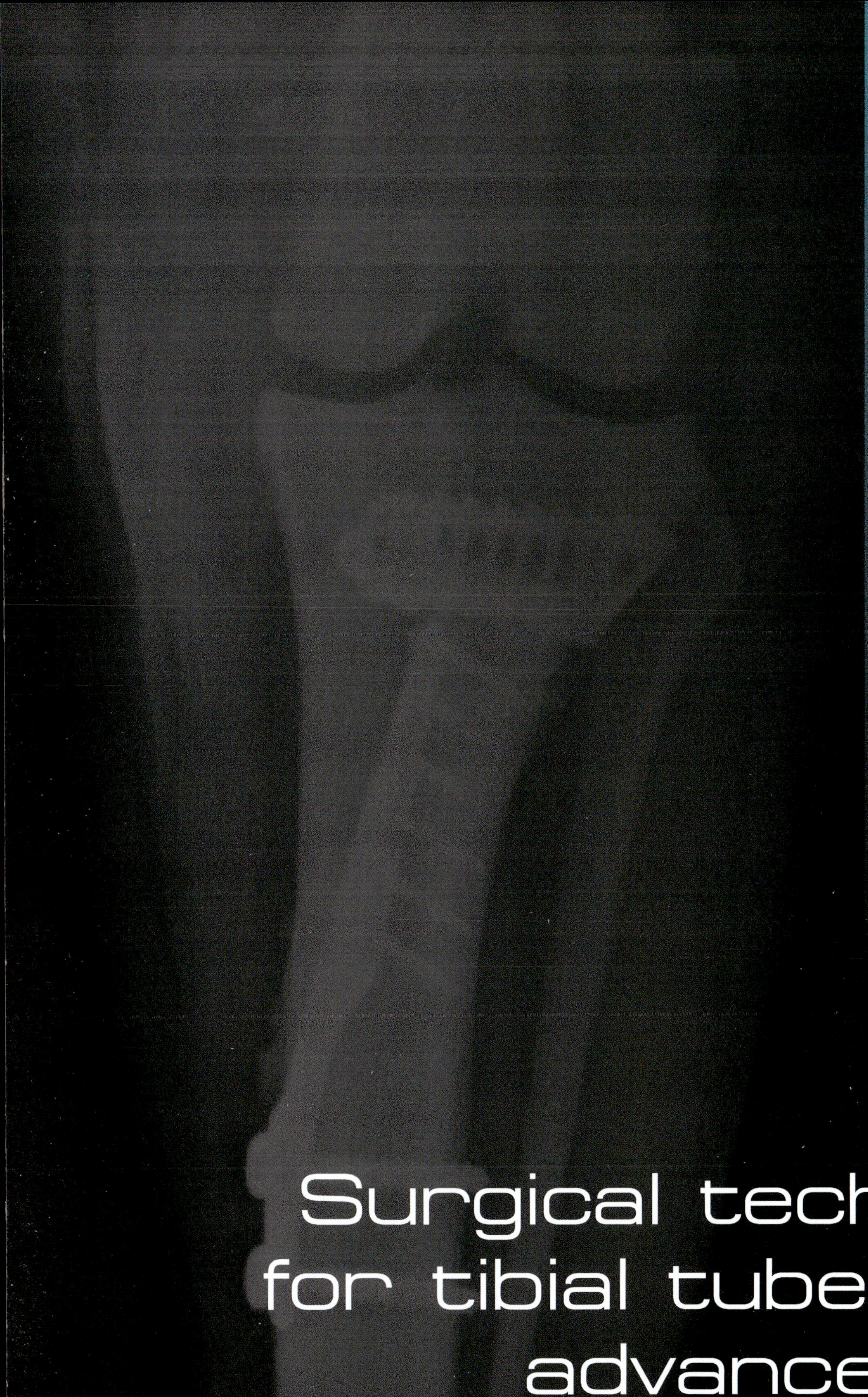

CHAPTER

8

Surgical technique for tibial tuberosity advancement

Introduction

ACL rupture is one of the most common causes of lameness in the hind limb in dogs and the most common cause of secondary degenerative osteoarthritis in the stifle joint.

For reasons that are not entirely understood, the ACL undergoes a degenerative process resulting in its partial rupture, then its complete rupture. Age, overweight, immune-mediated diseases, an excessive slope of the tibial plateau and other structural abnormalities are some of the proposed causes of this disease.

The high incidence of ACL disease in dogs has led to the development of many surgical techniques in an attempt to improve clinical results, particularly in dogs belonging to large breeds.

Conventional procedures sought to replace and/or reinforce the injured ACL. Current techniques tend to modify the anatomical geometry of the proximal tibia so as to neutralise the cranial thrust causing ACL rupture in the tibiofemoral joint and thus offset the ACL deficiency (Figs. 1 and 2). The ACL is not replaced, but when the shear forces causing it to rupture are nullified, the stifle joint will be dynamically stable; that is, it will not subluxate when the animal bears weight.

Basic biomechanics

In 1978, Henderson and Milton introduced the concept of cranial thrust. The supposed cause of this force is an excessive slope of the tibial plateau relative to the femur. Based on this theory, Slocum developed TPLO, the objective of which is to place the tibial plateau perpendicular to the axis of the tibia and thus eliminate the shear forces responsible for ACL rupture. Recent studies have not documented any difference in this angle between healthy dogs and dogs with an ACL deficiency.

Different biomechanical theories postulate that, in canine stifle joints and human knees, the resulting joint force is approximately parallel to the patellar ligament, and that an angle of more than 90° between the tibial plateau and the patellar ligament during the weight-bearing phase would be responsible for producing cranial thrust in the tibiofemoral joint. This cranial thrust overloads the ACL. If the angle between the patellar ligament and the tibial plateau is 90° during the weight-bearing phase (when the ACL is responsible for maintaining stability on the craniocaudal plane), there is no shear component in the overall force of the joint and no tension on the cruciate ligaments.

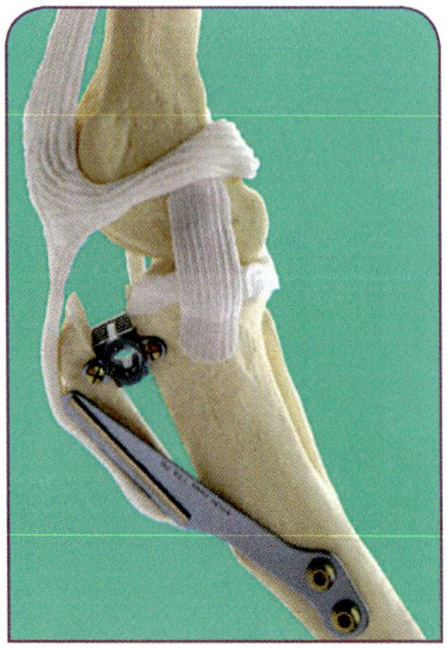

FIGURE 1. Image illustrating the fundamentals of the surgical technique of tibial tuberosity advancement.

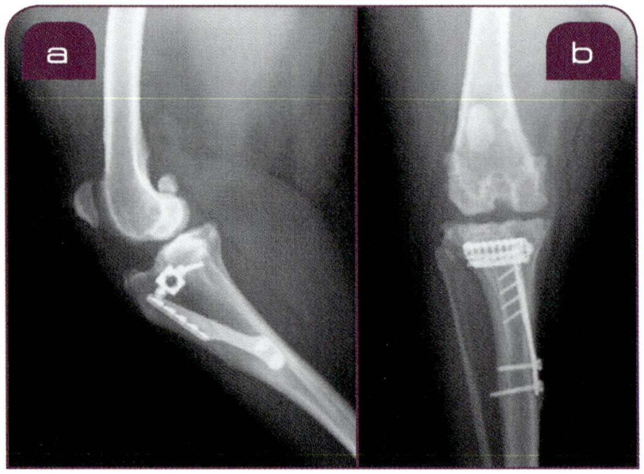

FIGURE 2. Lateral X-ray (a) and craniocaudal X-ray (b) of a Boxer following TTA.

It is possible to modify these tibiofemoral forces of cranial thrust by changing the geometry of the proximal tibia. This can be achieved by levelling the slope of the tibial plateau (Fig. 3) or advancing the tibial tuberosity (Fig. 4). In both cases, shear forces are displaced from the ACL towards the PCL and this ligament becomes the main stabiliser of the canine stifle joint. To prevent damage to this ligament, a proper preoperative plan must be made. The tibial tuberosity must not be advanced any more than strictly necessary. Similarly, the tibial plateau must not be rotated any more than strictly necessary.

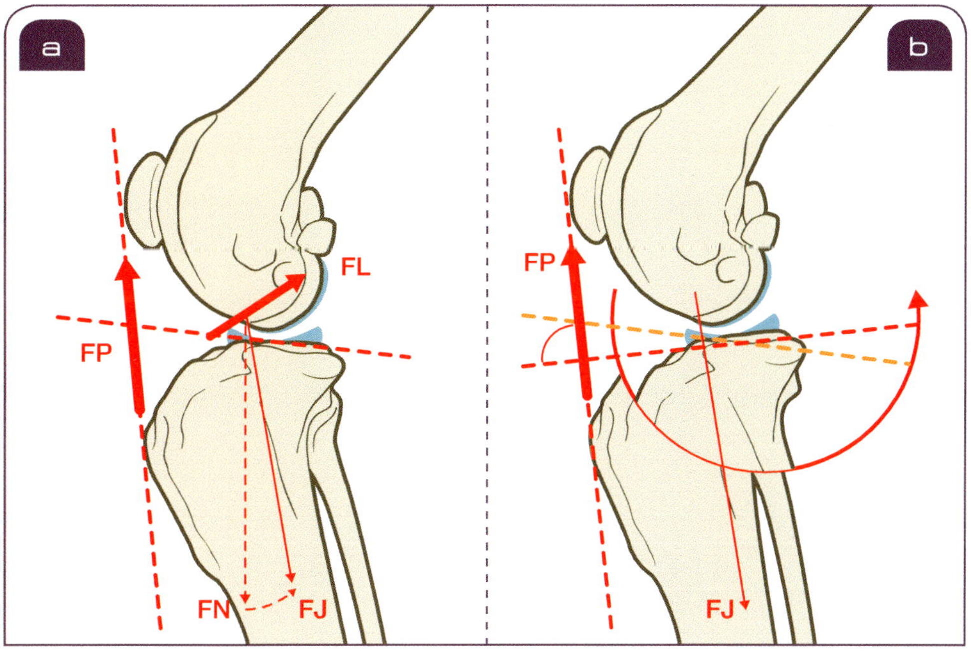

FIGURE 3. Diagrams showing the forces that act on the stifle joint before (a) and after (b) performing a TPLO. Once the tibial plateau has been levelled, the angle between the patellar ligament and the tibial plateau is 90° and there is no shear component in the overall force of the joint and no tension on the cruciate ligaments.

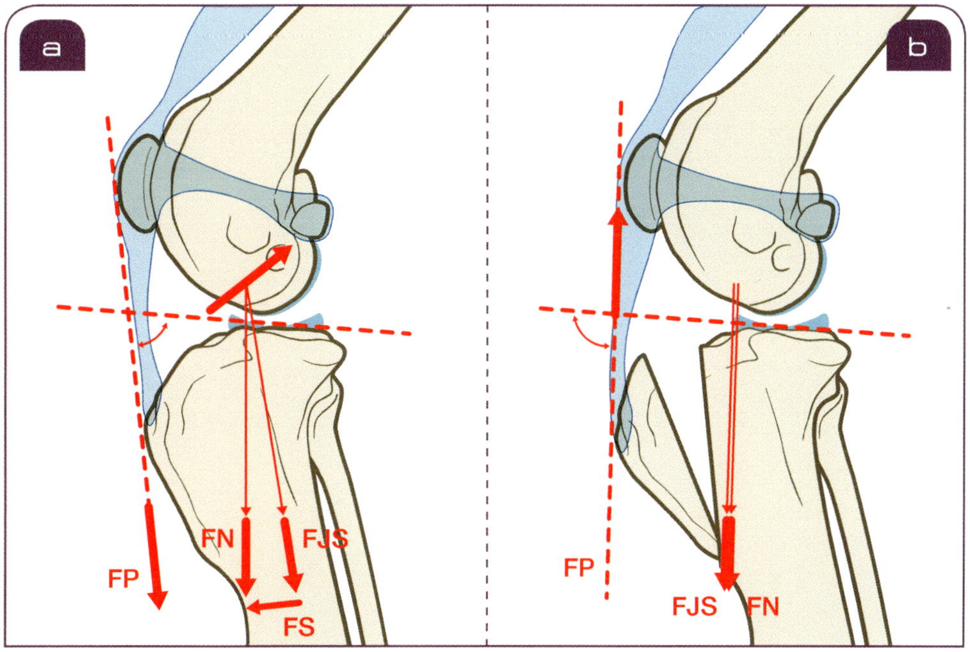

FIGURE 4. Diagrams showing the forces that act on the stifle joint before (a) and after (b) performing TTA. Once the tibial tuberosity has been advanced, the angle between the patellar ligament and the tibial plateau is also 90°, as it is after performing a TPLO, and there is no shear component in the overall force of the joint and therefore no tension on the cruciate ligaments.
The goal is to make the FP force perpendicular to the tibial plateau and to eliminate the FS force by superimposing FJS on FN. TTA allows the overall force parallel to the patellar ligament to be determined. If the patella and the tibial plateau are perpendicular then there is no component of rotation over the cruciate ligament.

Preoperative plan

The TTA technique requires a preoperative plan based on mediolateral X-rays of the stifle joint in extension and avoiding cranial subluxation of the tibia in complete ACL rupture. The patellar ligament is represented by its cranial edge and the orientation of the tibial plateau is represented by a line that passes over the tibial points of insertion of both cruciate ligaments (Fig. 5).

Next the distance of cranial advancement required to place the patellar ligament perpendicular to the tibial plateau is measured. This movement is centred on the patella to thus maintain its original position in the trochlea of the femur.

The preoperative plan for the advancement needed is made using a transparent template (Fig. 6) superimposed on X-rays. The size of the plate is also determined using the same template (Figs. 7 and 8).

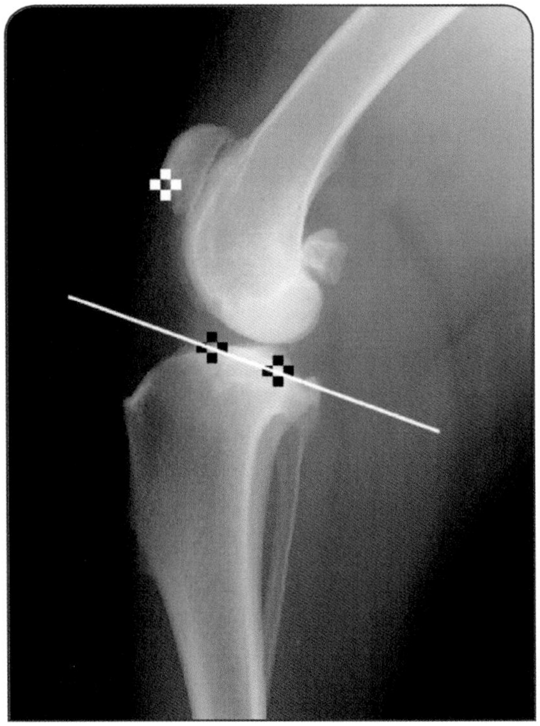

FIGURE 5. Determination of the tibial plateau and point of insertion of the patellar ligament.

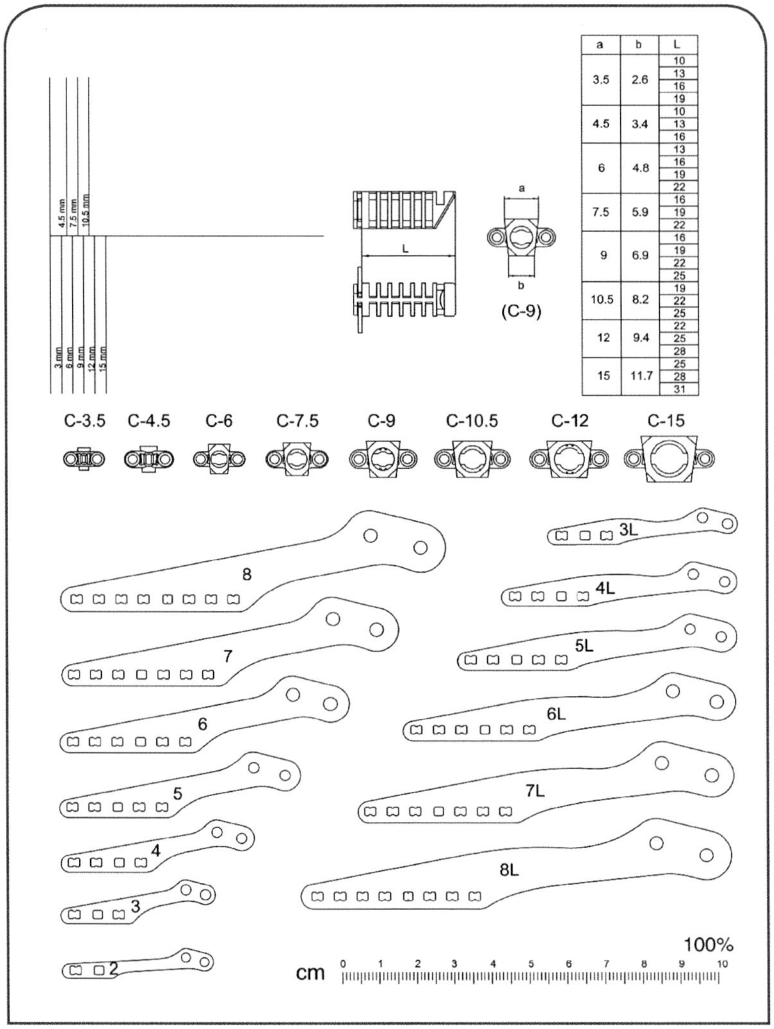

FIGURE 6. Detail of the TTA template (KYON Veterinary Surgical Products, Technoparkstrasse 1, Zurich, Switzerland).

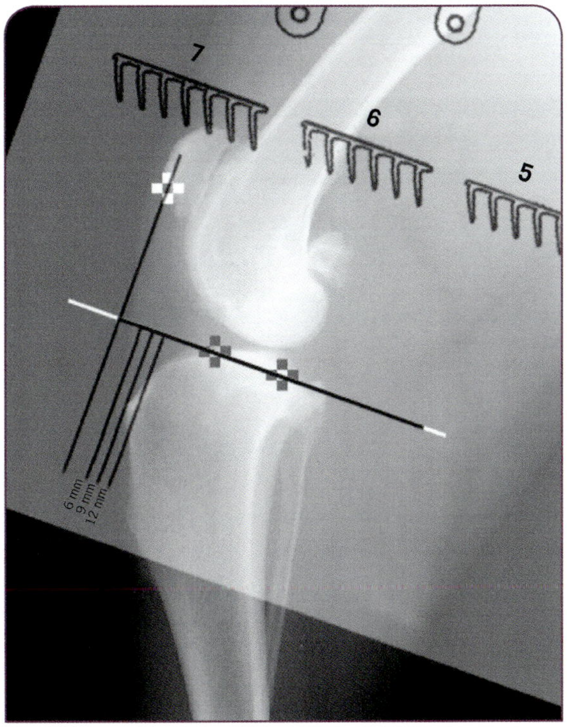

FIGURE 7. Detail of the calculation of the advancement needed on an X-ray of the stifle joint in mediolateral projection. In this case a 9 mm advancement is required.

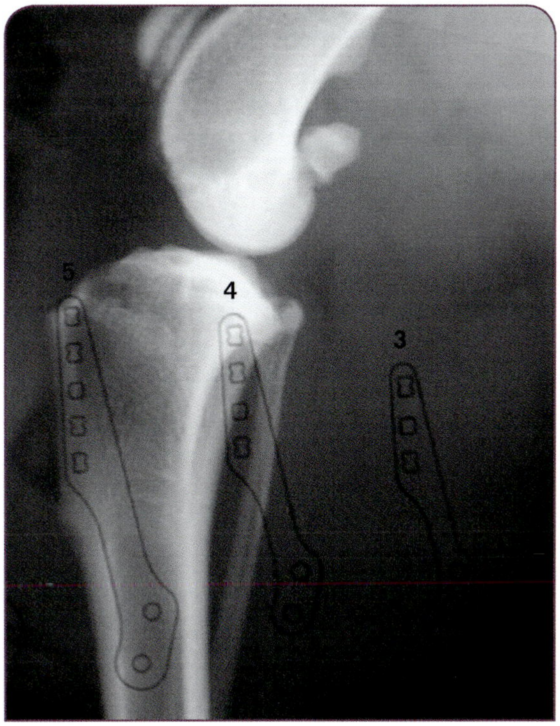

FIGURE 8. Detail of the selection of the necessary plate and forks. In this case five-prong forks and their corresponding plate are needed.

Implants

All implants used are made of pure titanium. They consist of plates with two to eight holes and their corresponding forks which may be used on either the left or right tibia, and cages with widths of 3, 4.5, 6, 7.5, 9, 10.5, 12 and 15 mm and different lengths to be inserted in the osteotomy and counteract compression force (Fig. 9).

The different implants are fixed with self-tapping titanium screws. Cages are fixed with 2.4 mm screws, plates with two to five holes are fixed with 2.7 mm screws and plates with six to eight holes are fixed with 3.5 mm screws.

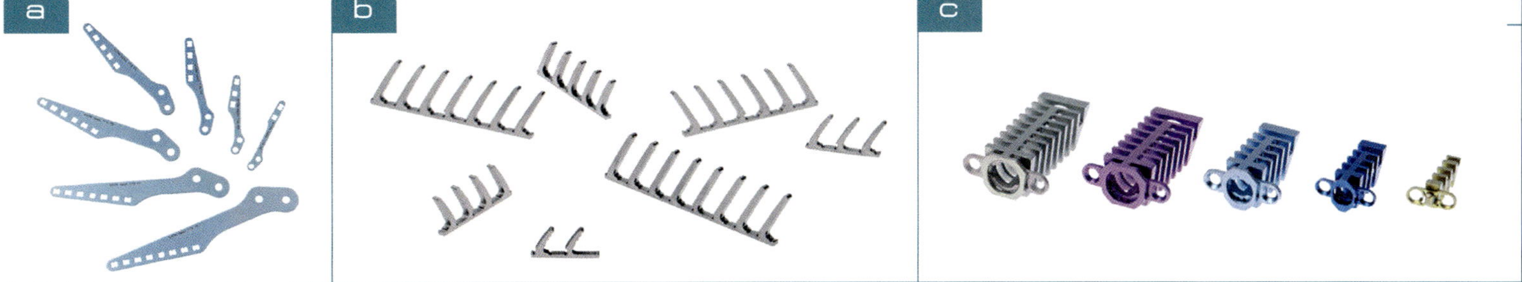

FIGURE 9. Detail of the plates (a), forks (b) and cages (c) used for TTA (KYON Veterinary Surgical Products, Technoparkstrasse 1, Zurich, Switzerland).

Surgical technique

An arthroscopy or a medial or mediocaudal arthrotomy can be performed to diagnose and treat potential injuries of the menisci in complete ACL rupture.

First, access is made medial to the proximal tibia, from the cranial part of the medial meniscus to the saphenous vein distally. The pes anserinus is cut and elevated carefully. The medial collateral ligament and the insertion of the patellar ligament with its synovial bursa are left intact.

The number of holes desired to place the plate with its teeth are made using a special drill guide (Fig. 10) and a 2.0 mm drill bit. The holes are immediately caudal to the cortex of the tibial crest (*margo cranialis*). The first hole is made at the level of the tibial tuberosity, medial to the tibial insertion of the patellar ligament, and the drill guide is secured by passing an anchor peg through this hole. Next the more distal hole is drilled and also secured with an anchor peg. Thus the drill guide is secure and the intermediate holes can be drilled (Figs. 11 and 12). Once all the fork holes have been made, the drill guide is removed and the two anchor pegs are replaced in the most distal and most proximal holes of the tuberosity so as not to lose track of their position (Fig. 13).

The next step consists of performing a transverse osteotomy of the tibial tuberosity, starting at a midpoint between the tibial crest and the body of the tibia and proceeding towards the cranial part of the extensor groove (called Gerdy's tubercle in humans) (Fig. 14). The osteotomy is bicortical up to the most proximal hole of the tibial tuberosity. Proximal to this, it is monocortical. Once the plate and forks have been fixed to the tibial tuberosity this portion is finished.

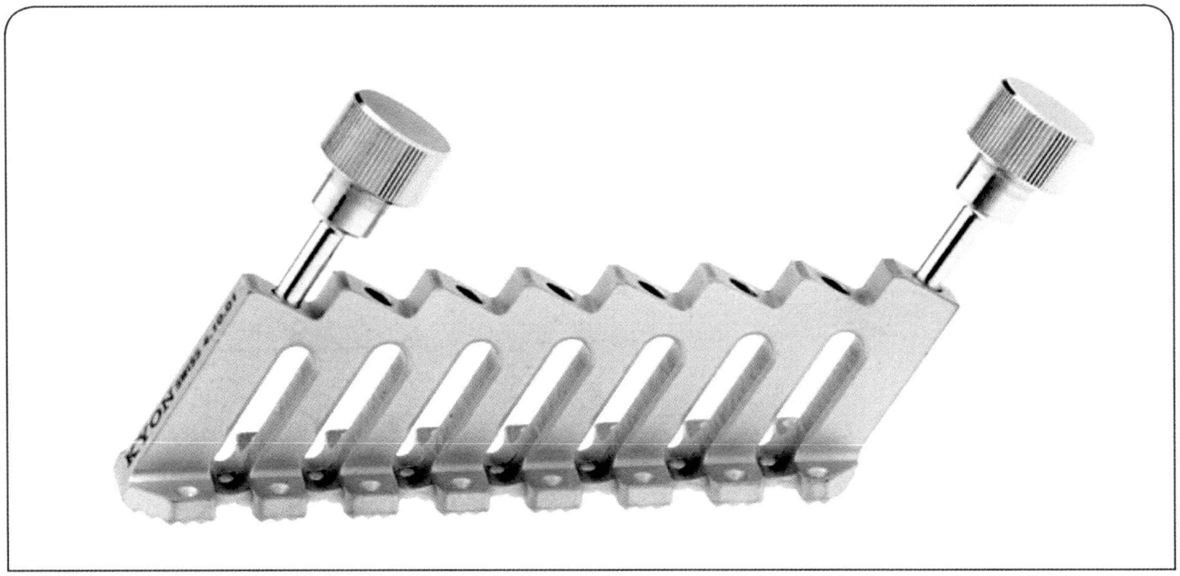

FIGURE 10. Detail of the special drill guide used to create the holes of the forks over the tibial tuberosity (KYON Veterinary Surgical Products, Technoparkstrasse 1, Zurich, Switzerland).

A very common error is a very cranial osteotomy. This often causes tibial tuberosity fractures. This can be prevented by measuring the distance from the tibial tuberosity to the planned osteotomy line on X-ray and transferring this to the bone, or palpating the cranial horn of the medial meniscus. This may be the best option. The skin is open, and the meniscus is very easily palpated. Keeping cranial to it should prevent problems.

Next, if necessary, the plate is gently moulded so that it conforms to the medial surface of the tibia (Fig. 15) and then the plate–fork set is fitted to the impacting tool (Fig. 16). Once the forks have been inserted into the bone (Figs. 17 and 18), the osteotomy is finished proximally and its width is measured in order to select a spacer of a suitable length (Fig. 19). The tibial tuberosity is moved cranially and proximally. Cranial displacement is determined by the cage. Proximal displacement is performed in order to maintain the position of the femoropatellar joint and prevent distal displacement of the patella. This displacement is approximately half of the given advancement (for example, if a 9 mm cage is placed, then the tibial tuberosity is displaced proximally around 4-5 mm).

Next, a cage of a suitable width and length is placed to maintain the distraction obtained and the assembly is kept in position using pointed reduction forceps. The cage and plate are fixed with screws (Figs. 20 and 21).

The defect created in the osteotomy can be filled in with a spongy bone graft if desired.

A recent study compared using a bone graft to not using a bone graft and found no differences in terms of healing times.

Finally, the fascia, subcutaneous tissue and skin are sutured and the wound is covered with a dressing or bandage.

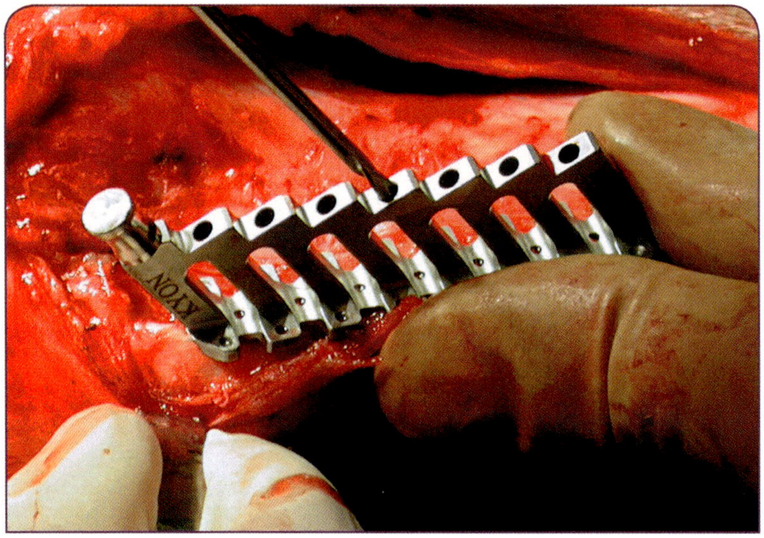

FIGURE 11. Intraoperative view of the drill guide fixed to the tibial tuberosity by the proximal anchor peg.
At this time the most distal hole is drilled.

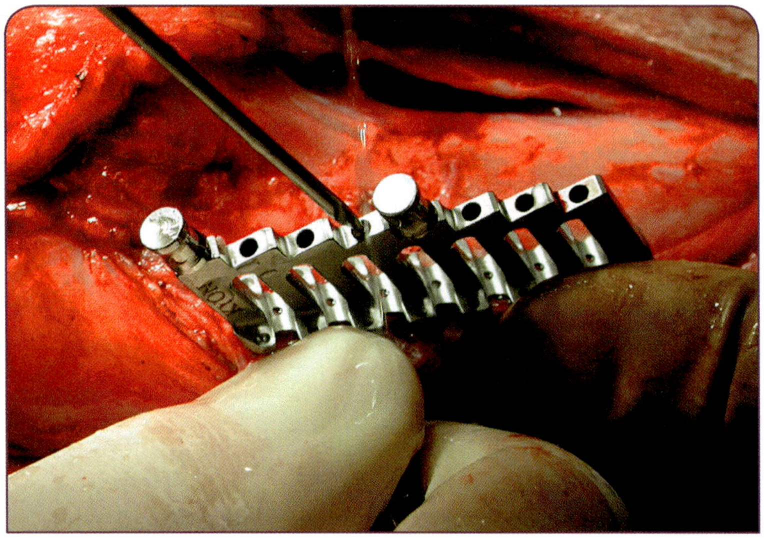

FIGURE 12. The intermediate holes are made after the proximal and distal holes have been drilled and the drill guide has been fixed with the anchor pegs.

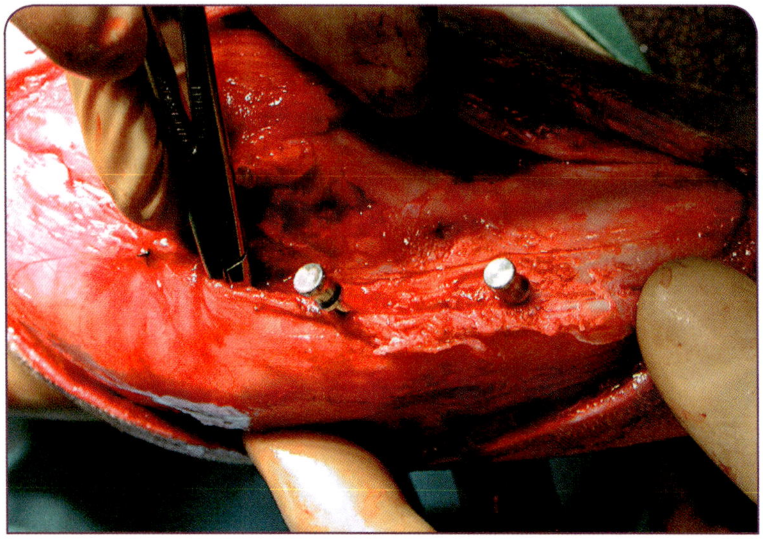

FIGURE 13. Once the holes have been drilled, the drill guide is removed and the anchor pegs are left in place. Next, straight haemostatic forceps are placed cranial to the medial meniscus to mark the direction of the osteotomy.

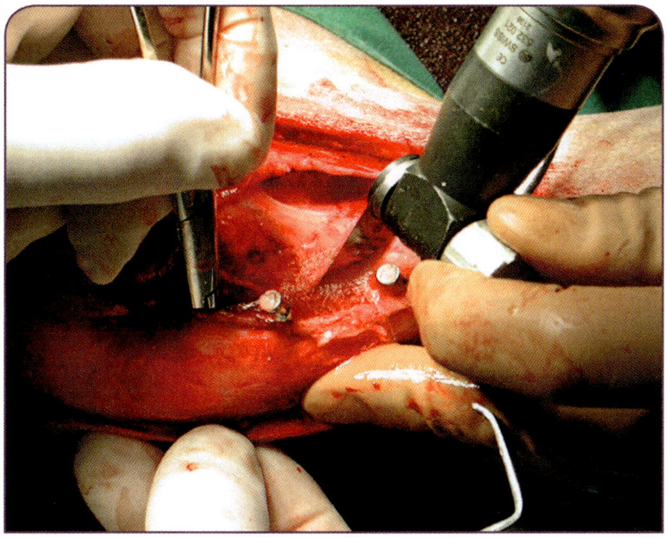

FIGURE 14. The osteotomy is performed from the distal area to the proximal area. Its most distal part is bicortical. The portion proximal to the holes is incomplete in order to keep the tibial tuberosity connected to the body of the tibia and thus facilitate insertion of the forks into the tibial tuberosity.

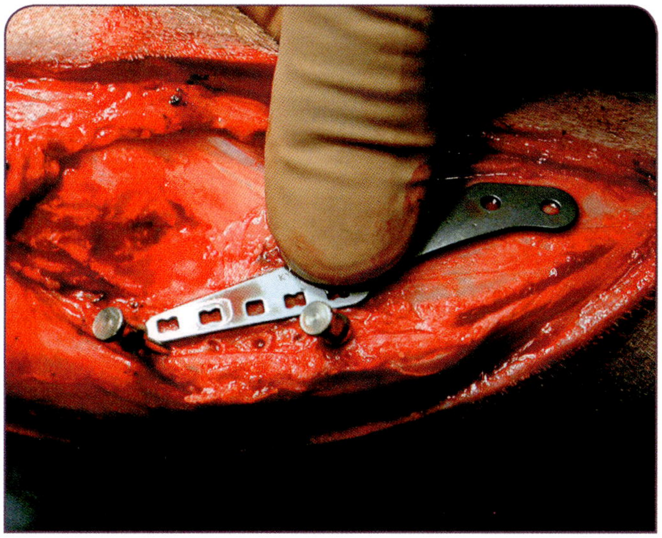

FIGURE 15. The plate is superimposed on and, if necessary, slightly moulded to the proximal part of the tibia.

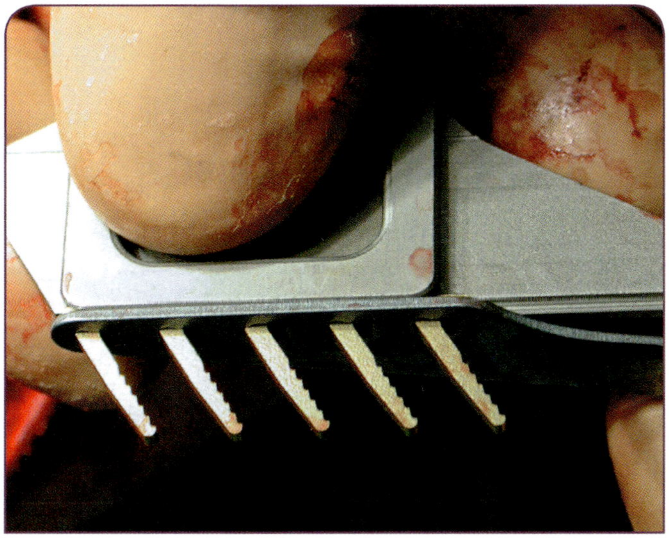

FIGURE 16. Detail of the plate with the forks and impacting tool.

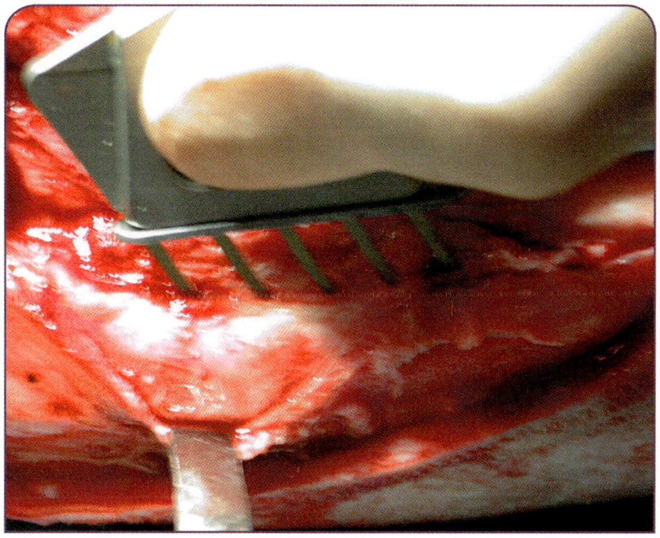

FIGURE 17. The set consisting of a plate, forks and impacting tool is placed over the holes and then impacted.

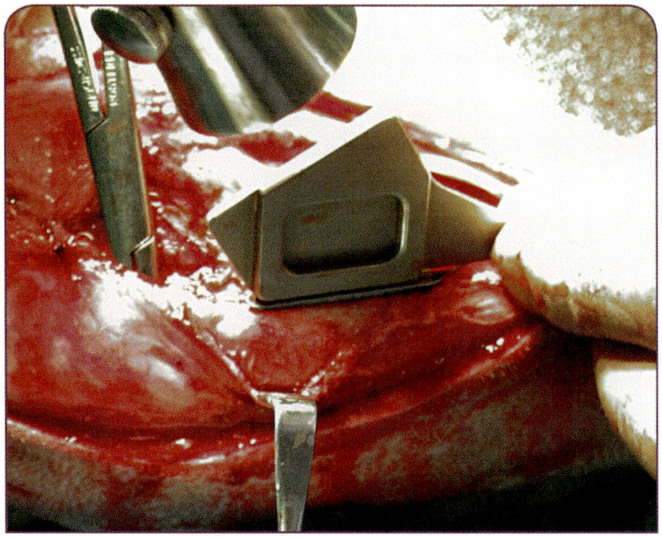

FIGURE 18. The forks are completed inserted and gently pounded.

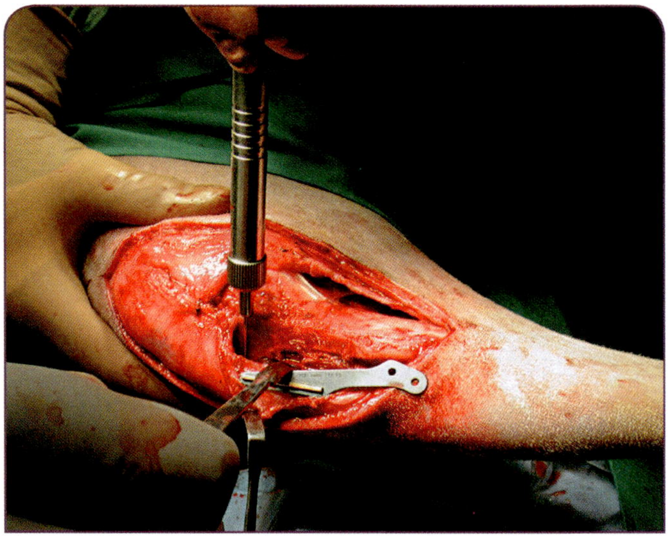

FIGURE 19. Once the plate has been impacted, the osteotomy is finished. The width of its most proximal part is measured and a cage of a suitable length is selected.

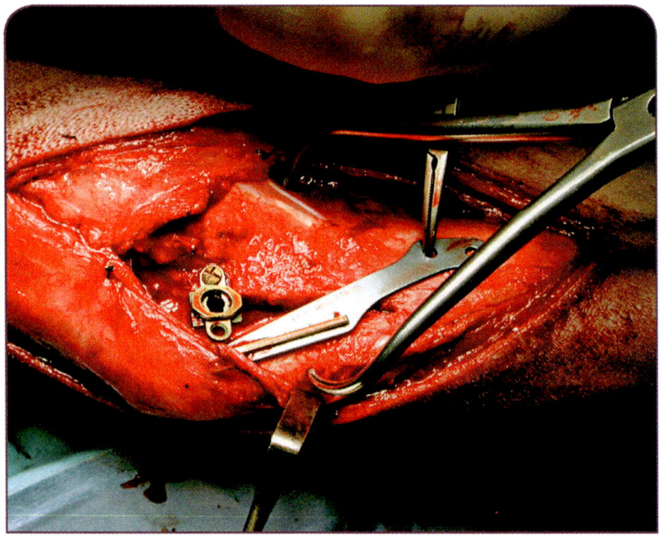

FIGURE 20. The cage is placed, the assembly is kept in place with forceps and the cage is fixed to the body of the tibia with a 2.4 mm screw. This screw is directed caudally and distally so that it is not positioned in the stifle joint. The next screws fix the plate to the body of the tibia. They are 2.7 mm screws in plates with up to five holes and 3.5 mm screws in larger plates. The screw that fixes the cage to the tibial tuberosity is the last to be placed.

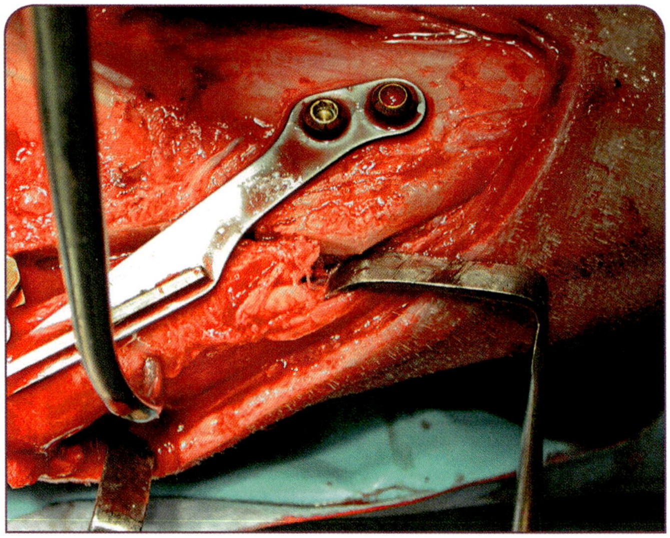

FIGURE 21. Detail of proximal displacement of the tibial tuberosity.

Postoperative radiographic monitoring

Once the surgery is complete X-rays are taken in mediolateral and craniocaudal projections while the patient is still anaesthetised (Figs. 22 and 23). These projections serve as a point of reference for subsequent radiological studies and enable evaluation of the following:

- Mediolateral projection:
  - Direction of the osteotomy.
  - Reduction of the osteotomy.
  - Proper position of the screws.
  - Advancement achieved of the tibial tuberosity and confirmation of its new location between the tibial plateau and the patellar ligament (90°).
- Craniocaudal projection:
  - Suitable placement of the cage and forks and confirmation that none is overly long.
  - Suitable placement of the plate fixation screws.

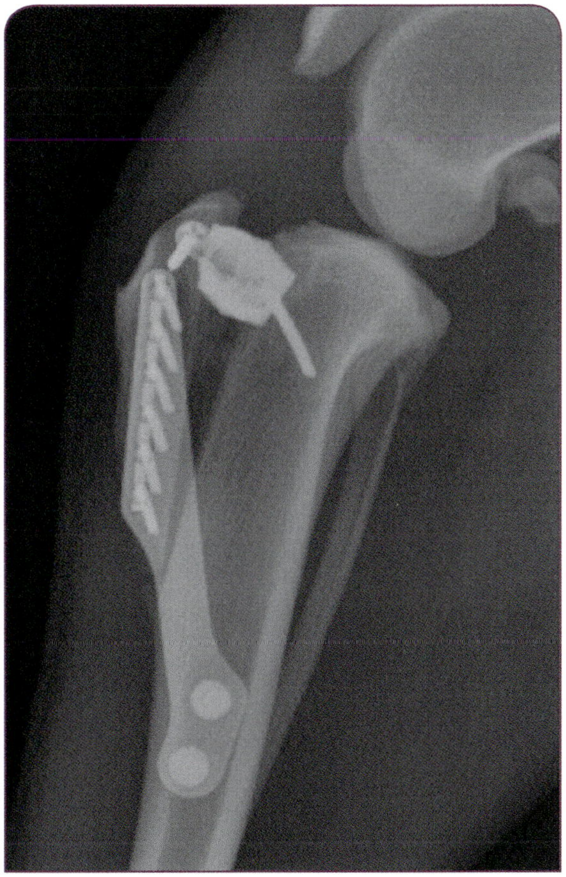

FIGURE 22. Postoperative examination of the stifle joint that has undergone surgery (mediolateral projection). This projection enables evaluation of the proper positioning of the implants and the advancement achieved.

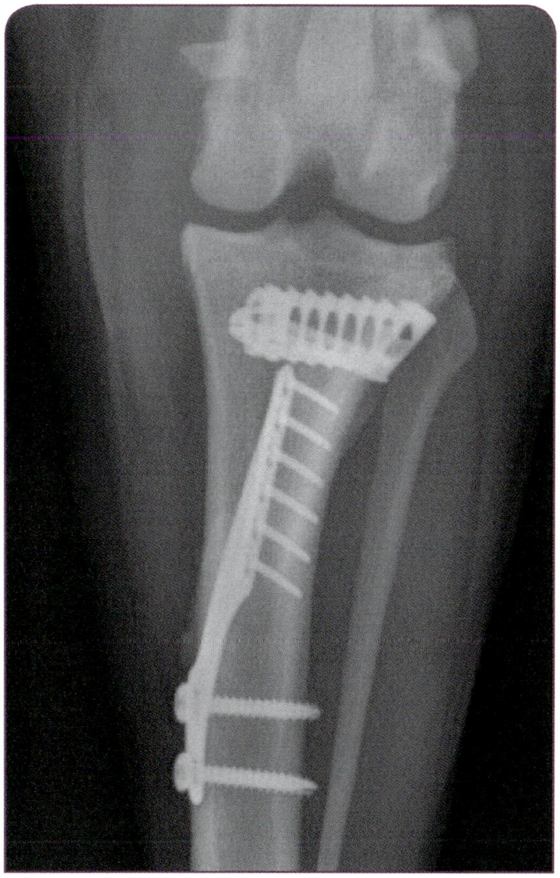

FIGURE 23. Postoperative examination of the stifle joint that has undergone surgery (craniocaudal projection). The length of the cage, the proper insertion of the forks, the length of the screws that fasten the plate to the tibia and the alignment of the patellar ligament are examined on this X-ray.

Postoperative care

Patients that undergo TTA do not require hospitalisation; however, hospitalisation is recommended to optimally monitor their vital signs and postoperative pain during the first 24 hours.

A Robert Jones bandage is placed for 24 to 48 hours. The patient is provided with non-steroidal anti-inflammatory drugs (NSAIDs) and analgesics to treat inflammation and pain. Analgesics are to be administered during the first 24 hours, and NSAIDs are to be administered for five to 10 days following surgery.

The first radiological examination is performed six to eight weeks after surgery to confirm that healing of the osteotomy has occurred (Fig. 24). If it has not then the examination is repeated every four weeks until it is confirmed. Healing is not complete after six weeks, but it is generally sufficient to provide suitable stability.

If the radiological examination confirms that healing is progressing properly then walks are lengthened up to normal.

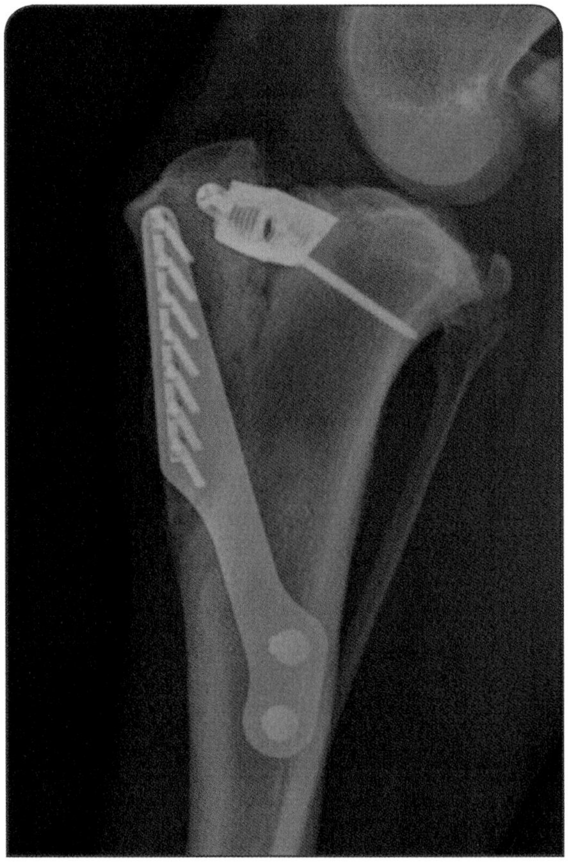

FIGURE 24. Mediolateral projection of the stifle joint six weeks after surgery. Partial healing of the osteotomy is observed.

CHAPTER

9

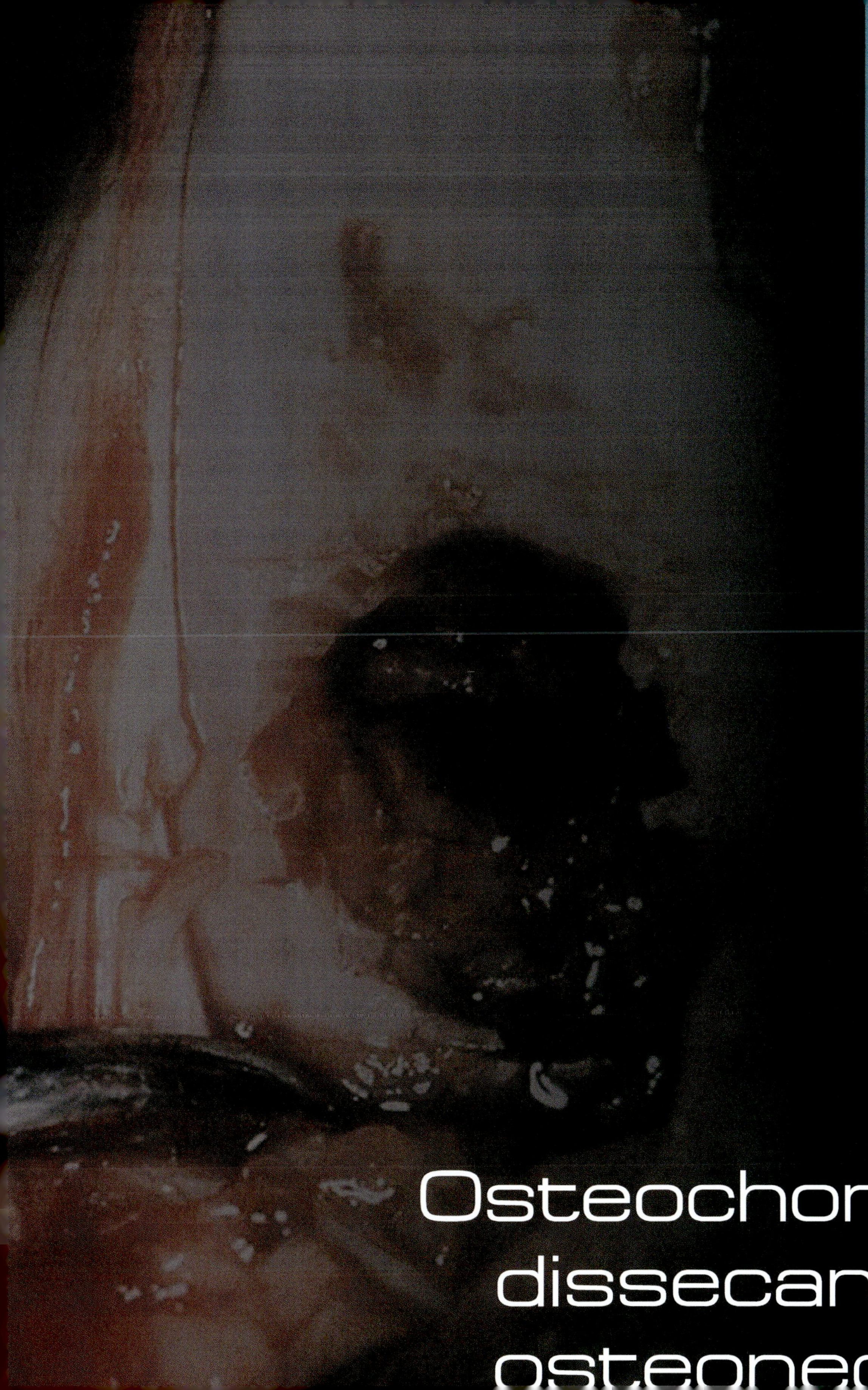

Osteochondritis dissecans and osteonecrosis

Osteochondritis

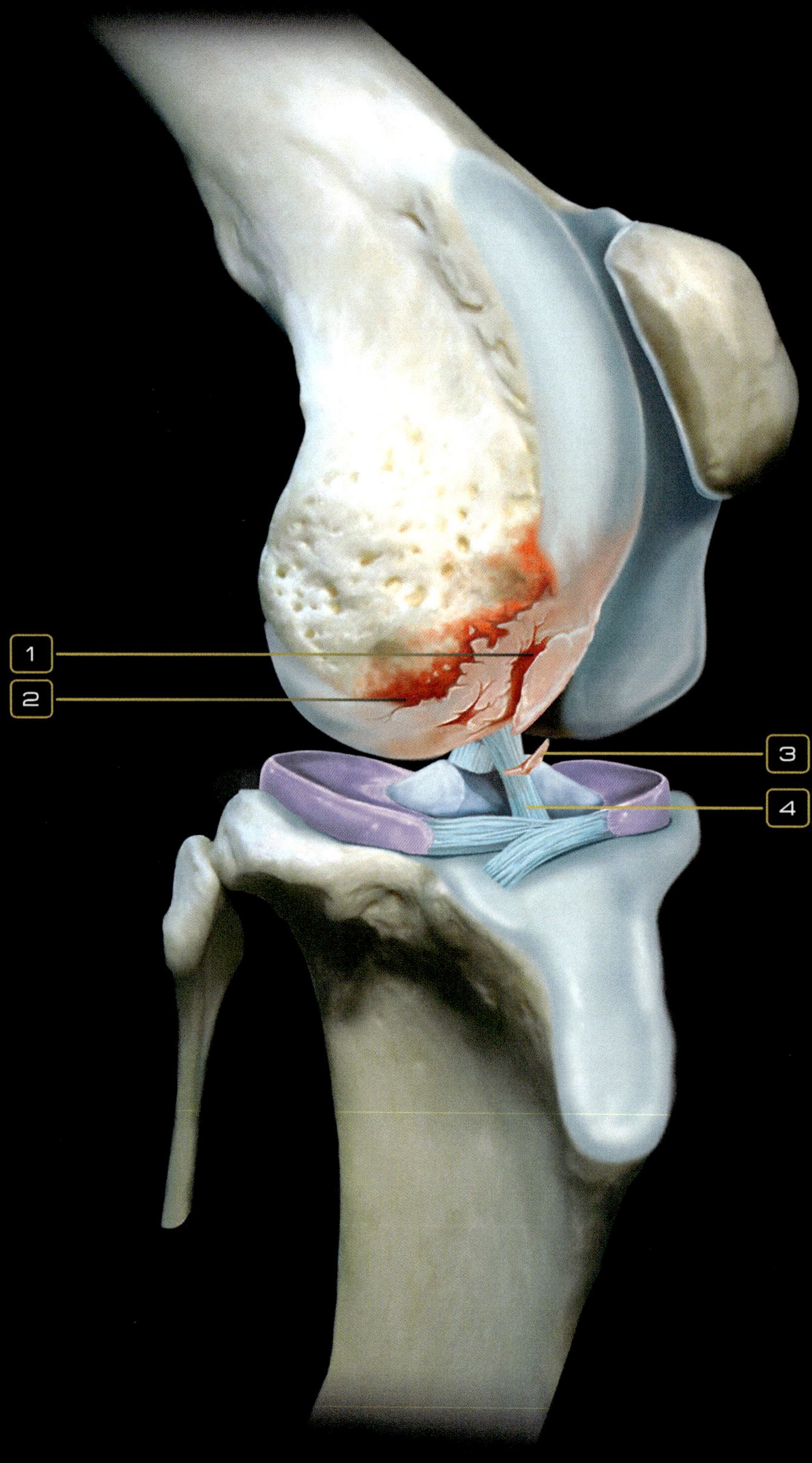

LATERAL VIEW

1 Cartilage destruction

2 Osteoarthritis and bone sclerosis

3 Separation of osteochondral fragments

4 Abnormality of ligaments (mainly the ACL)

Osteochondritis dissecans

Introduction

Osteochondritis dissecans consists of a joint injury characterised by the separation of a cartilage fragment with its corresponding subchondral bone. It was first recorded in humans and was given its name at the end of the 19th century by König, a German surgeon. Although injuries of this nature can be found in various joints, particularly in the shoulder but also in the hip, elbow and tarsus, the stifle joint is the most commonly affected joint. It is the most common cause of intra-articular loose bodies in young patients. It is also one of the causes of gonarthrosis.

Aetiopathogenesis and location

It is more common in males (in a 3:1 ratio) and tends to clinically manifest at five to seven months of age. It has a characteristic but not exclusive location. In 85 % of cases, injuries are on the lateral femoral condyle. In 70 % of cases, injuries are on the lateral edge of the lateral femoral condyle, in the intercondylar area; this is called the “classic area”.

Factors cited as responsible for osteochondritis dissecans include bone infarction due to embolism; abnormalities in the ossification process, which may or may not be related to endocrine diseases; and other systemic and traumatic diseases in very young animals.

Certain systemic diseases such as systemic lupus erythematosus (SLE), certain haemoglobin diseases and hyperadrenocorticism involve similar osteocartilaginous detachment injuries. However, in these diseases the bone bed is part of an extensive area of adjacent osteonecrosis, while in osteochondritis dissecans the osteochondral segment is separated by fibrous tissue of the underlying condylar bone, which is well vascularised.

Moreover, several recent observations have attempted to link osteochondritis dissecans to preceding trauma:

- First, arthroscopic observation of these injuries has revealed that, except in extremely rare cases of multiple epiphyseal dysplasia associated with osteochondritis dissecans, classically described juvenile epiphyseal disorders appearing on X-ray do not correspond to true separations.
- Second, injuries similar to those found in osteochondritis dissecans have been experimentally reproduced in knees of cadavers subjected to rotation and compression in the “classic area”.
- Finally, the medical histories of patients with osteochondritis dissecans indicate traumatic events in 45 % of cases and sporting practice in 60 % of cases. In fact, in many groups studied, 10 % of cases can be classified as acute osteochondral fracture. It must be borne in mind that German Shepherds are among the most commonly affected animals. This is a classic breed to subject to agility tests and strenuous exercise starting from a very young age.

Diagnosis

Osteochondritis dissecans manifests differently depending on the extent and progression of the injury. Concerning progression, the osteochondral fragment may remain stable and be movable without completely detaching from its bed or turn into an intra-articular loose body.

When the fragment is stable, osteochondritis dissecans manifests with variable, sometimes sporadic pain occasionally accompanied by moderate articular effusion. Different authors have reported in these patients a characteristic gait in external rotation of the tibia, probably as a result of irritation of the ACL, whose insertion is close to the “classic area” of osteochondritis dissecans. It has also been reported that when the stifle joint is extended in internal rotation in these patients, pain occurs around 30° before reaching full extension and remits in external rotation.

If the fragment is unstable, osteochondritis dissecans manifests with popping and a feeling of instability and locking.

When the osteochondral fragment completely detaches, it manifests as a "joint mouse", which can be palpated at the bases of the sac and increases the frequency of locking. Other causes of an intra-articular loose body are, in young animals, a rare disease called synovial osteochondromatosis (in which chondroid metaplasia of the synovial membrane produces many nodules which break off and become loose in the joint) and, in adult animals, osteochondral injuries caused by constant friction which become degenerative in osteoarthritis.

The diagnosis is confirmed by a plain X-ray. Craniocaudal and lateral projection and a projection of the intercondylar space should be ordered. Both CT and MRI scans (the latter earlier) support the diagnosis (Figs. 1 and 2). Arthroscopy is very useful to determine the location, size and stability of the injury and is key to making treatment decisions.

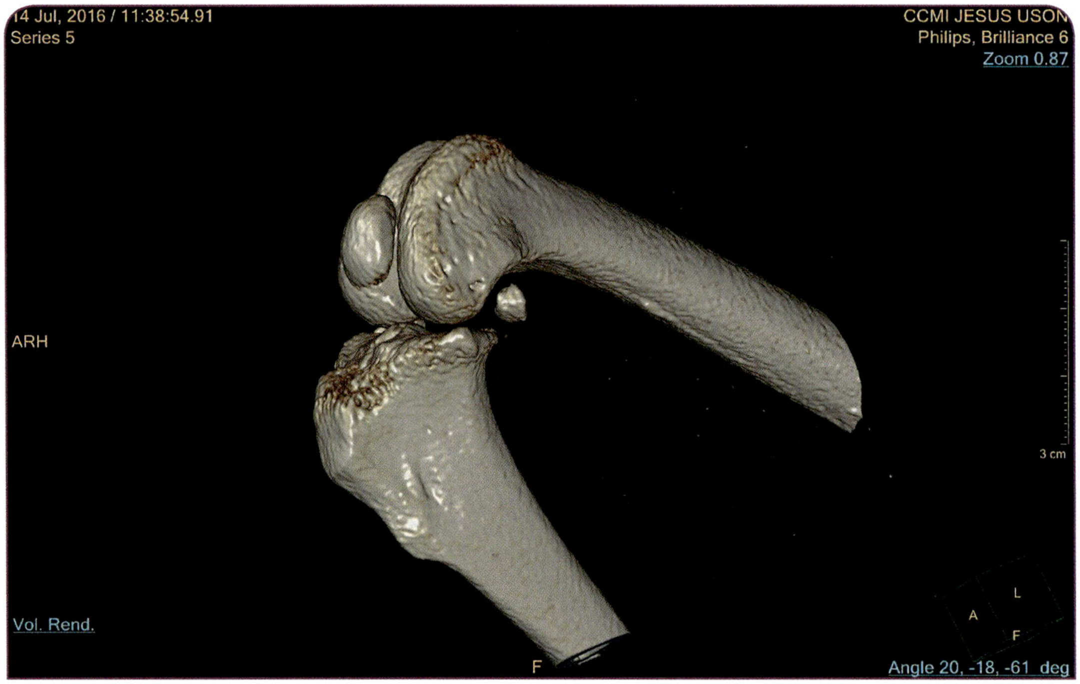

FIGURE 1. Three-dimensional CT scan. Osteochondritis in the right stifle joint.

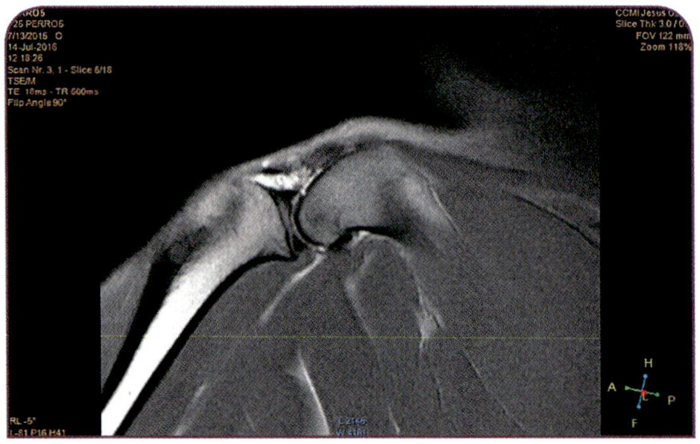

FIGURE 2. MRI scan. Osteochondritis in the right stifle joint.

Treatment

In patients under 18 months old, the injury may end up spontaneously healing. Therefore, conservative treatment with no weight-bearing, rest and analgesics, as dictated by the symptoms of the animal, is initially indicated. The course of the injury is monitored, clinically and on X-ray, for eight to 10 weeks, and if symptoms persist once this time has elapsed, an arthroscopy is indicated to make perforations over the injuries in order to stabilise them by stimulating union (forage). In animals belonging to giant breeds, unstable flaps can even be fixed with pins (preferably made of biodegradable polymers) and free flaps can be removed.

Treatment consists of an arthrotomy and meticulous examination of the abnormal cartilage (Fig. 3). The sclerotic bone which is now uncovered is perforated with a fine drill bit to facilitate its revascularisation. If an abnormality of the lateral meniscus is observed it is advisable to do a partial resection.

The prognosis is always guarded as in these cases a serious deforming joint disease often develops.

In summary

- This disease is particularly seen in giant breeds. The authors often diagnose it in German Shepherds.
- The first symptoms appear at five to seven months old.
- An inflamed stifle joint, pain in extension and muscle atrophy are observed.
- X-rays should be taken in craniocaudal, caudocranial and mediolateral projections.
- The changes observed are obvious and are always located on the lateral condyle.

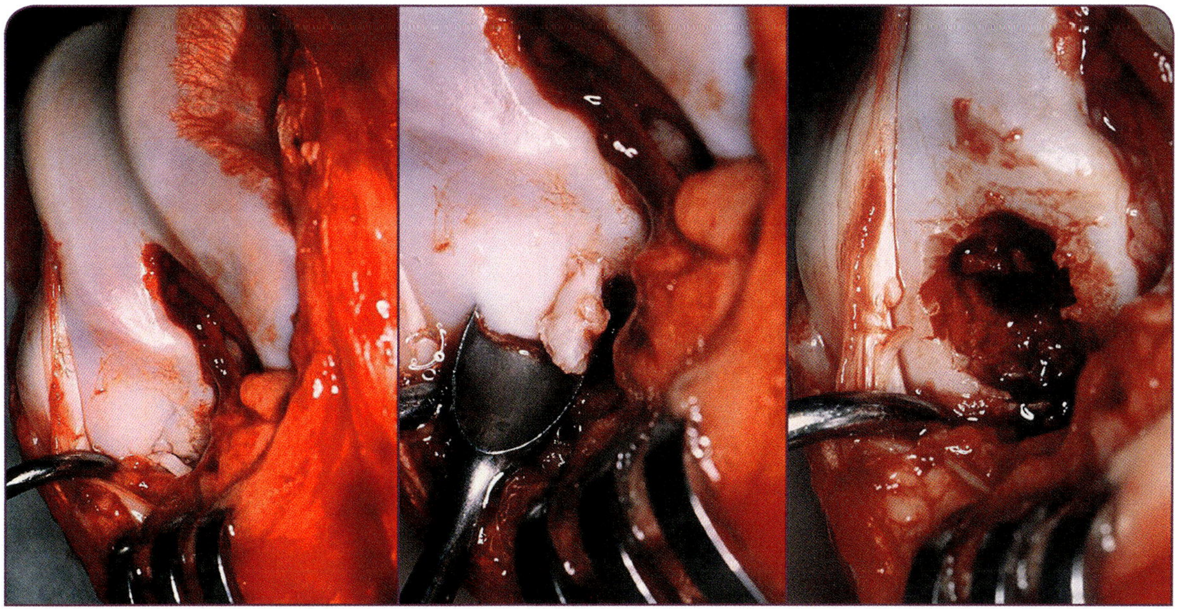

FIGURE 3. Osteochondritis dissecans of the lateral condyle of the femur.

Osteonecrosis

Aetiopathogenesis

Osteonecrosis in adults is most often located on the head of the femur (Legg–Calvé–Perthes disease), where it has significant clinical repercussions. Osteonecrosis in the stifle joint also has significant clinical repercussions. It results from generalised processes in adults with stifle joint pain or is idiopathic.

The onset of ischaemic injuries in various places on articular surfaces, which are accompanied by trabecular collapse and demarcation of osteochondral areas that clearly differ from healthy tissue, has already been mentioned as a process associated with systemic lupus erythematosus and endogenous or iatrogenic hyperadrenocorticism. This secondary osteonecrosis tends to be bilateral and surprisingly asymptomatic. It also tends to affect multiple joints and have an atypical location.

Attempts have been made to explain the idiopathic form with a vascular hypothesis (this is difficult to support given the abundance of radially distributed intraosseous anastomoses in the typical location) and a traumatic hypothesis (this is based on biomechanical studies and the fact that it often co-occurs with osteoporosis); increased intraosseous pressure probably plays a role. This injury has not been experimentally reproduced.

Epidemiology and location

This predominantly occurs in females (in a 3:1 ratio) and elderly animals over nine years old in 80 % of cases. It is diagnosed *post mortem* in 90 % of cases and the initial diagnosis is osteoarthritis in the same percentage of cases. One in every five cases is bilateral. The injury usually is in the lower weight-bearing area of the medial femoral condyle but sometimes is on the lateral femoral condyle or medial tibial plateau.

Diagnosis

Osteonecrosis tends to initially manifest with severe pain of sudden onset that is well delimited in a specific area (unfortunately this pain tends to be attributed to osteoarthritis). It is typically accompanied by a variable degree of articular effusion as well as pain and muscle contracture which translate to significantly limited mobility. In this initial phase, X-ray is not helpful and provides no findings beyond an image easily mistaken for osteoarthritis. This, together with pseudo-locking, which manifests with an intermittent antalgic gait, and the location of the pain often lead the clinician to suspect an arthritis injury and/or an injury of the medial meniscus. If these signs and symptoms are present and an arthroscopy is performed, it most likely does not reveal bone disease and does reveal some partial ACL rupture or meniscal degeneration due to the advanced age of these animals. This leads the clinician to perform a TPLO or TTA together with a partial meniscectomy.

This unjustified therapeutic activity unfortunately not only does not lead to any improvement but also amounts to unnecessary surgery. Sadly, the animal does not improve and the owner becomes mistrustful. However, if this process is known to be present, the owner may be informed of such a possibility. If this process is not known to be present, then the owner may be informed that Tc ^{99m} (sodium pertechnetate) scintigraphy or MRI, which would reveal the presence of an ischaemic injury in the corresponding location, must be ordered so as to rule it out. This earns the respect and esteem of the owner.

In any case, observation of the injury after at least six months is considered to be justified. This observation must be done by means of an arthroscopy for surgical evaluation, and must always be done before performing ACL surgery with the new techniques which, while a blessing, serve to treat an ACL mechanism injury, not any problem that may occur in the stifle joint, as novices in this discipline tend to believe.

Later on X-ray findings are as follows:

- A slight flattening of the subchondral plate.
- A limited area of lower density.
- A greater flattening delimited by a dense rim of sclerosis.
- Secondary osteoarthritis of the medial femorotibial area.

The severity of the clinical manifestations corresponds to the stage of the injury and two X-ray parameters:

1. The product of the craniocaudal dimensions and the lateral dimensions, obtained with craniocaudal and lateral projections.
2. The relationship in craniocaudal projection between areas of necrosis and width of the condyle: less than 3.5 cm^2 and 40 %, respectively, are believed to represent a good prognosis and require conservative treatment, while more than 5 cm^2 and 50 %, respectively, are believed to require surgical treatment.

Osteonecrosis requires a differential diagnosis essentially with meniscal injuries, gonarthrosis and osteochondritis dissecans. Table 1 shows the main differences between osteochondritis dissecans and osteonecrosis.

Treatment

Cases that have a good prognosis and are unlikely to progress to gonarthrosis must be treated conservatively by taping, NSAIDs and physiotherapy. In cases that have a poor prognosis, local procedures, mainly forage (perforation) by a conventional arthroscopy or arthrotomy, fail to yield consistently satisfactory or predictable outcomes.

Moreover, the role of stem cells is under review, since the short-term outcomes are inconsistent and there is little long-term case-based reasoning or parallel research. For this reason, in patients under nine years old with genu varum, a valgising osteotomy above the tibial tuberosity should be performed with a TPLO using Slocum's technique to treat animals that are "crooked" (this word is commonly used in clinical practice to refer to animals with both varus and valgus deformities of the hind limb).

In the authors' opinion, an initial arthrodesis should be performed in cases with a very poor prognosis, provided that the injury is very extensive and the animal is very elderly, has a poor quality of life and does not respond to medical treatment.

TABLE 1. Main differences between osteochondritis dissecans and osteonecrosis.

Parameters	Osteochondritis dissecans	Osteonecrosis
Age	Puppy or young adult	Over 8-9 years old
Sex	Male	Female
Traumatic event	In approximately 50 % of cases	Very rare
Onset	Gradual	Sudden
Location	• Lateral condyle • Intercondylar	• Medial condyle • Weight-bearing area • Also on lateral condyle and tibial plateau
Anatomical pathology	Vascular bed	Ischaemic bed
Radiology	Delimitation with loose bodies	Collapse without loose bodies
Scintigraphy	Hypouptake	Hyperuptake

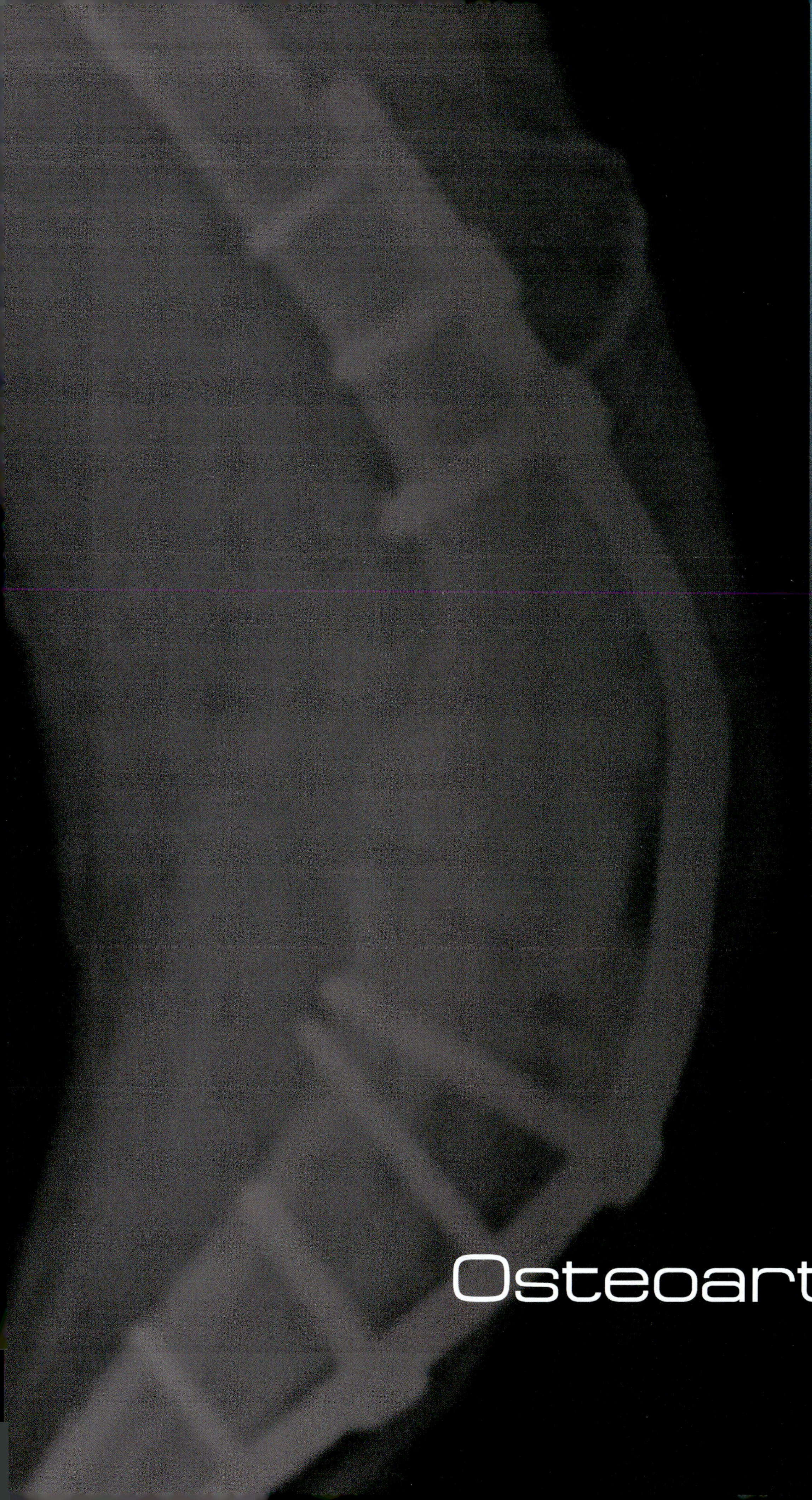

CHAPTER 10

Osteoarthritis

Osteoarthritis

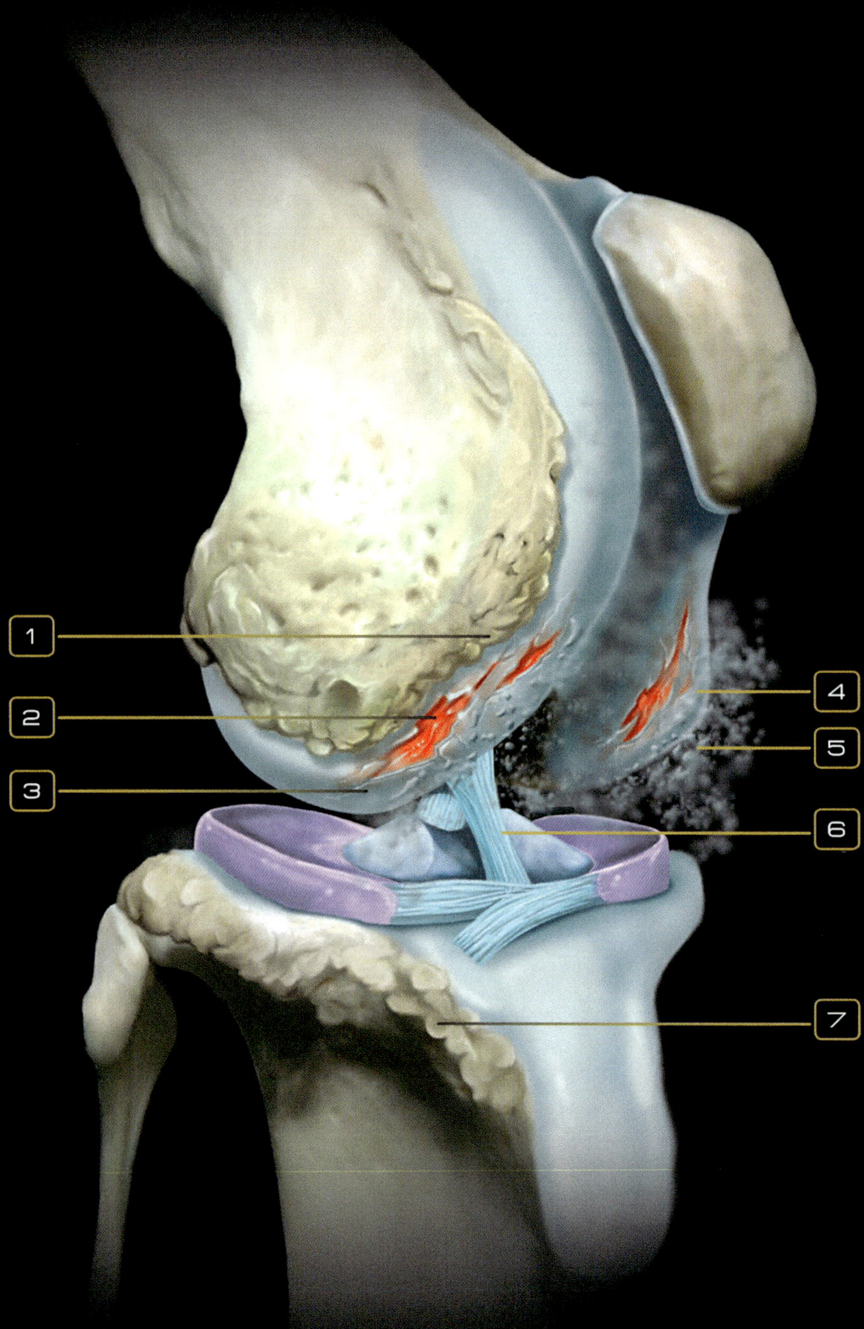

LATERAL VIEW

1 Microfractures and sclerosis of the subchondral bone

2 Vascular penetration of the area

3 Chondral fibrosis

4 Articular cartilage destruction

5 Separation of cartilage fragments

6 Abnormality and weakness of muscles, tendons and ligaments

Introduction

This chapter comprehensively analyses joint diseases in dogs. The term osteoarthritis (OA) refers to a group of non-inflammatory joint diseases. Although the pathophysiology of the disease generally involves an inflammatory component, it is accepted that the initial events are mechanical.

As an anecdotal detail, osteoarthritis was first diagnosed in animals even before it was first diagnosed in humans. The finding of signs of spondyloarthritis dates back to Neanderthals (around 40,000 years ago). This disorder has been observed in the spinal column of some dinosaurs that are phylogenetically more ancient than humans. Therefore, it is nothing new. Nevertheless it remains an important issue for both the pharmaceutical industry and surgical clinical management in both humans and dogs.

It is the most common condition among connective tissue diseases and its prevalence increases with age. In dogs seven years old and older, 80 % of the population has radiological signs of osteoarthritis in at least one joint, although symptoms only significantly manifest in 25 % of those affected. Some studies have even affirmed that OA affects more than 20 % of the canine population over one year old and particularly affects certain breeds. Although clinical signs vary, pain always occurs. When pain is chronic it ends up modifying the behaviour of the animal. Thus it affects not only the quality of life of the animal itself, but also that of its owner, who is influenced by the daily dynamics of the pet (Figs. 1 and 2).

Definition

Osteoarthritis is defined as a slow-progressing, usually single-joint disease that may affect both small and large weight-bearing joints. It is clinically characterised by pain, deformity, limited mobility, focal erosive injuries, articular cartilage destruction, subchondral sclerosis and formation of cysts and osteophytes.

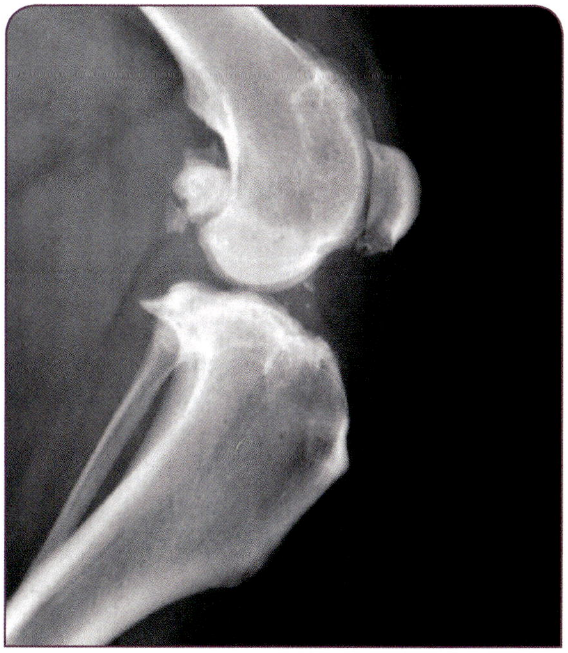

FIGURE 1. Moderate arthritis.

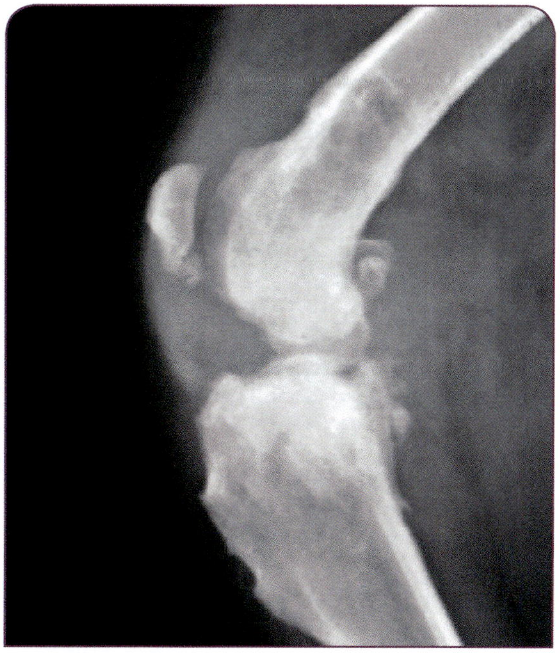

FIGURE 2. Serious chronic arthritis associated with a degenerative rupture.

The disease appears to start in the articular cartilage. Changes in this tissue, which are virtually pathognomonic, worsen with age. Any abnormalities that occur in the underlying bone and the synovial membrane are considered to be secondary. No systemic abnormalities have been confirmed; however, research is being conducted in search of blood markers allowing dogs that belong to breeds with a genetic predisposition to be screened and diagnosed early.

> Although, as mentioned, osteoarthritis generally occurs in elderly animals, its specific characteristics must be distinguished from joint changes that are a part of normal tissue involution.

Normal joint ageing involves the onset of chondral fibrosis and marginal osteophytes, but significantly differs from genuine osteoarthritis with respect to water and proteoglycan content and distribution. This will be discussed later on in relation to nutraceutical treatment of these diseases. In terms of pathology there is fibrillation and fragmentation, vascular penetration of the limiting highly basophilic area (tidemark), uniform staining of the matrix and densely clustered cell groups. Water content increases and proteoglycan concentration decreases. Collagen fibres are compacted but otherwise minimally affected. There is a marked increase in both catabolic and anabolic processes. The quality and nature of the products synthesised are abnormal in terms of composition and distribution of macromolecules, capacity for aggregation, and formation of non-collagen proteins such as chondronectin.

Aetiopathogenesis

Although osteoarthritis is multifactorial in aetiology, two well defined types are recognised based on the clinical course of the disease:

- **Primary osteoarthritis:** no pre-existing joint abnormality that may lead to the onset of osteoarthritis is identified.
- **Secondary osteoarthritis:** there is a clear history of a traumatic event (joint fracture or dislocation), an inflammatory event (septic or aseptic arthritis, birth defect or incongruity, or hip dysplasia), deforming juvenile diseases in dogs (Legg–Calvé–Perthes disease or epiphysiolysis) or mechanical abnormalities in axes that constitute longitudinal deformities of long bones in dogs (genu varum or genu valgum).

Recently it has been noted that some locations classified as primary could be caused by minimal changes in the signs and symptoms listed, which are clinically latent for years but end up causing disease through joint incongruity for which they are responsible. An example that may illustrate this point is articular incongruity of the elbow in dogs. In fact, many clinical and experimental observations point to the mechanical factor as the main cause of osteoarthritis.

The effects on articular cartilage of both experimental compression impact and experimental shear impact have been studied and found to be comparable to the action of repeated forces and the concentration of pressure created in limited areas by articular incongruity. Abnormalities due to wearing out of chondral structural macromolecules and the subsequent subchondral bone reaction (microfractures, repair and sclerosis) have been shown to lead to a reduction in the cushioning properties of the subchondral cartilage–bone

Osteoporosis versus osteoarthritis

Hip, spine and wrist fractures are strikingly uncommon in patients with osteoarthritis, and inversely, osteoarthritis is strikingly rare in patients with osteoporosis, in whom those traumatic injuries often occur. The greater bone elasticity of the latter group and the greater bone density and stiffness of the former group may explain the difference and support the theory put forward by Radin (1976) that the osteoarthritis process starts in subchondral sclerosis.

system and thus increase demand for greater mechanical activity which starts the process.

Ultimately, new avenues for studies on osteoarthritis associated with biochemical disorders such as ochronosis and haemochromatosis are opening up in view of the evidence of intrinsic enzyme abnormalities connected to many systemic, synovial and chondral mediators. This attracted the interest of the researchers Bonastre et al. (2013). It should be noted that no studies have conclusively found these to be primary phenomena so much as phenomena consecutive to initial mechanical abnormality. In any case, research is ongoing.

Basic mechanisms associated with the start of the process

These mechanisms, which have clearly been confirmed to be involved in secondary forms and may be involved in the primary form, are as follows:

- Direct injury of cartilage tissue and probably subchondral bone in displaced joint fractures, osteochondral defects, and chondrolysis due to inflammatory synovitis in aseptic arthritis or to enzyme aggression in septic arthritis.
- Mechanical overload due to articular congruity defects, as in hip dysplasia, Legg–Calvé–Perthes disease, epiphysiolysis, poorly reduced acetabular fractures and inactive arthritis sequelae with morphological deterioration of the bone ends.
- Abnormalities in bone vascularisation or the underlying bone structure (ischaemic bone necrosis) and in bone densification due to overload.

In any case, the changes initially detected are believed to be failures in collagen mesh and degradation of interstitial matrix aggregates. Collagen fibres form a three-dimensional structure that traps and compresses proteoglycans. These in turn keep the collagen fibre matrix taut by virtue of their water content. Given the subtle interaction between the three elements, any failure in one of them is understood to disrupt the balance maintaining the physical, chemical and mechanical properties of cartilage. Weakening of the cross-links between collagen fibres seems to precede failure in mesh traction, with first rupture and then collagen fibre fragmentation. This allows more water to penetrate the lattice and the resulting turgidity further weakens the tissue. Mechanical overload of chondrocytes has been shown to lead chondrocytes to release proteolytic enzymes (metalloproteoglycanases). These in turn worsen collagen and proteoglycan abnormalities (Fig. 3).

The role of certain cytokines and growth factors that appear to be involved in both homeostasis of the normal matrix and osteoarthritis is being studied. Some are involved in the pathogenesis of osteoarthritis, such as interleukin 1 (IL-1) (which has been found to be increased in osteoarthritis, inflammatory joint diseases and rheumatoid arthritis) and tumour necrosis factor α (TNF–α), since they stimulate the production of proteases from synovial chondrocytes and fibroblasts. These enzymes can break down the matrix of collagen and proteoglycans and suppress their synthesis. Other factors such as transforming growth factor β (TGF-β) are capable of counteracting the effects of these cytokines.

The injury sequence regardless of onset is presumed to be as explained in Box 1.

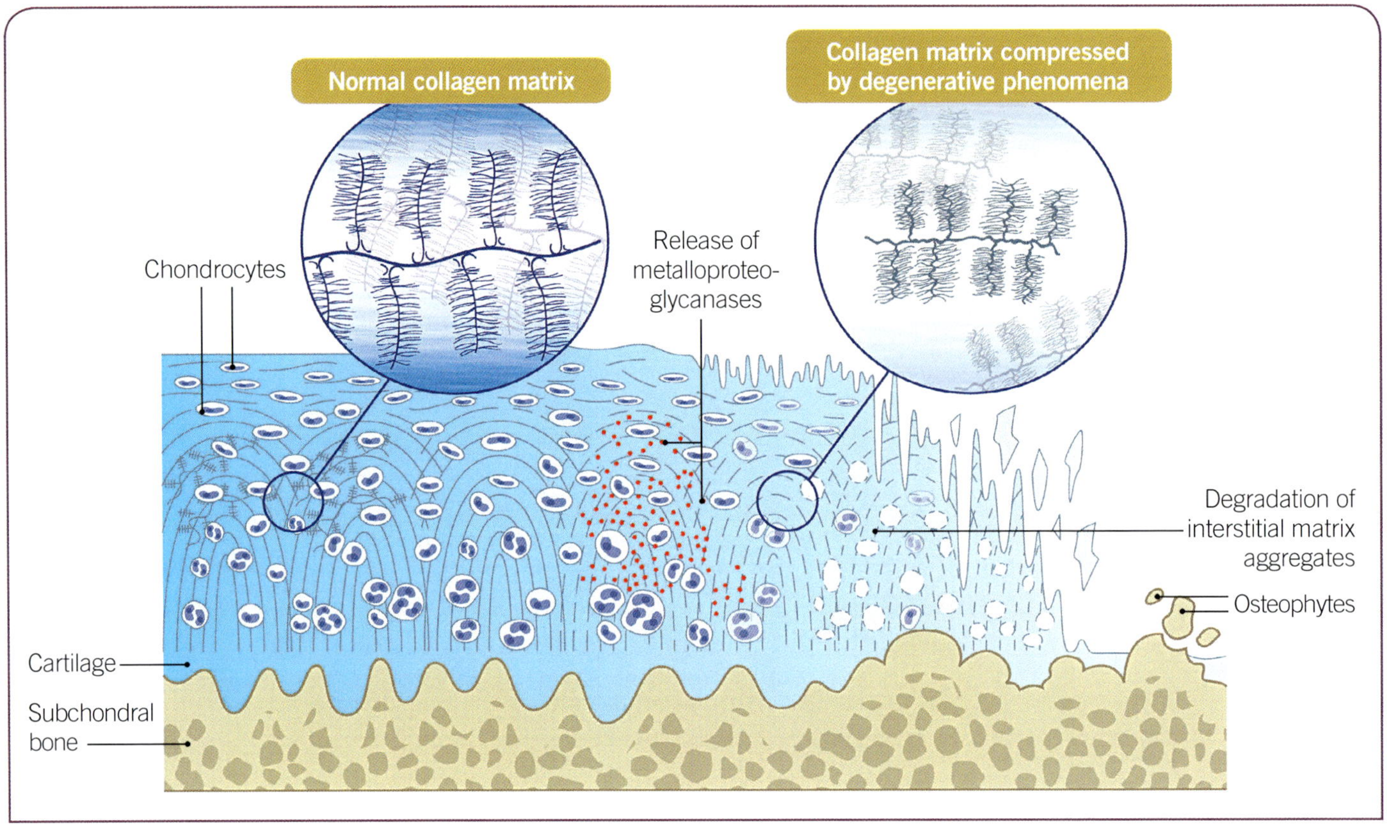

FIGURE 3. Abnormality of the physical, chemical and mechanical properties of cartilage leads to its deterioration and also impairment of adjacent joint and bone structures.

BOX 1

Injury sequence of osteoarthritis.

Cell proliferation in clones or clusters

↓

Increase in the reparative response (accelerated but lower-quality synthesis of structural macromolecules)

↓

Simultaneous degradation reaction which ultimately exceeds the above reaction (release of lysosomal and cartilaginous enzymes)

↓

Incompetence of the subchondral cartilage-bone system + inflammatory synovial reaction secondary to absorption of cartilaginous particles

↓

Acceleration of the destructive process

Clinical implications

Pain

From a clinical perspective, the various joint tissues mentioned (to which is added the accompanying muscle contracture) are believed to be involved in the genesis of pain, which is a fundamental characteristic of the condition. In effect, capsuloligamentous distension, synovial and soft tissue inflammation, and denudation of surfaces touching bone tissue are believed to be its main causes. Furthermore, there is a known link to hyperaemia, stagnation and bone densification in cases of a clear predominance of pain (osteoid osteoma).

Limited mobility

Limited mobility, another clinical characteristic, is due to fibrosis and capsulosynovial adhesions as well as the bony protuberances for which osteophytes and marginal reactions are responsible. Although normal joint lubrication mechanisms are obviously lost in the joint with osteoarthritis, this factor has a minimal impact on movement restriction compared to those mentioned above. Localised joint stiffness tends to occur when getting up in the morning and after a period of inactivity during the day.

In addition, bone destruction, osteophytes and capsuloligamentous and muscle retractions lead to common deformities (genu varum and genu valgum).

Osteoarthritis pain

Osteoarthritis pain is classically defined as pain of insidious onset occurring when the joint is used and remitting when the joint is at rest which later on, with disease progression, persists even at rest or occurs with small movements. The pain follows the typical "osteoarthritis pattern" being more severe when starting to walk, decreasing with walking and then worsening.

Joint abnormalities

Physical examination shows a swollen joint with no articular effusion, a hard consistency on palpation due to osteocartilaginous proliferation and pain on passive mobilisation. It is normal to detect crepitation and crunching during movement.

Plain X-rays reveal the macroscopic appearances described in cartilage (erosion and ulceration) and bone (subchondral sclerosis, osteophytes and cysts) as well as joint deformities.

It must be emphasised once again that scintigraphy studies are nonspecific in nature and lead to erroneous diagnosis of bone necrosis in incipient forms with somewhat atypical X-ray manifestations of osteoarthritis or joint inflammation due to other causes.

It goes without saying that laboratory studies should be used to rule out other diseases, since osteoarthritis has no systemic repercussions and therefore no typical laboratory findings.

Treatment

Both osteoarthritis and arthritis are multi-joint diseases and that is why this section does not only cite the stifle joint. However, this does not mean that the objective of this text is not to take a holistic approach to the stifle joint.

Medical treatment

The biomechanical and biochemical processes described can carry on cyclically to the point of complete joint destruction, since, as noted, the tissues themselves lack sufficient capacity for repair.

Initial treatment measures are based on improving mechanical conditions (in terms of magnitude and distribution of weight borne) and relieving pain in its different tissue components (inflammation, muscle contracture, joint distension and hyperaemia). As a result, control of weight overload, administration of analgesics and occasionally anti-inflammatory drugs, rest (not immobilisation) in phases of exacerbation, modification of usual function, and owner education help relieve the clinical signs and symptoms of the animal.

Until not long ago treatment was limited to pain relief. Different molecules intended to modify the course of the disease and restore function to the joint have recently been developed.

Box 2 shows the most commonly accepted therapeutic classification for pharmaceutical products to fight against osteoarthritis.

Most of these chondroprotective substances are complex sugars available in oral, intramuscular and intra-articular presentations.

The most common oral presentations contain glucosamine and chondroitin sulphate, in combination or alone. Products for injection include polysulphated glycosaminoglycans, which may be administered intramuscularly or intra-articularly, and pentosan polysulphate, which has an effect similar to that of polysulphated glycosaminoglycans. Pentosan polysulphate in particular has pleiotropic effects on joint tissues and may improve degeneration of joint cartilage by either delaying it or even preventing it, depending on the case and the response of the patient. Therefore it may be a useful supplement in preventing and treating OA.

Finally, hyaluronic acid is an important component of synovial fluid. It is administered intra-articularly and protects the cartilage by lubricating the joint and preventing leukocyte extravasation into the joint.

BOX 2

Therapeutic classification of pharmaceutical products.

Symptomatic fast-acting drugs

- Analgesics.
- NSAIDs.
- Corticosteroids.

Symptomatic slow-acting drugs for osteoarthritis (SYSADOAs)

- Hyaluronic acid.
- Chondroitin sulphate.
- Glucosamine.

Disease-modifying osteoarthritis drugs (DMOADs)

- Hyaluronic acid.
- Chondroitin sulphate.

Surgical treatment

Surgical treatment depends on the extent and pattern of the disease and the symptoms of the patient. Interventions in this regard may be classified as symptomatic, pathophysiological or suppressant. Symptomatic interventions include articular lavage and muscle releases. Pathophysiological interventions include interventions intended to modify abnormal weight-bearing conditions in the joint, perforations of subchondral bone (forage) and stem cell use (which had a promising start that was not supported by results and was gradually abandoned). Suppressant interventions include both excision and replacement arthroplasties as well as arthrodesis.

Changes in the dynamics of joint weight-bearing

The two procedures performed on joints with osteoarthritis to decrease or redistribute weight borne by the joint are muscle releases and osteotomies.

Muscle releases performed by means of cuts in contractured musculature around the joint decrease pain and to some extent increase mobility. However, they also represent an assault on the stability of the joint which could end up being very harmful in a potential joint replacement.

Osteotomies, like muscle releases, decrease pain and increase the articular space. Modification of at least one joint end by a properly guided osteotomy has yielded outcomes with satisfactory medium-term pain relief and an acceptable quality of life for the animal, especially in cases of TPO. The beneficial effect may be due to several factors:

- The mere fact of disrupting bone continuity triggers reparative tissue and vascular changes which may result in vascular normalisation.
- Better alignment of the limb improves capsuloligamentous distension and muscle contracture. Most importantly, it balances loads as it improves articular congruity by modifying the orientation of the articular surfaces, thereby reducing the biomechanical component of the osteoarthritis cycle.
- Finally, better apposition of articular surfaces covered in cartilage reduces friction between denuded bone surfaces. Although it has been suggested by some observations, the potential for actual recovery of the joint interline by means of fibrocartilaginous regeneration is doubtful. Images of perceptible widening in postoperative examinations are probably due to the new location of the cartilage fragments following the change in position occasioned by a realignment osteotomy.

Ultimately, osteotomy with good preoperative planning and good technique seems to be a very effective alternative in select patients, especially in young and active animals.

Arthroplasty

When osteoarthritis has reached a very advanced phase, if debilitating pain does not respond to conservative treatment and local conditions preclude the potential for a realignment osteotomy, the only option consists of nullifying the joint. This may be achieved by means of an arthrodesis, excision (resection) arthroplasty or replacement (prosthetic) arthroplasty.

- **Arthrodesis:** fixation in a functional position (specific to each joint) by means of fusion following excision of the articular surfaces of both bone ends. While it definitively eliminates pain, it still causes disability. This disability is substantial in the stifle joint and elbow; more acceptable in the hip, wrist and hock; and imperceptible in the short vertebral segments (instability and wobbler syndrome). In any case, it represents a high long-term risk due to overload of adjacent joints (Figs. 4-11).
- **Excision arthroplasty:** technique in which the joint ends are resected with or without soft tissue interposition, as in a hip arthroplasty. The disappearance of pain, once the tissues in which it originates have been removed, is accompanied by shortening, instability and loss of force.
- **Replacement arthroplasty:** technique in which the joint is removed by resecting the two articular surfaces and reconstructed by replacing them with metal-alloy, polymer or ceramic prosthetics. The use of this type of arthroplasty (which is total as it includes all surfaces) eliminates pain, maintains mobility and stability, and corrects alignment defects.

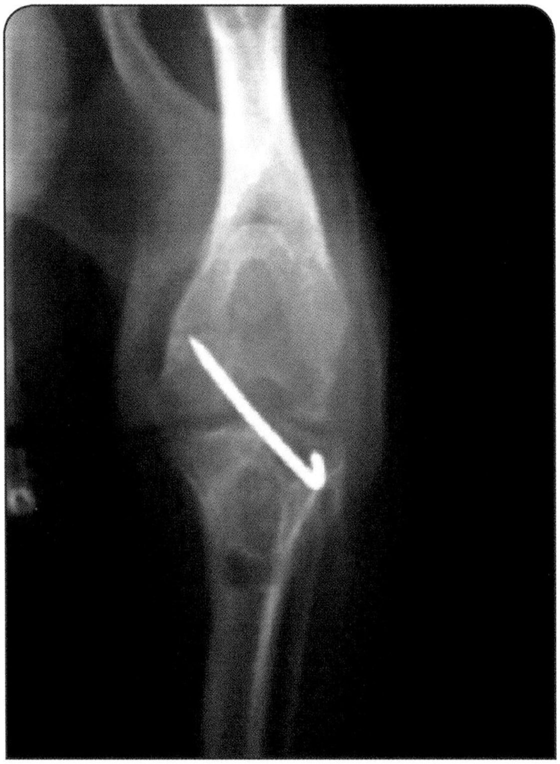

FIGURE 4. Surgical malpractice which causes not only defective surgical resolution but also iatrogenic joint disease.

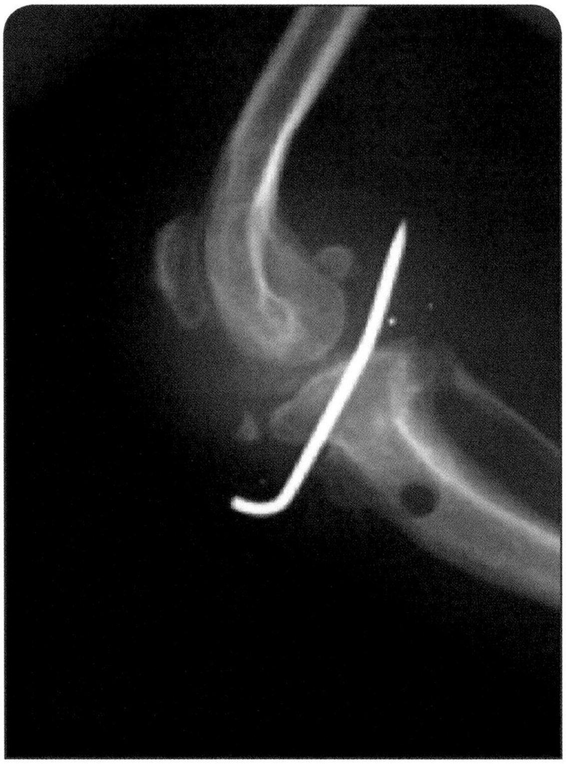

FIGURE 5. Laterolateral view of the previous case.

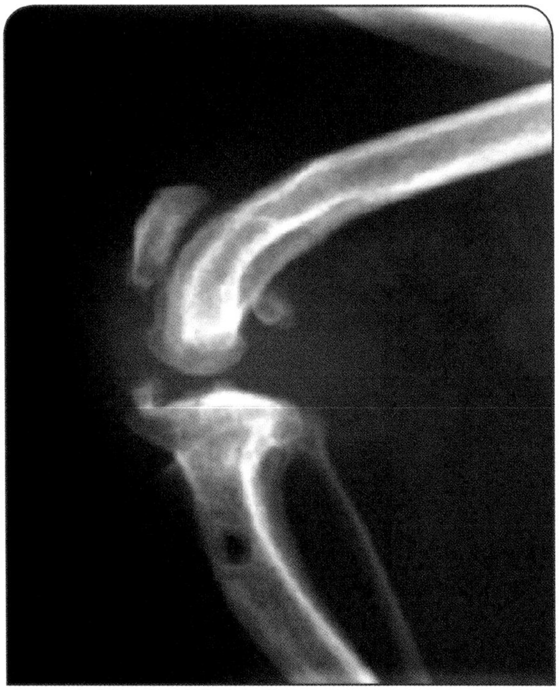

FIGURE 6. Image eight weeks after the implant from the previous figures has been removed and an arthrotomy with articular lavage, combined with an adjuvant medical treatment, has been performed.

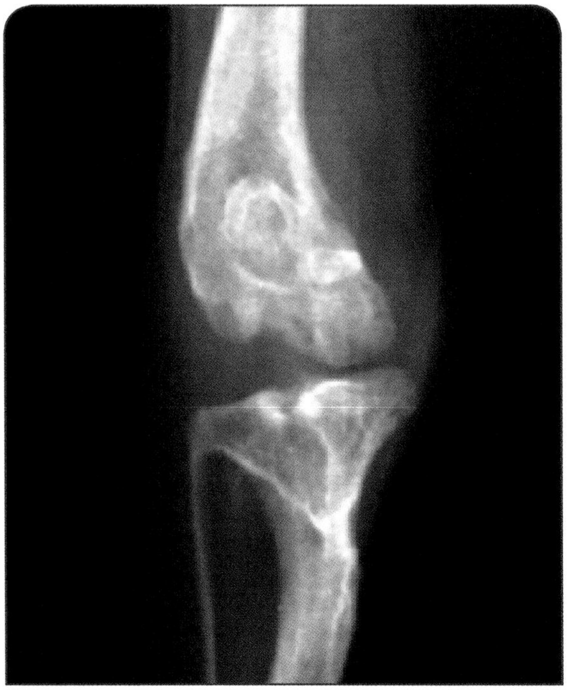

FIGURE 7. Craniocaudal view of the previous case. The patient is a candidate for arthrodesis.

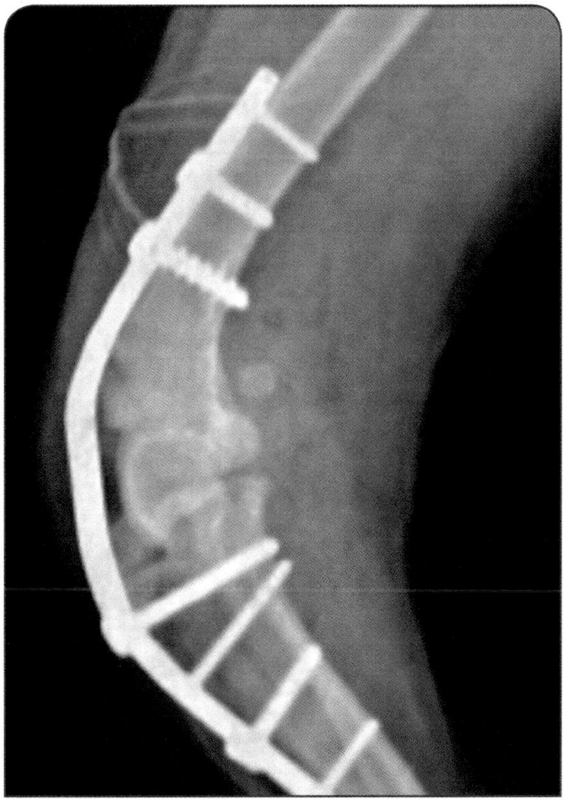

FIGURE 8. Postoperative arthrodesis.

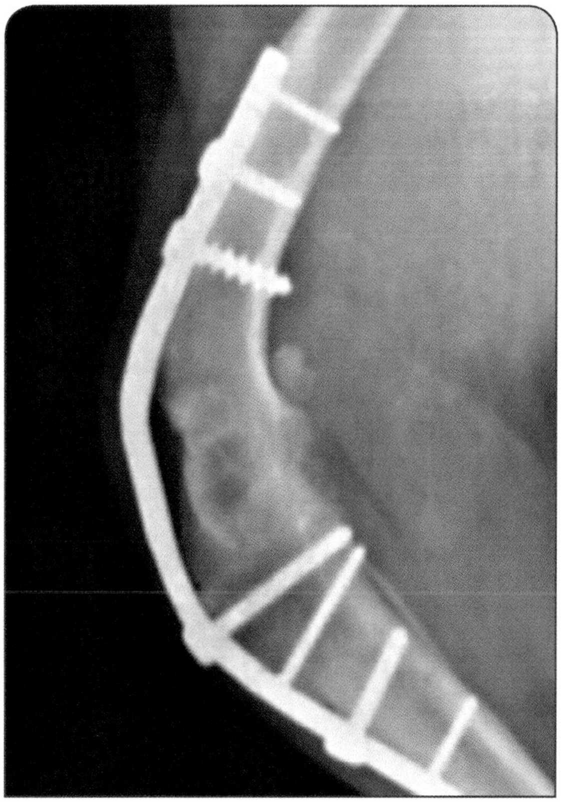

FIGURE 9. Case from the previous figure after 12 weeks.

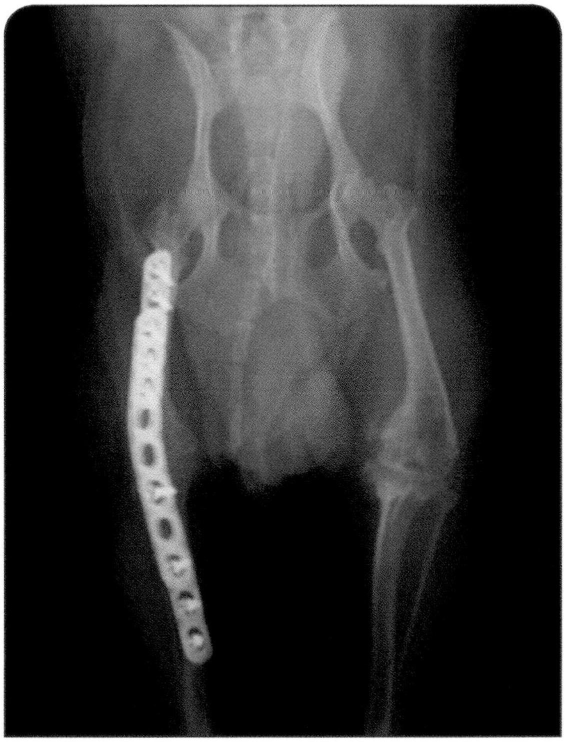

FIGURE 10. Craniocaudal view of arthrodesis with a double cuttable plate.

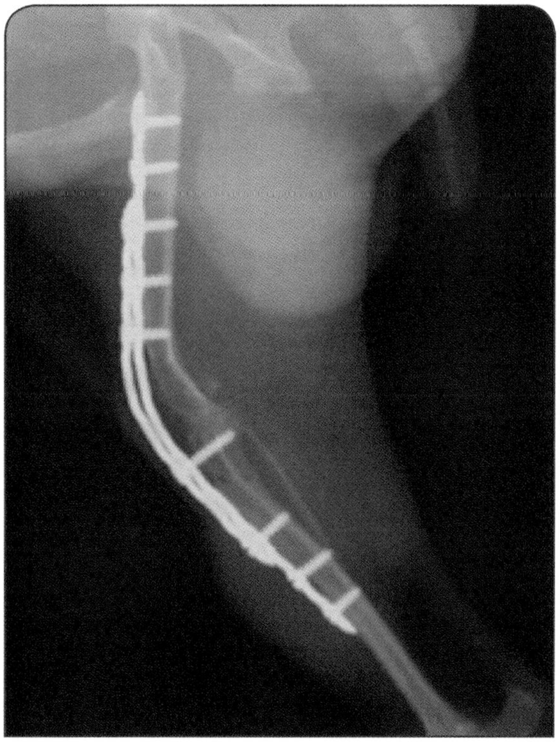

FIGURE 11. Lateral view of the previous case after 12 weeks.

Conclusions and recommendations on arthritis/osteoarthritis

Isolated aseptic arthritis is rare in small animals; polyarthritis is more common. Septic arthritis is even more common. It is caused by injecting corticosteroids, hyaluronic acid and so on without taking the necessary aseptic precautions.

In any case, subchondral and osteophytic reactions may be found to occur in bone remodelling in osteoarthritis.

Thus osteoarthritis may be considered to be a final collective phase of a heterogeneous series of aetiopathological conditions that affect joint tissues. These aetiological conditions are multifactorial and include biochemical, enzyme, genetic and biomechanical factors.

The characteristic pathology results include narrowing of the articular space, peripheral osteophytes, subchondral bone sclerosis and formation of cysts.

Although it is commonly considered to be a disease that mainly affects cartilage, some studies have proposed variable repercussions for synovial fluid, muscle, ligaments and bone. It has been suggested that changes in subchondral bone play a significant role as an aetiological factor in the early development of degenerative joint disease.

In cases of arthritis, the authors generally perform an arthrotomy with joint lavage and then put on an immobilising cast. Anti-inflammatory and nutraceutical medication can also be used as adjuvant treatment.

In chronic degenerative cases, a combination of drugs based on NSAIDs and chondroprotective agents is initially administered, and surgery is performed in the stages in which the patient experiences claudication depending on the requirements of the case and the characteristics of the owners.

This surgical treatment has a variable functional prognosis. Depending on both the joint and the surgical treatment used, it may be acceptable, poor or unknown. In the hip a replacement arthrotomy or, failing this, an excision arthrotomy is performed.

Physiotherapeutic exercises carefully performed by veterinary surgeons trained in musculoskeletal physiotherapy may be useful. These exercises are intended to strengthen the periarticular soft tissues, fight against muscle contracture and decrease mechanical overloads that pass through the articular surface.

Novel surgical techniques such as sliding humeral osteotomy (SHO) have been propounded for the elbow. The authors propose studying their effects on other joints to resolve diseases such as osteochondritis of the stifle joint or humerus to reduce the mechanical load on the damaged part of the joint by diverting the biomechanical axis of the affected limb to a location that is more comfortable for the animal.

CHAPTER

11

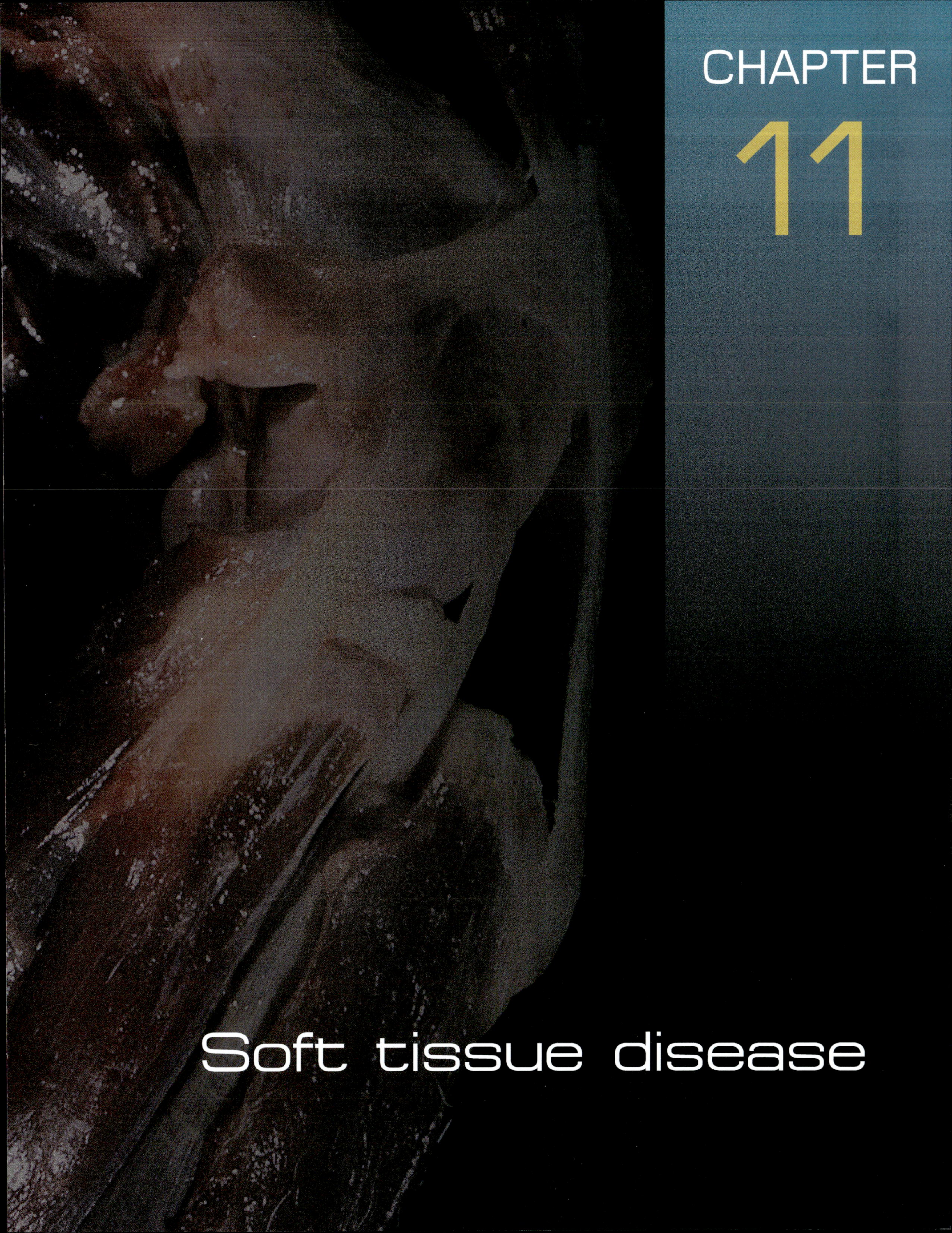

Soft tissue disease

Introduction

This chapter presents the most important painful conditions of the stifle joint. Some of the injuries described here have already been discussed, but the authors believe that it is very educational to include all of them in a single "soft tissue" summary to which the reader may refer when no other injuries are present or to make a differential diagnosis.

The chapter starts by analysing the differential diagnosis of the painful and inflamed stifle joint (see the next page). This description encompasses all processes that may affect the stifle joint and not just the soft tissues, as well as the steps involved in the diagnostic approach in general.

An algorithm of the diagnostic and therapeutic plan for chronic swelling of the stifle joint can be seen in Chapter 2 (page 33).

Intra-articular diseases

Injury in the synovial folds or plicae

There are three synovial folds in the patellar joint: suprapatellar, mediopatellar and infrapatellar. According to some authors, mechanical irritation of these folds due to pinching causes painful signs and symptoms which may be mistaken for meniscal injuries or femoropatellar disease. However, efforts to attribute pain behind the patella to a fold must only be made once other more common causes have been ruled out.

Bursitis and pain in the infrapatellar fat pad

There are three types of prepatellar bursae: subcutaneous, subfascial and subtendinous. There is also the distal infrapatellar bursa, between the patellar ligament and the tibia. The subcutaneous type is most problematic as it is a common site of chronic inflammation accompanied by bursitis in animals which experience pressure and friction in their stifle joints. This tends to occur in dogs subjected to agility tests and large dogs that live on cement or similar surfaces and experience continuous microtrauma which ends up causing this disease. It is also common in the elbow.

In the stifle joint, the distal infrapatellar bursa, located between the caudal aspect of the patellar ligament and the proximal tibial epiphysis, together with the nearby infrapatellar fat pad, may be the origin of insidious chronic local pain which may cause sudden changes in the temperament of the animal.

Reflex sympathetic dystrophy

The stifle joint is one of the most common sites of this disease. It may result from trauma or surgical procedures, especially patellofemoral surgical procedures. From a clinical perspective, it manifests much as it does in other sites, with signs of pain, reddening and oedema followed by stiffness and atrophy.

To date it has rarely been identified in animals. Since physiotherapy in animals has come into play it has facilitated the diagnosis of these and other diseases hitherto unknown to veterinary clinicians.

The most effective therapeutic measure is lumbar sympathectomy. This requires equipment that determines evoked potentials and proven experience (available in university hospitals) and can be combined with physiotherapy, drugs and transcutaneous electrical nerve stimulation (TENS).

Syndrome of joint pain and inflammation

The clinical presentation of all conditions to be described is similar, and is characterised by pain and inflammation. Sometimes the characteristics and location of the syndrome enable a diagnosis to be made and confirmed with complementary methods (usually plain X-ray). However, in many cases the pain is widespread or poorly localised. This requires the clinician to systematically examine the animal as explained below. It must be borne in mind that most considerations in this section also apply to examination of other joints.

Presentation in one or more joints

In isolated impairment of the stifle joint the presumptive diagnoses are as follows:

- Traumatic injury of menisci, ligaments or articular surfaces.
- Infection.
- Osteonecrosis.
- Joint disease.

Obviously, some of these diseases sometimes concomitantly affect other joints just as some diseases that characteristically affect multiple joints initially only appear in one joint.

Clinical course

The clinical course also aids in identifying the underlying disease: signs and symptoms of sudden onset suggest a mechanical or infectious aetiology, and episodic or recurrent signs and symptoms suggest a degenerative injury, a joint disease or chronic meniscal or ligament injuries.

Many of these clinical signs and symptoms are characteristic of certain ages. For example, osteochondritis dissecans and injuries of the infrapatellar fat pad are typical in young animals, injuries of the menisci and ligaments are typical in young adult animals and osteoarthritis is typical in elderly patients.

Certain diseases are more common in one sex or the other; thus, osteochondritis dissecans is more common in males, while arthritis secondary to SLE and osteonecrosis predominantly occur in females.

Accompanying clinical manifestations

Other symptoms associated with pain and inflammation also have significant diagnostic value. For example, fever is typical of infectious arthritis and SLE, and certain skin injuries also suggest SLE. In addition, gastrointestinal and urological signs and symptoms are associated with some of these diseases (e.g. stomatitis with SLE).

Complementary diagnostic methods

Imaging techniques (especially plain X-ray) often provide decisive data. In articular effusion, studying fluid extracted by puncture also informs diagnosis. Finally, certain laboratory tests support the clinical diagnosis in diseases such as SLE (antinuclear antibodies) and spondyloarthropathies. A synovial biopsy rarely has diagnostic value, while biopsies of other tissues (skin, muscle, nerve, etc.) may have a great deal of clinical value to diagnose myositis, etc.

Musculotendinous diseases

Many of these diseases have already been discussed in other chapters and are summarised here in this section specific to soft tissue injuries in the stifle joint.

Rupture of the tendon of the quadriceps femoris muscle

This is uncommon. It tends to occur in young animals as a result of traumatic wounds, accidents, falls, etc. It also occurs as a result of sudden muscle contraction in old animals with degenerative tendon abnormalities, sometimes in relation to repeated injections of corticosteroids for osteoarthritis and in animals with concomitant systemic diseases such as diabetes, chronic kidney failure and hyperthyroidism. On the rare occasions when it occurs due to this type of degenerative injury, the distal end of the tendon of the quadriceps femoris often brings with it a piece of bone from the proximal end of the patella.

In partial rupture, the problem often goes unnoticed and undiagnosed. In complete rupture, with injury of the four tendon layers and the synovial membrane of the retropatellar bursa, a fissure is detected between the muscle and the proximal end of the patella, with pain at this level and inability to actively fully extend the joint. This is seen after different tests (such as the direct extensor reflex and the cruciate extensor reflex) have been performed on these patients and have yielded no results, due not to a neurological injury, but to a lack of mechanical capacity. Furthermore, all this must occur in the absence of haemarthrosis, since its presence reveals a traumatic rather than degenerative aetiology. Obviously, these case reports require good communication between the veterinary internist and the orthopaedic surgeon.

Partial rupture can be treated by immobilisation in extension for at least four to six weeks (the older the animal, the longer the time of immobilisation) (Fig. 1). This must be done using a Robert Jones bandage, which allows weight-bearing by providing pressure, since a bandage in flexion on an adult animal for so many weeks will lead to loss of muscle mass as well as loss of function, which amounts to the same thing.

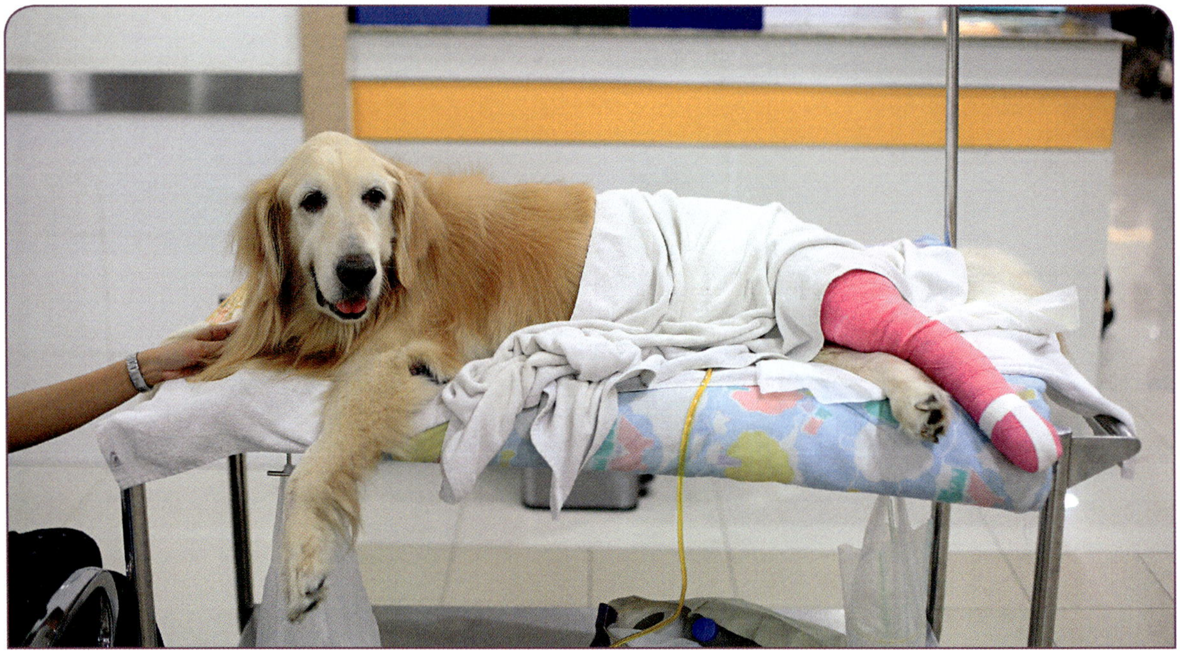

FIGURE 1. Bandage on the hind limb in extension (Blanscape, Shutterstock.com).

Complete rupture requires surgical repair by means of direct suture and reinforcement thereof with a flap from the aponeurosis of the quadriceps, as well as a Type II transarticular external fixator for three weeks. Adding stem cells to this specific type of surgery initially showed extraordinary results; however, expectations in this regard have decreased over the years. This exciting topic is explored no further in this textbook which humbly aspires to serve as a practical guide for clinical veterinary surgeons.

Contracture of the quadriceps femoris muscle

This disease with an unfavourable prognosis has two different types of causes: iatrogenic and traumatic. Iatrogenic disease in turn has two different types of causes: malpractice and calcium injection treatments in the first few months of life. Paradoxically, most clinicians are unaware of this, and ever since compound feeds were developed and calcium injection treatments in young animals lapsed into disuse, iatrogenic disease has been uncommon in the western world. This may not be true elsewhere. In any case, the problem tends to appear in the first 18 months of the life of the animal due to repeated administration of intramuscular injections.

In traumatic disease, damage may be accidental; however, unfortunately, no less often it is iatrogenic due to inexpert surgery. In the latter case the surgeon exclusively focuses on repairing the bone and is not concerned with "pampering" the muscle that enables caudal extension of the limb. Significant contracture with joint stiffness tends to occur and also tends to be accompanied by regular or permanent chronic dislocation of the patella cranially and proximally by the action of the contracture. The joint stiffness is correlated to fibrosis of the vastus intermedius muscle and the chronic dislocation is correlated to fibrosis of the vastus lateralis muscle. In both cases treatment is surgical and consists of correcting the shortening of the part of the quadriceps muscle involved by means of lengthening, disinsertion and tenotomy procedures. Capsular plication or movement of the patellar ligament must be performed if dislocation of the patella is seen.

Contracture is commonly observed in very advanced ages and is associated with complex fractures of the middle and distal third of the femur. It results from the development of fibrosis and adhesions between the deep aspect of the muscle and the subtendinous bursa and the tendons of insertion of the quadriceps femoris muscle in the area distal to the focal point of the fracture. It limits sliding and leads to stiffness in extension. Treatment is surgical and consists of disinserting the muscle subperiosteally, from the distal portion to the proximal portion, until 90° of flexion are obtained. Continuous passive mobilisation must be used during the postoperative period to prevent recurrences. The prognosis has improved somewhat since physiotherapy has come into play as a veterinary specialisation. Realistically, however, in the authors' opinion it remains poor in a very high percentage of cases.

Rupture and injury of the patellar ligament

Injuries of the patellar ligament are uncommon. Ruptures tend to actually be avulsions of the proximal or distal insertion of the ligament into bone. Those that occur in the thickness of the tendon appear almost exclusively in athletes with a history of local inflammation with corticosteroids.

Complete rupture leads to proximal patellar displacement and inability to actively fully extend the stifle joint. Such a case requires surgical treatment, which consists of fixing the detached bone fragment or suturing the thickness of the tendon by reinforcing it with fascia lata or another structure. Usually these techniques are complemented with a wire handle crossed on the cranial aspect of the patella, which reduces local tension and facilitates healing.

Patellar tendinitis

The unique biomechanical features of the extensors of the stifle joint account for injuries as a result of repeated microtrauma. These are diagnosed with increasing frequency and their nature varies depending on the age of the animal: patellar tendinitis develops in adults, while true traction apophysitis develops in young animals.

Patellar tendinitis in adults is called "jumper's knee" due to the frequency with which this condition develops in animals that jump regularly. It is common in German Shepherds and other dogs that compete in agility events (Fig. 2). Usually it responds well to rest, modification of activity and sometimes local injections. Empirical surgery is performed on an exceptional basis. It involves splitting, a technique based on surgical incisions in the tendon.

Osgood-Schlatter disease

Osgood-Schlatter disease is the most characteristic form of apophysitis in young animals. It generally develops when an animal is two years old and results from negative effects exerted by the extensors on the cranial part of the growth plate of the tibial tuberosity. It is characterised by pain that occurs in the area mentioned during and after activity, remits with rest and is sometimes accompanied by swelling and irregularities in ossification and radiotransparent areas, which are seen on X-ray of the stifle joint in lateral projection. Rest for several weeks and immobilisation with a Robert Jones bandage in extreme cases solve the problem.

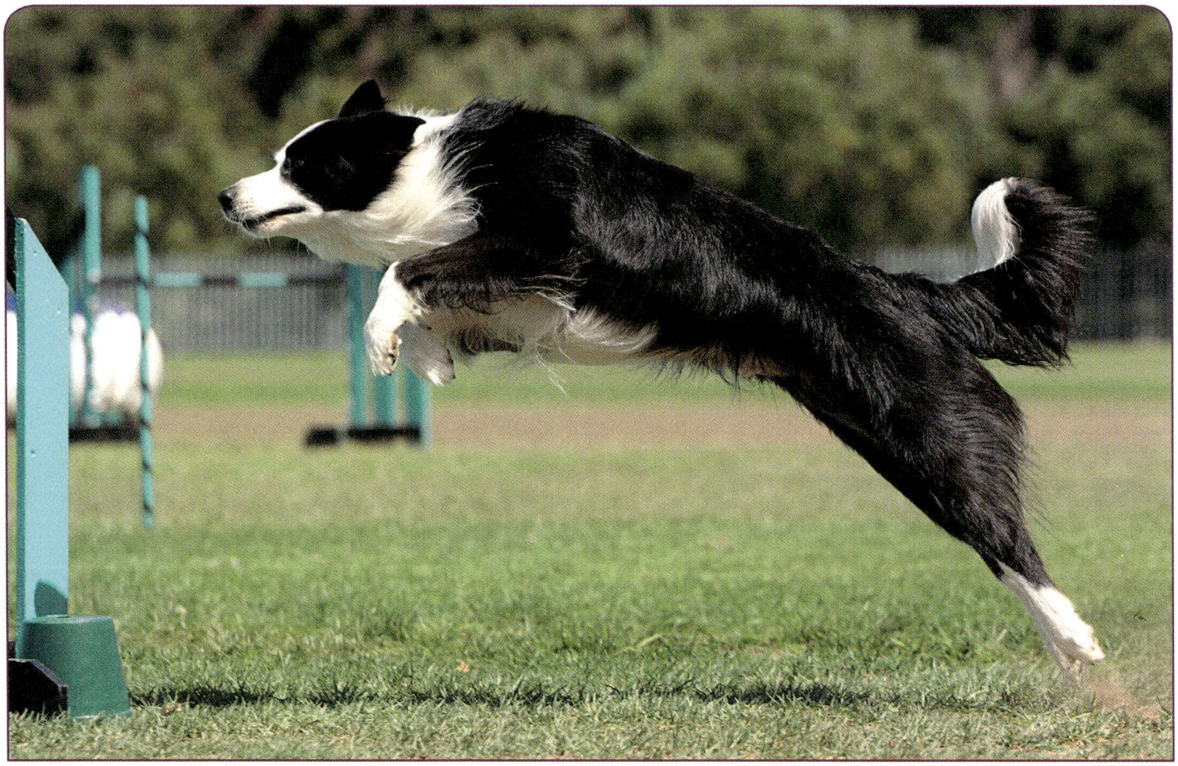

FIGURE 2. Border Collie in an agility competition (Mackland, Shutterstock.com).

Periarticular injuries

As occurs in painful femoropatellar conditions, periarticular injuries that cause pain are often related to mechanical overloads. Pain in the cranial, caudal, medial or lateral aspects of the stifle joint suggests a certain disease.

Cranial aspect

Patellar bursitis

This is mentioned above. It tends to respond to treatment with a Robert Jones compression bandage, rest and NSAIDs. Puncture is recommended if the bursa is very enlarged or an infectious aetiology is suspected. Surgical excision of the bursa may be indicated in the event of multiple recurrences.

Caudal aspect

Semimembranosus bursitis

The subtendinous synovial bursa of the semimembranosus muscle may become inflamed and cause pain on the caudal aspect of the proximal area of the tibia, close to the joint interline. If the pain does not remit with NSAIDs, rest and physiotherapy, injections with a local anaesthetic and corticosteroids may be indicated.

Popliteal cyst

In young animals, a popliteal cyst appears as a painless swelling on the medial side of the popliteal fossa, close to the tendons of the pes anserinus. It is filled with a mucinous substance and, in half of cases, connected to the joint. Its cause is unknown, and very often it spontaneously resolves after a few years. Therefore, except on very rare occasions, it requires no treatment in addition to observation.

In adults it presents as an obvious swelling on the popliteal fossa, close to the tendons of the pes anserinus. If there is any doubt puncture can be performed to demonstrate the presence of fluid. This injury should be considered to be symptomatic, that is to say, secondary to some intra-articular disease (meniscal injury, osteoarthritis or a type of chronic synovitis such as rheumatoid arthritis). If an adult animal has a popliteal cyst it is essential to identify and treat the disease responsible for it, since merely removing the cyst does not solve the underlying problem. Sometimes, especially in animals with arthritis due to SLE, the cyst spontaneously ruptures and clinical signs and symptoms of swelling and distal oedema occur. These signs and symptoms remit with treatment with a Robert Jones bandage, rest, local heat and administration of NSAIDs.

Fabella syndrome

The sesamoid bone located in the proximal tendon portion of the lateral gastrocnemius muscle (fabella) may cause pain on the caudolateral aspect of the stifle joint in animals whose growth plates are closing or as a result of extracapsular ACL surgeries (Olmstead's technique). The pain is aggravated by extension of the stifle joint. If the signs and symptoms do not remit with rest and NSAIDs, injections of anaesthetic and corticosteroids are administered; if discomfort persists after six to eight weeks have elapsed, the fabella may be removed.

Medial aspect

Pes anserine bursitis

The most common cause of pain on the medial aspect of the stifle joint is inflammation of the serous bursa of the pes anserinus. This anatomical structure consists of the tendons of the sartorius (caudal portion), gracilis and semitendinosus muscles at their insertion into the medial aspect of the proximal end of the tibia. The pes anserinus is fundamentally important in TPLO surgery.

These signs and symptoms often occur in athletic dogs (racing dogs) but are also seen in animals with osteoarthritis. Pes anserine bursitis requires a differential diagnosis with meniscal injuries, osteonecrosis and stress fractures. It tends to respond to treatment with rest, local heat and NSAIDs. Injections of local anaesthetic and corticosteroids are sometimes needed.

Medial collateral ligament bursitis

This is caused by inflammation of a subligamentous synovial bursa located deep to the medial collateral ligament. This causes pain in the medial region of the stifle joint accompanied by swelling around this ligament. The pain increases with hyperextension, valgus and external rotation and tends to respond to conservative treatment.

Saphenous nerve entrapment

This sensitive nerve may become entrapped at its exit from the adductor canal. Pain and paraesthesia insidiously occur on the medial aspect of the stifle joint. The pain tends to be aggravated by activity and persists at rest. In examination, there is pain on palpation over the adductor canal. If conservative treatment with rest, NSAIDs, local cold and ultrasounds fails, nerve blocks with local anaesthetic may be performed. In rare cases surgical release of the nerve is required.

Lateral aspect

Popliteus tendinitis

Sporting activities (for example in Greyhounds) may also cause tenosynovitis of the tendon of origin of the popliteal muscle, which starts on the lateral epicondyle of the femur and passes through the popliteal hiatus on the caudolateral aspect of the lateral meniscus (deep to the lateral collateral ligament). Thus there is pain with lameness of insidious onset after the animal has been exercising for a while. As opposed to a cranial condition, the animal usually cannot continue the activity. The pain is more severe in flexion and during the initial phase of stepping. It is reproduced by pressing on the tendon immediately in front of the lateral collateral ligament and above the joint interline with the stifle joint flexed. Popliteus tendinitis responds to conservative treatment, including modifications of physical activity.

Proximal tibiofibular joint dislocation

Forced torsion of the leg with the stifle joint in flexion can cause subluxation or even dislocation of this joint. The injury is more common in animals with ligament hyperlaxity and often goes unnoticed as a cause of persistent pain. Manual mobilisation of the upper end of the fibula reproduces the pain, and X-rays taken for comparison to the opposite side reveal that the head of the fibula is abnormally positioned relative to the fibular articular aspect of the tibia. Usually the dislocation is manually reduced under muscle relaxation. It is a common injury following repair of ACL rupture with the technique of fibular head transposition.

Biceps femoris tendinitis

This tendon is also a common site of inflammation due to overload on animals subjected to strenuous exercise. Symptoms usually remit with conservative treatment.

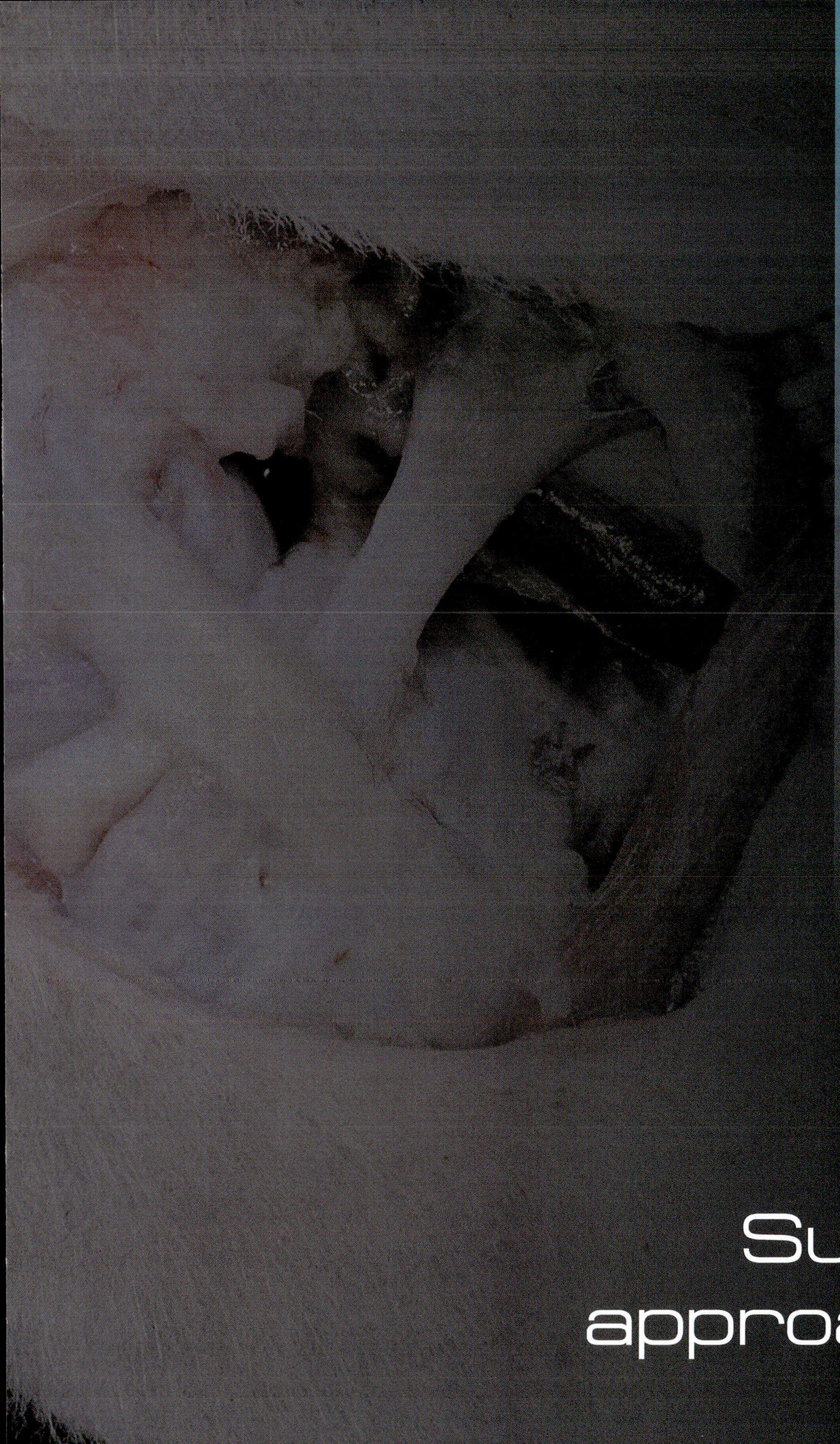

ANNEX

Surgical approaches

Approach to the distal portion of the femur and stifle joint through a lateral incision

Indications

- Diagnostic arthrotomy of the stifle joint.
- Open reduction and fixation of condylar, supracondylar and intercondylar fractures.
- Medial and lateral dislocations of the patella.
- Repair of rupture of the cranial cruciate ligament.
- Examination and partial resection of the lateral meniscus.

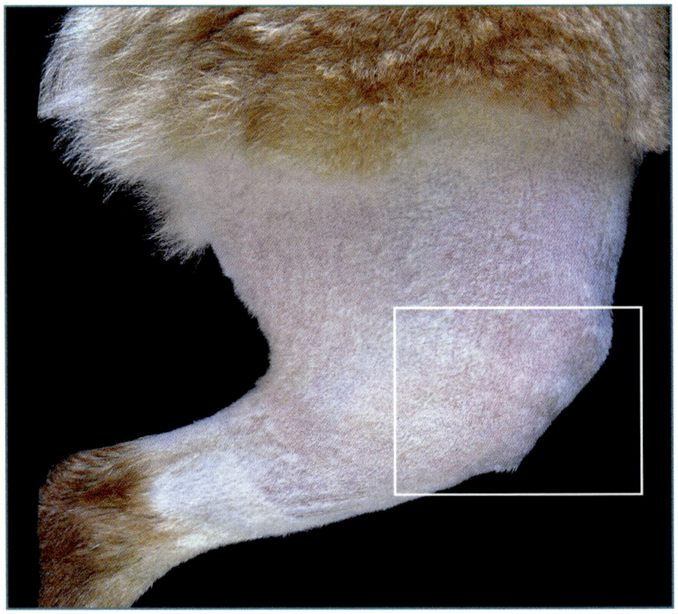

1 The approach starts with an incision from the tibial tuberosity to the patella, projected to the distal third of the femur. This arc-shaped skin incision extends from the distal third of the femur to the proximal third of the leg and passes over the lateral epicondyle of the femur.

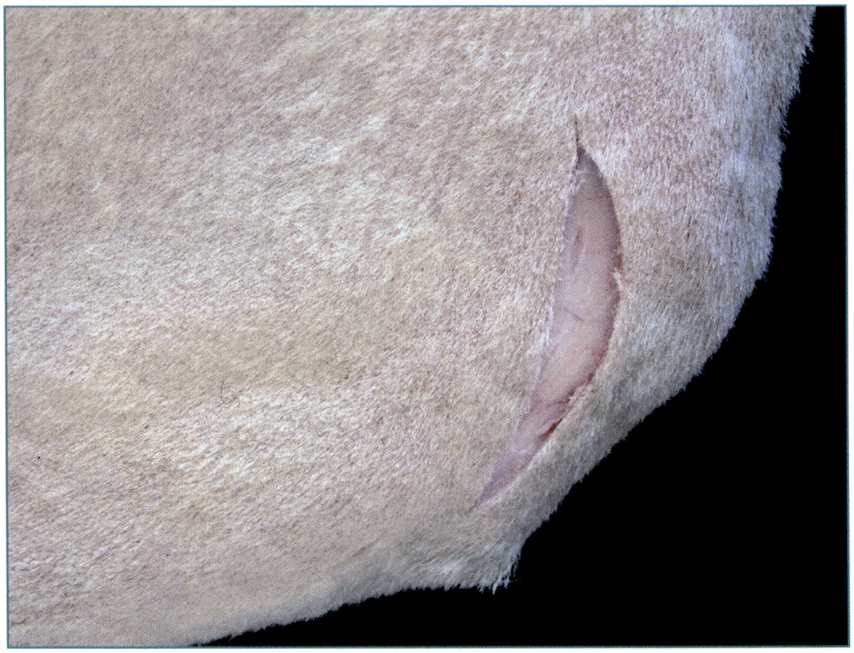

2 Once the edges of the skin incision have been retracted the fascia lata muscle and the fascia of the stifle joint are identified. An incision is made cranial to the biceps femoris muscle. Distally the fascia of the stifle joint is cut parallel to the patella and patellar ligament.

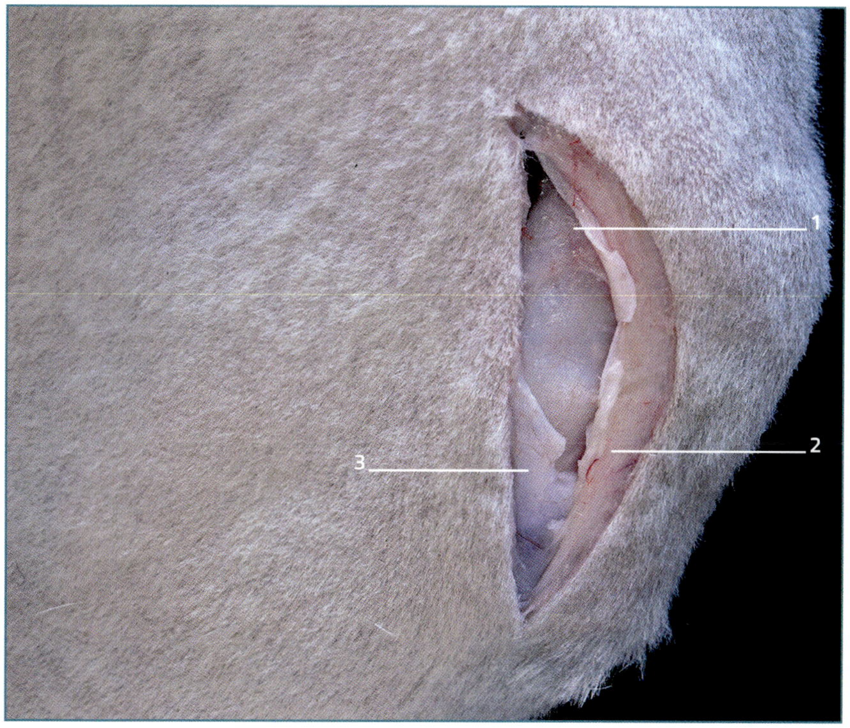

1 Fascia lata
2 Fascia of the stifle joint
3 Biceps femoris m.

3 The section between the insertions of the biceps femoris muscle and the quadriceps femoris muscle allows the stifle joint capsule to be identified and sectioned parallel to the patellar ligament.

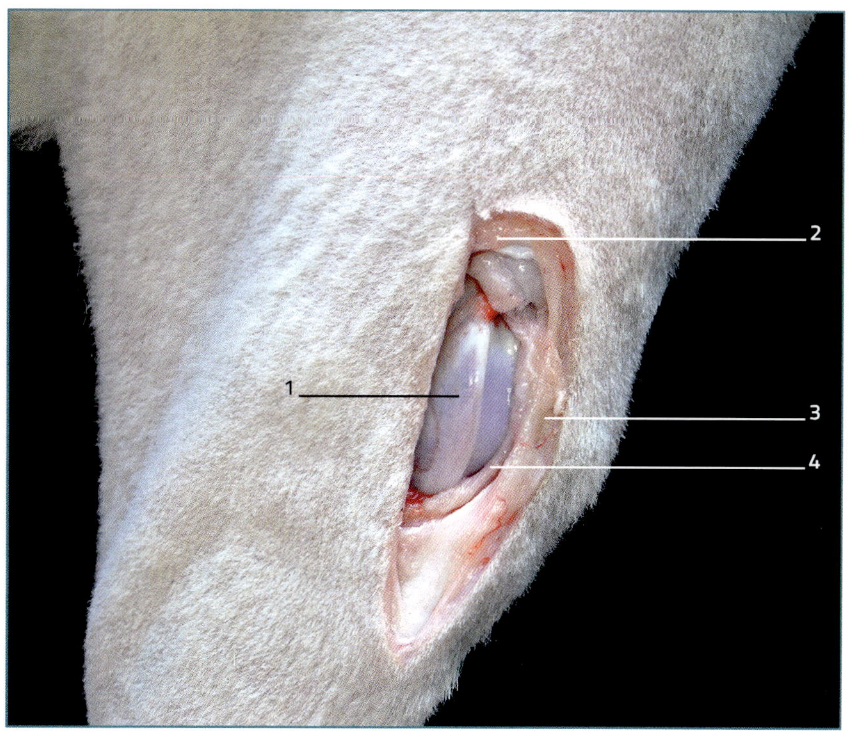

1 Trochlea of the femur
2 Tendon of the quadriceps femoris m.
3 Fascia lata
4 Patellar ligament

4 Once the stifle joint capsule has been sectioned and the tendon of the quadriceps femoris muscle has been forcibly moved towards the medial area, the patella is dislocated and thus the inside of the joint is exposed. The tendon of origin of the long digital extensor muscle and the infrapatellar fat pad which partially covers the cruciate ligaments are seen in the distal area of the joint.

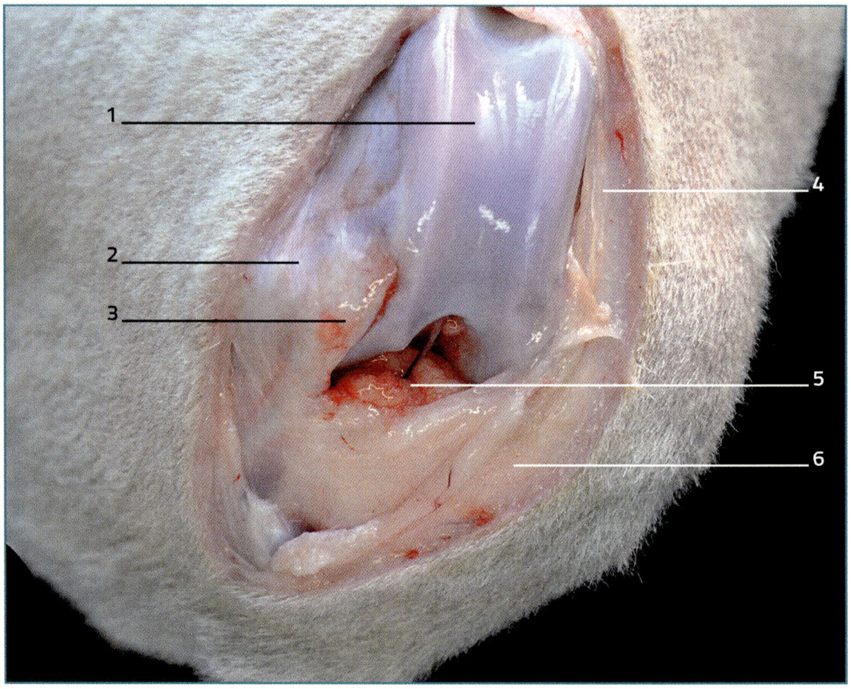

1 Trochlea of the femur
2 Condyle of the femur
3 Tendon of the long digital extensor m.
4 Joint capsule
5 Infrapatellar fat pad
6 Patellar ligament

5 After the infrapatellar fat pad has been forcibly retracted, the cranial cruciate ligament and the lateral meniscus can be identified.

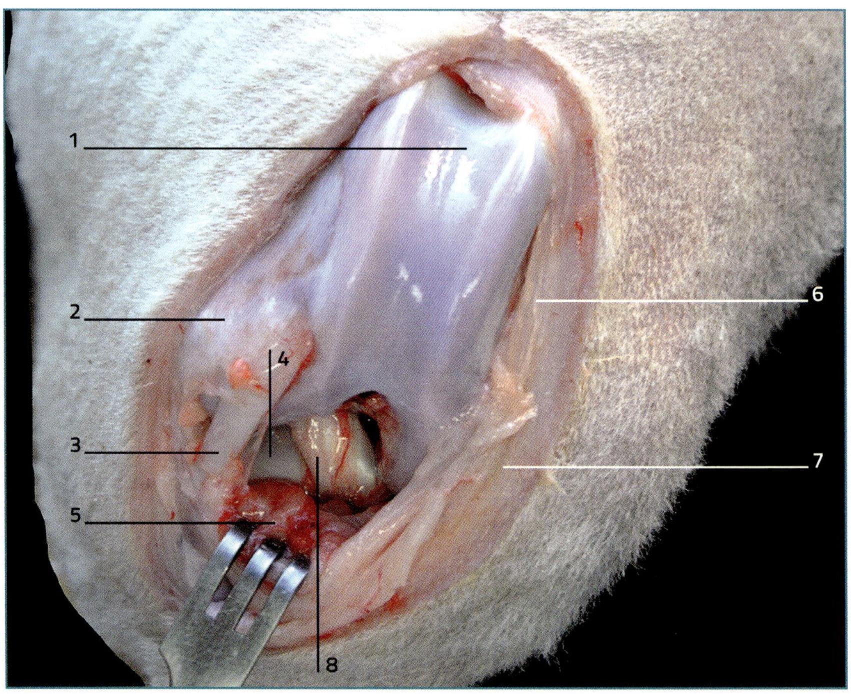

1 Trochlea of the femur
2 Condyle of the femur
3 Tendon of the long digital extensor m.
4 Lateral meniscus
5 Infrapatellar fat pad
6 Joint capsule
7 Patellar ligament
8 Cranial cruciate ligament

Approach to the medial collateral ligament and caudomedial region of the stifle joint

Indications

- Diagnostic arthrotomy.
- Repair of rupture of the medial collateral ligament.
- TPLO technique to treat rupture of the cranial cruciate ligament.
- TTA technique to treat rupture of the cranial cruciate ligament.
- Examination and partial resection of the medial meniscus.
- Open reduction and fixation of fracture of the medial condyle of the femur.
- Detachment of the medial head of the gastrocnemius muscle.

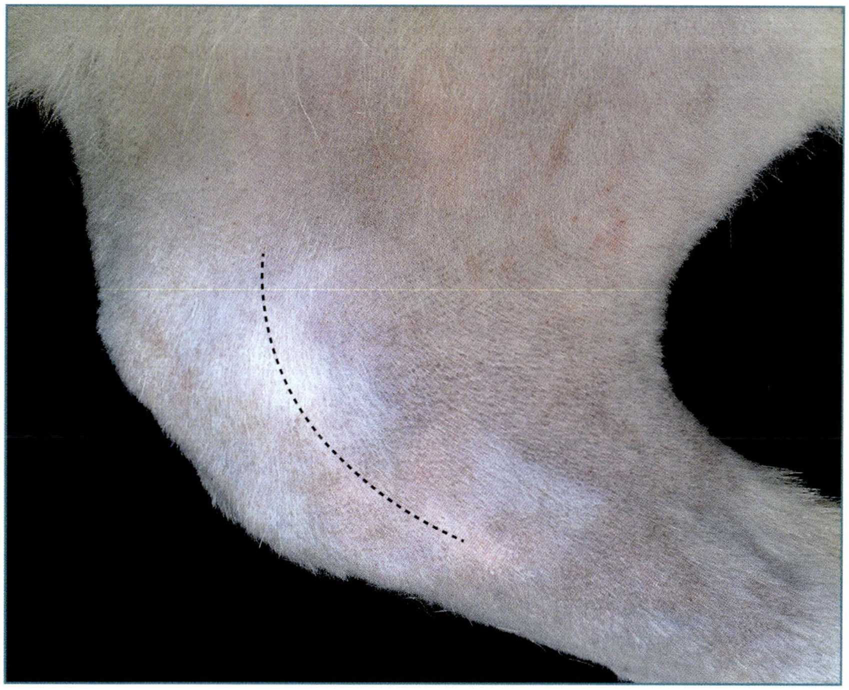

1 The required placement is in lateral decubitus with the contralateral limb in abduction. The skin incision is made over the medial epicondyle of the femur and extended proximally and distally.

2 Following separation of the skin edges in the cut area, the fascia of the stifle joint and the insertion of the caudal portion of the sartorius muscle are identified.

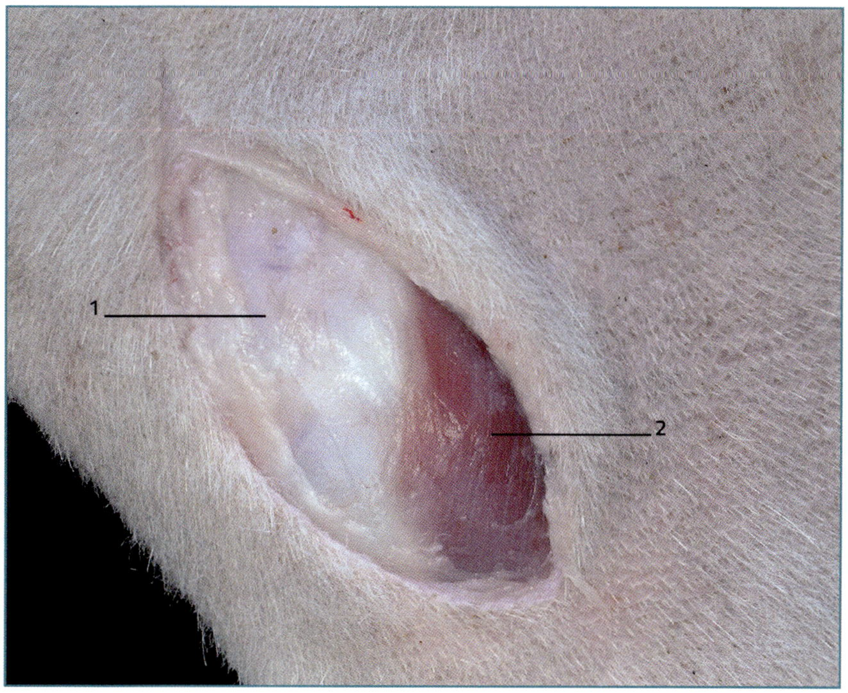

1 Fascia of the stifle joint
2 Sartorius m. (caudal portion)

3 Once part of the medial fascia of the stifle joint has been cut and retracted, the insertion of the caudal portion of the semimembranosus muscle and the medial collateral ligament of the stifle joint are identified.

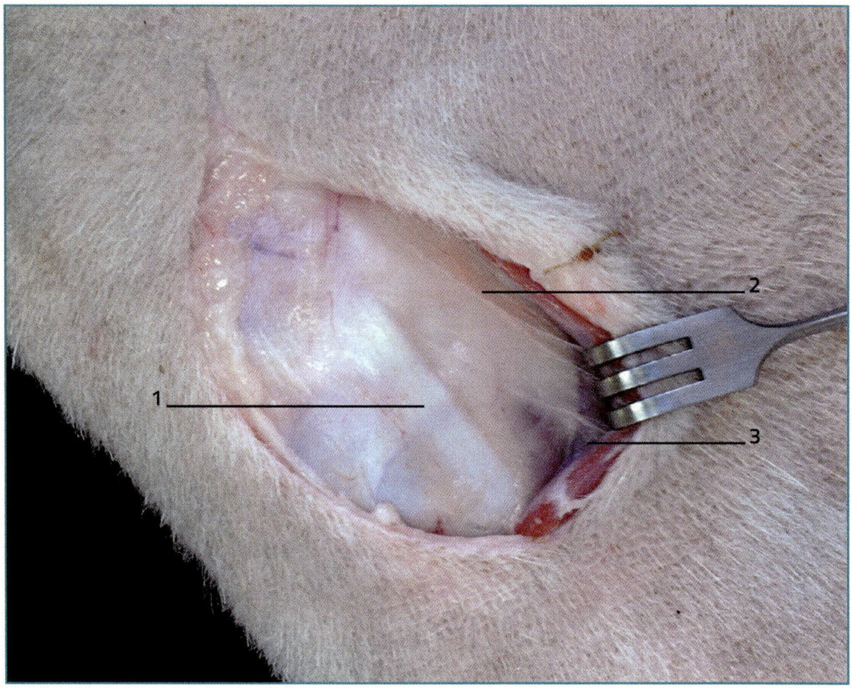

1 Medial collateral ligament
2 Semimembranosus m. (caudal portion)
3 Sartorius m. (caudal portion)

4 Caudal movement of the caudal portion of the sartorius muscle enables identification of the insertion of the two portions of the semimembranosus muscle.

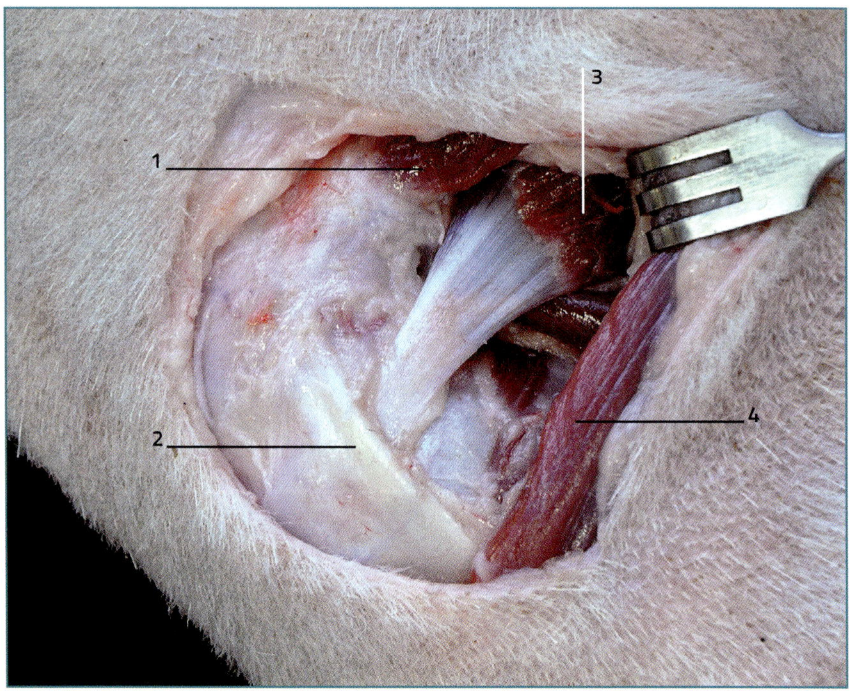

1 Semimembranosus m. (cranial portion)
2 Medial collateral ligament
3 Semimembranosus m. (caudal portion)
4 Sartorius m. (caudal portion)

5 Widening of the space delimited by the cranial and caudal portions of the semimembranosus muscle exposes the joint capsule in relation to the medial condyle of the femur, which is easy to identify once the joint capsule has been sectioned.

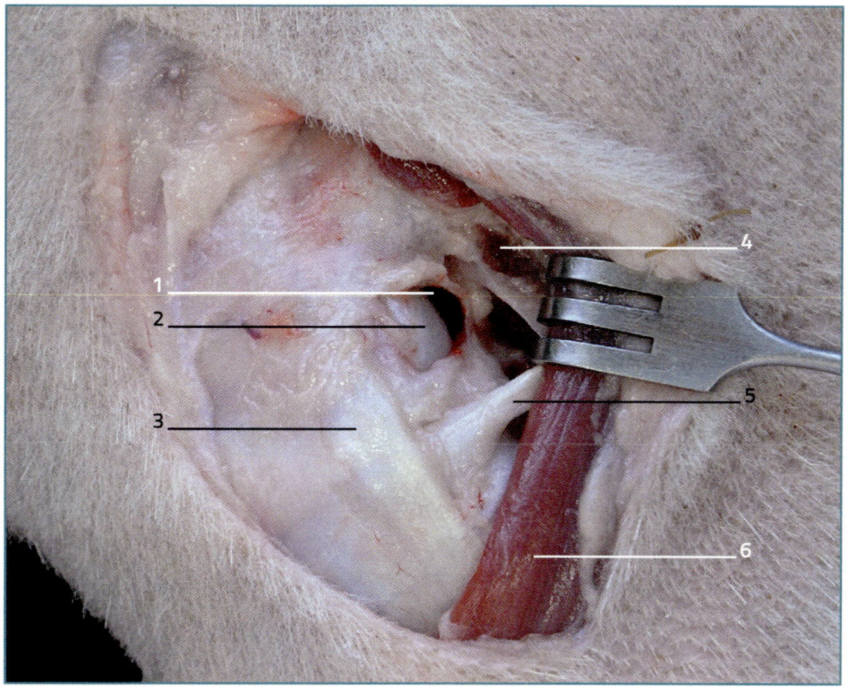

1 Joint capsule
2 Medial condyle of the femur
3 Medial collateral ligament
4 Gastrocnemius m. (medial portion)
5 Semimembranosus m. (cranial portion)
6 Sartorius m. (caudal portion)

6 In this dissection quite a bit of the joint capsule has been removed. This allows the topography of the medial meniscus and its relationship to the tendon of insertion of the caudal portion of the semimembranous muscle and the medial collateral ligament to be clearly identified.

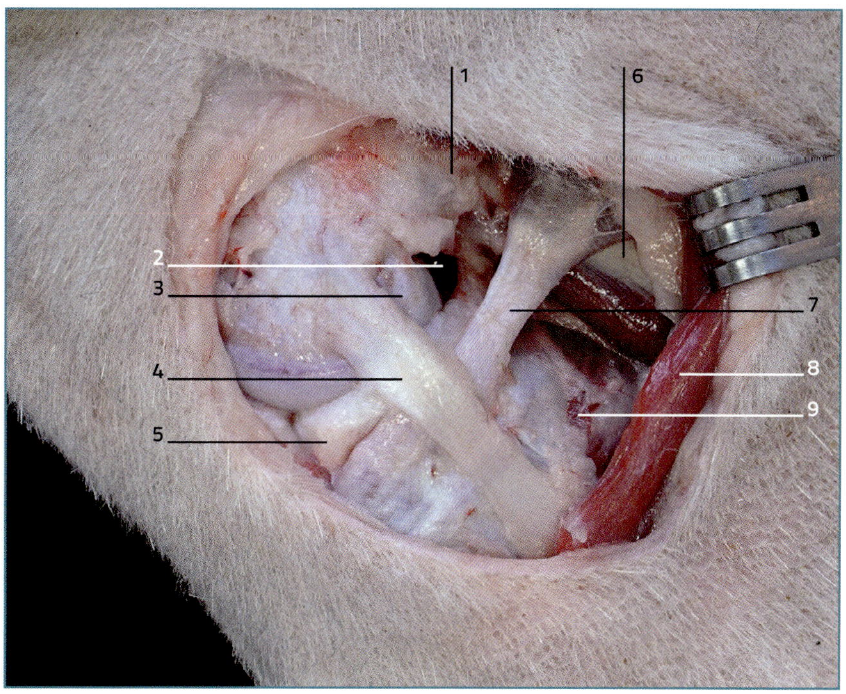

1 Semimembranosus m. (cranial portion)
2 Joint capsule
3 Medial condyle of the femur
4 Medial collateral ligament
5 Medial meniscus
6 Gastrocnemius m. (medial portion)
7 Semimembranosus m. (caudal portion)
8 Sartorius m. (caudal portion)
9 Popliteus m.

Approach to the lateral collateral ligament and caudolateral region of the stifle joint

Indications

- Diagnostic arthrotomy.
- Repair of rupture of the lateral collateral ligament.
- Detachment of the lateral head of the gastrocnemius muscle.
- Technique of fibular head transposition to treat ACL rupture.
- Examination and partial resection of the lateral meniscus.
- Open reduction and fixation of fracture of the lateral condyle of the femur.

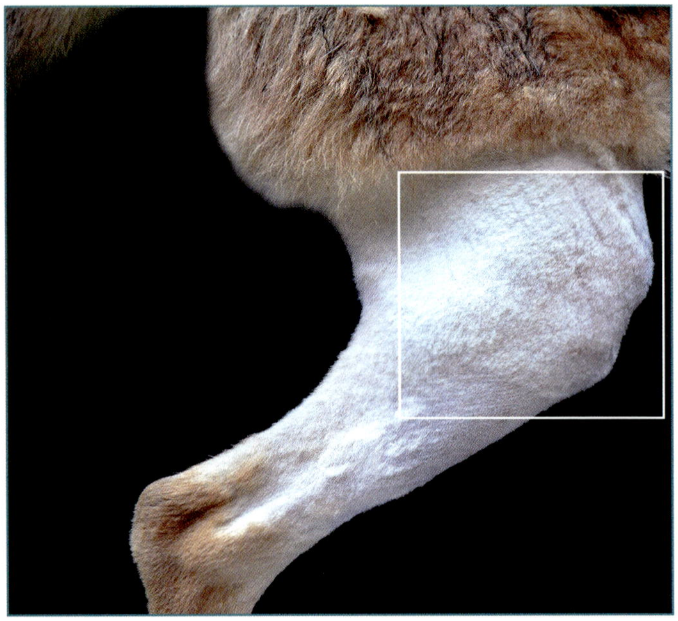

1 The approach starts with a skin incision from the lateral epicondyle of the femur towards the proximal end of the tibia and towards the distal end of the femur.

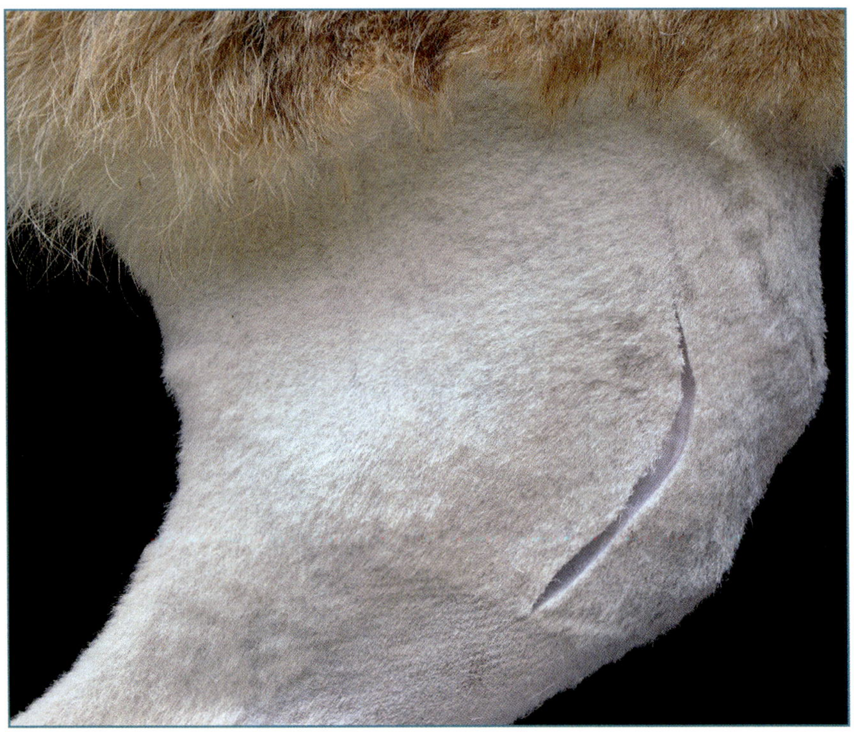

2 Once the skin has been retracted, the fascia of the stifle joint and the aponeurotic insertion of the biceps femoris muscle into this fascia are identified.

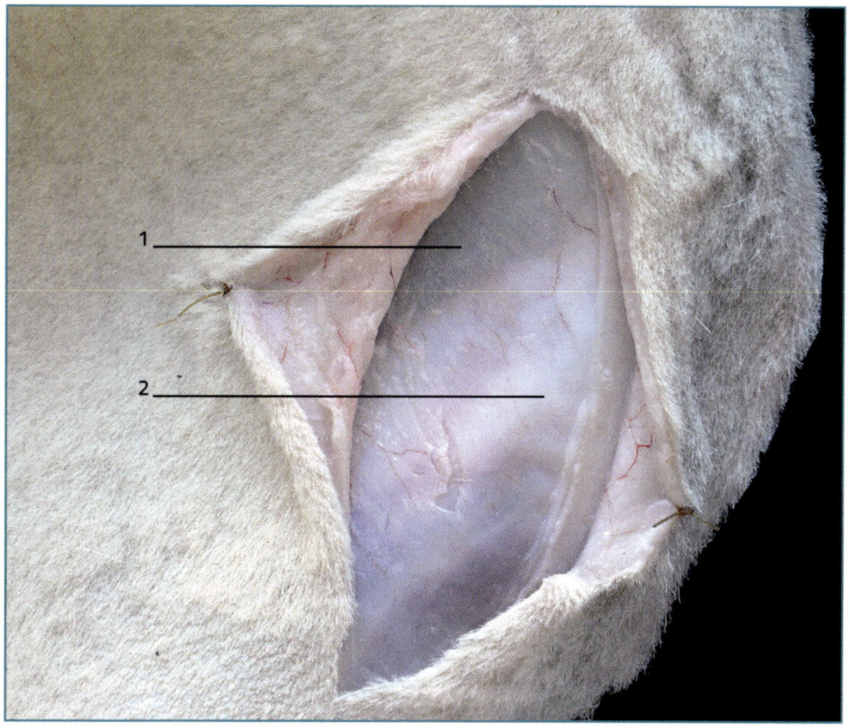

1 Biceps femoris m.
2 Fascia of the stifle joint

3 After the fascia of the stifle joint has been sectioned and the biceps femoris muscle has been moved caudally, the space between the gastrocnemius muscle (lateral head) and the lateral collateral ligament is identified. Special care must be taken not to disturb the path of the common peroneal nerve, located between the biceps femoris and gastrocnemius muscles.

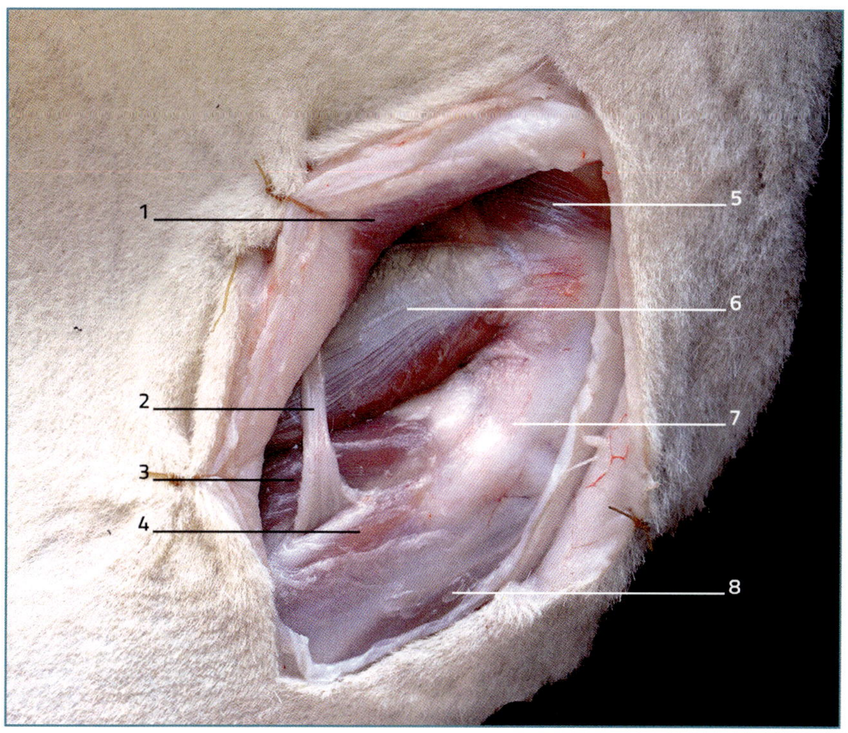

1 Biceps femoris m.
2 Common peroneal nerve
3 Lateral digital flexor m.
4 Long peroneal m.
5 Vastus lateralis m.
6 Gastrocnemius m. (lateral head)
7 Lateral collateral ligament
8 Tibialis cranialis m.

4 After the gastrocnemius muscles (lateral head) and the popliteal muscles have been delimited, the joint capsule and the lateral meniscus, covered by the tendon of origin of the popliteus muscle, are accessed.

1 Biceps femoris m.
2 Common peroneal nerve
3 Lateral digital flexor m.
4 Long peroneal m.
5 Gastrocnemius m. (lateral head)
6 Popliteus m.
7 Lateral collateral ligament
8 Lateral meniscus
9 Tendon of the long digital extensor m.
10 Tibialis cranialis m.

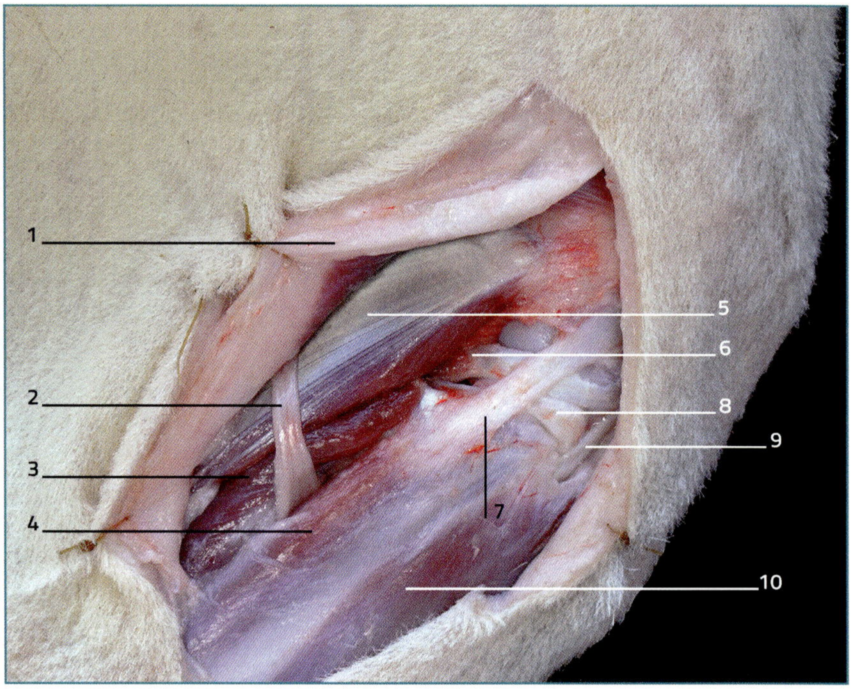

5 Forcing the tibia to rotate internally or medially relative to the femur reveals the relationship of the tendon of origin of the popliteus muscle to the eccentric edge of the lateral meniscus. In this dissection the tendon of origin of the long digital extensor muscle can be identified when the joint capsule is removed.

1 Biceps femoris m.
2 Common peroneal nerve
3 Lateral digital flexor m.
4 Long peroneal m.
5 Gastrocnemius m. (lateral head)
6 Popliteus m.
7 Lateral collateral ligament
8 Lateral meniscus
9 Tendon of the long digital extensor m.
10 Tibialis cranialis m.

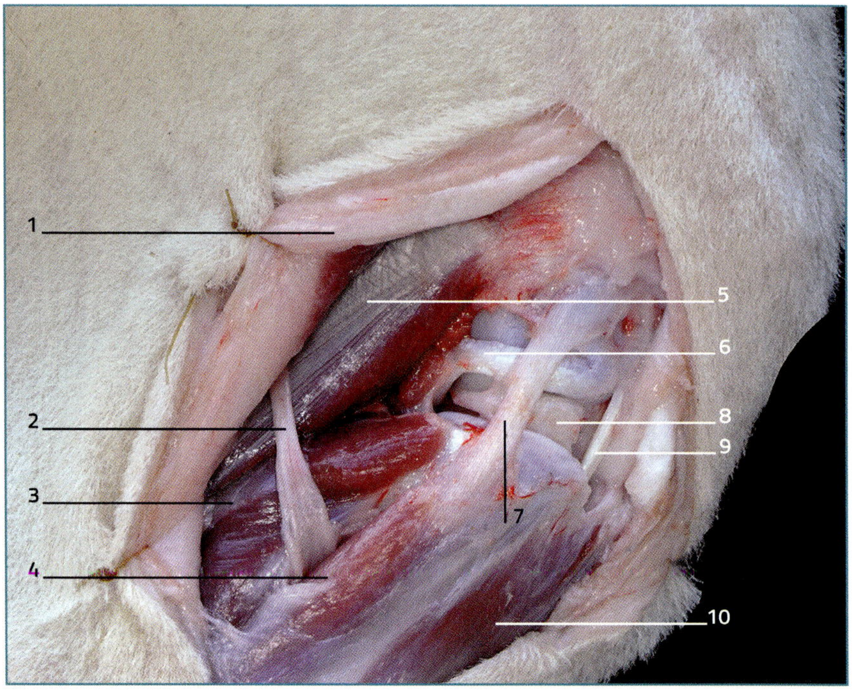

6 Forcible movement of the tendon of origin of the popliteal muscle towards the distal area, together with internal rotation of the tibia, exposes the lateral meniscus.

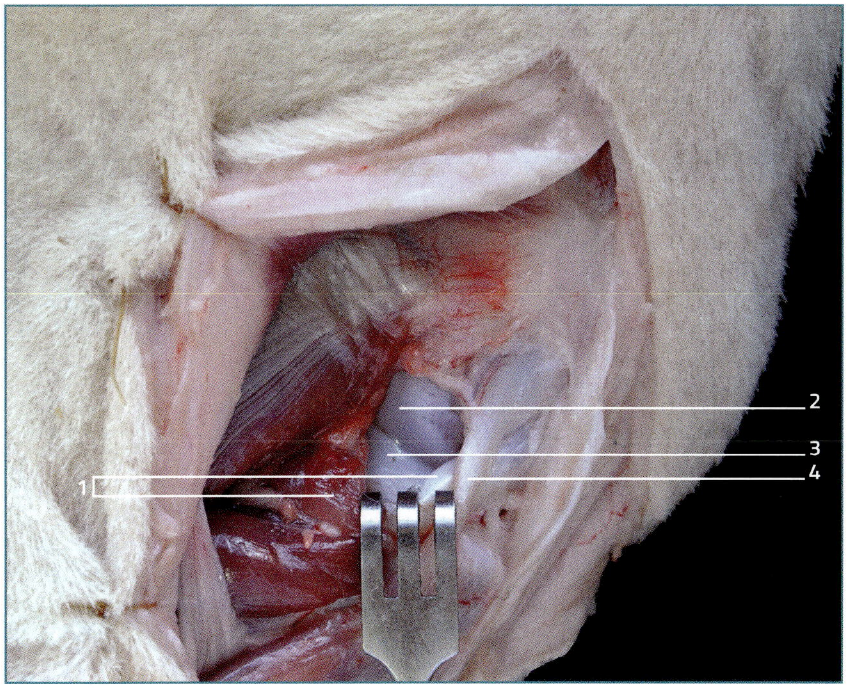

1 Popliteus m.
2 Lateral condyle of the femur
3 Lateral meniscus
4 Lateral collateral ligament

Approach to the proximal portion of the tibia through a medial incision

Indications

- Open reduction and fixation of proximal fractures of the tibia.
- Repair of rupture of the medial collateral ligament.
- TPLO technique to treat rupture of the cranial cruciate ligament.

1 The patient is placed in lateral decubitus with the contralateral limb in abduction. The skin incision extends from the distal end of the femur to the medial aspect of the tibia and passes over the medial epicondyle of the femur.

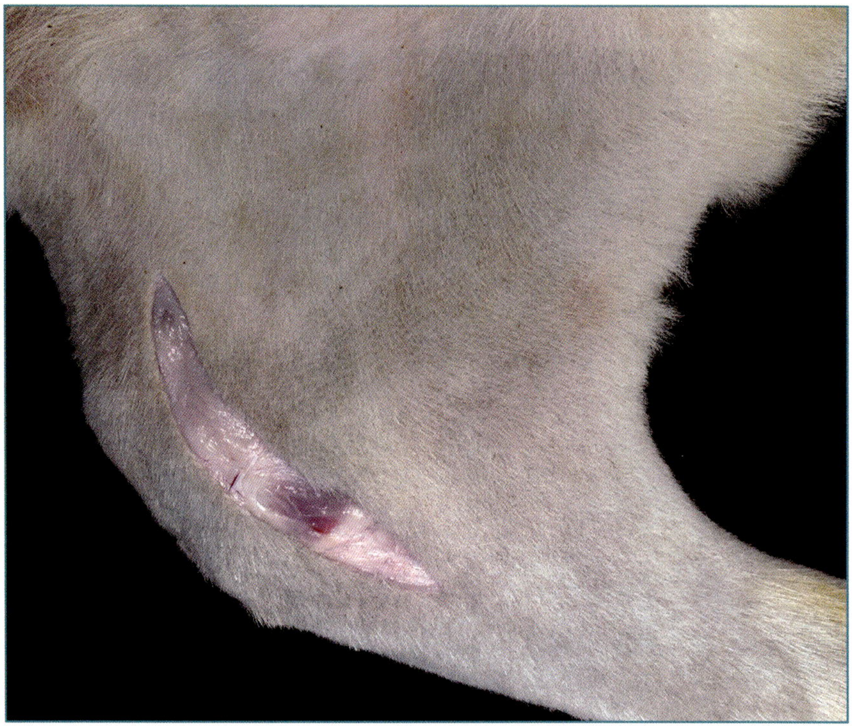

2 Once part of the fascia of the stifle joint has been dissected, the insertion of the caudal portion of the sartorius muscle, which must be sectioned, is identified. The tendon of insertion of the gracilis muscle can also be seen.

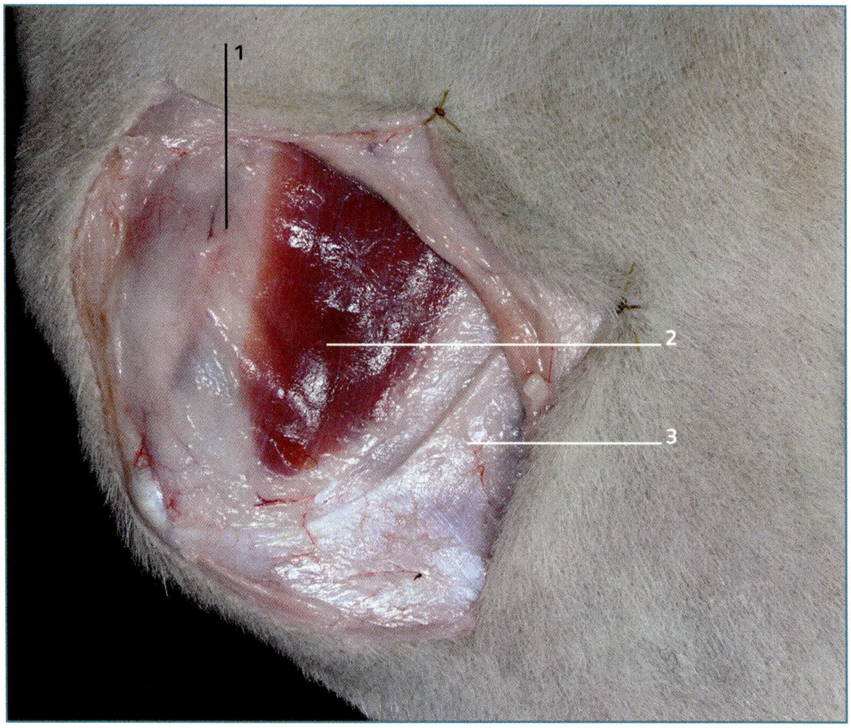

1 Descending artery and vein of the stifle joint
2 Sartorius m. (caudal portion)
3 Tendon of the gracilis m.

3 After the insertion of the caudal portion of the sartorius muscle has been sectioned, the medial collateral ligament is identified.

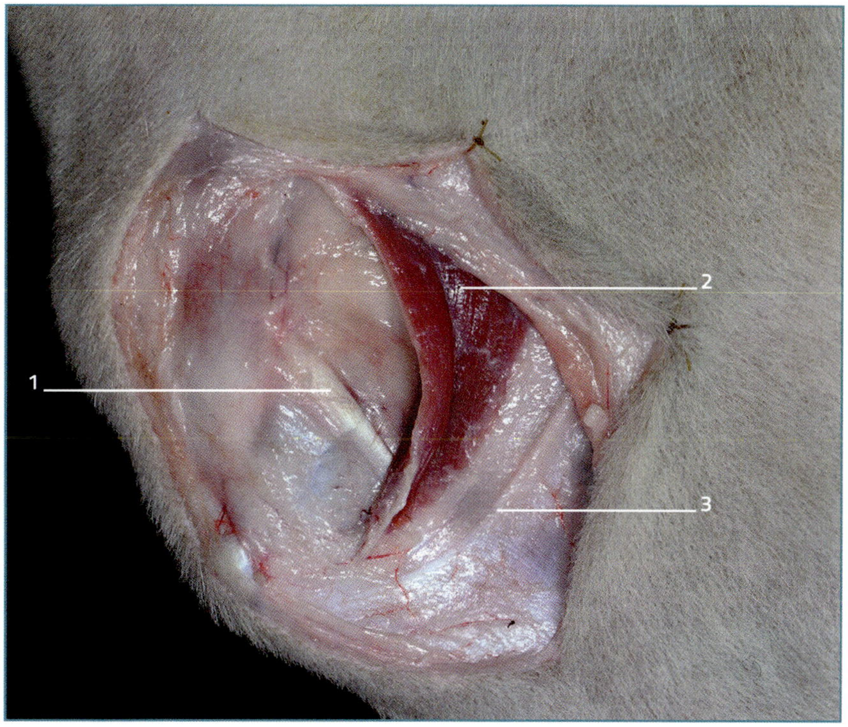

1 Medial collateral ligament
2 Sartorius m. (caudal portion)
3 Tendon of the gracilis m.

4 When the sartorius muscle is moved towards the caudal area, the insertion of the popliteus muscle is partially exposed, as is the insertion of the cranial and caudal portions of the semimembranosus muscle.

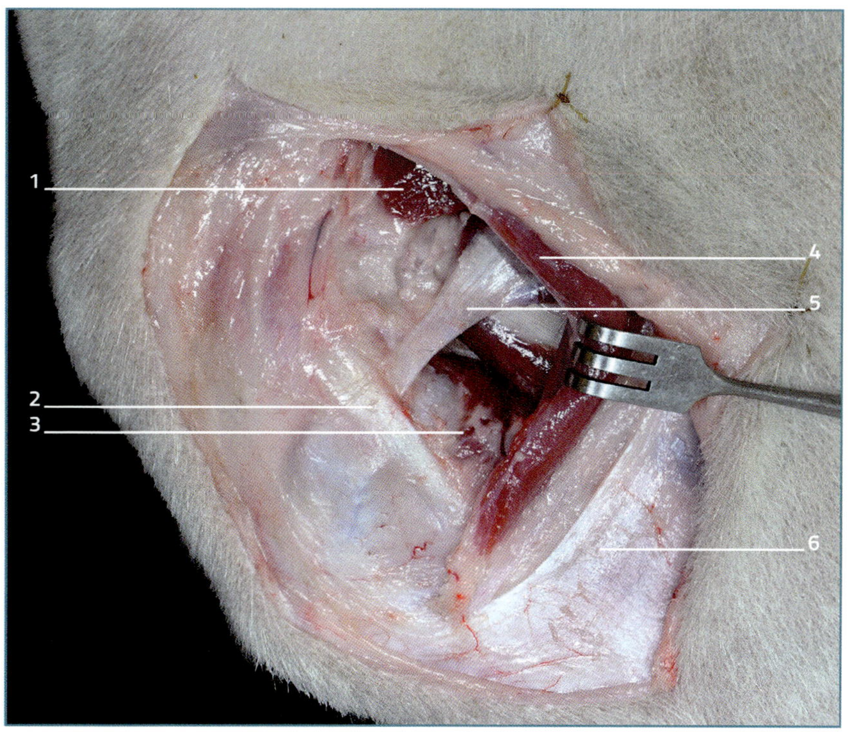

1 Semimembranosus m. (cranial portion)
2 Medial collateral ligament
3 Popliteus m.
4 Sartorius m. (caudal portion)
5 Semimembranosus m. (caudal portion)
6 Tendon of the gracilis m.

5 Caudal extension of the dissection partially exposes the insertion of the gracilis and semitendinosus muscles, which must be sectioned.

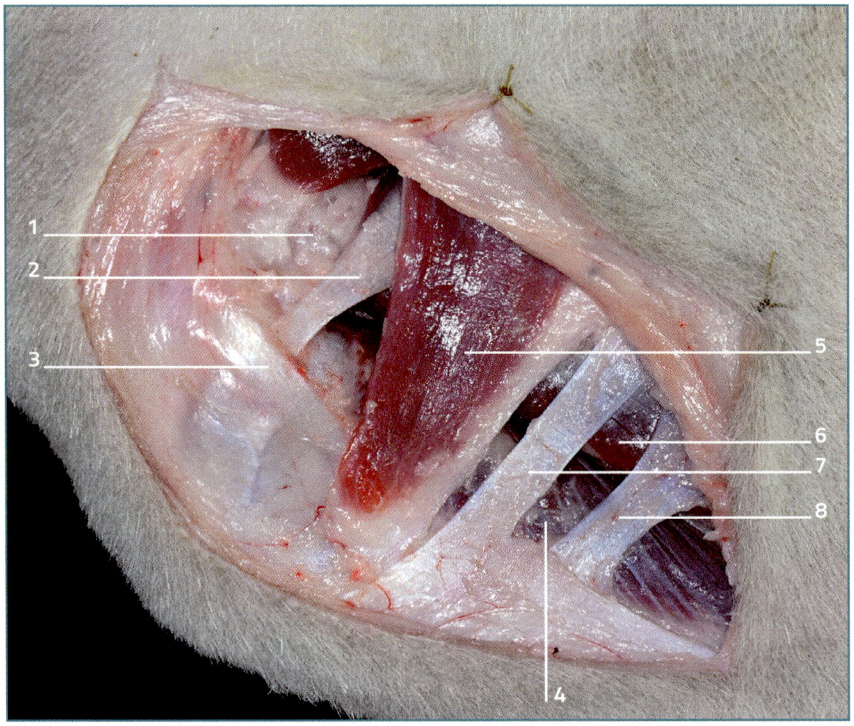

1 Semimembranosus m. (cranial portion)
2 Semimembranosus m. (caudal portion)
3 Medial collateral ligament
4 Popliteus m.
5 Sartorius m. (caudal portion)
6 Gastrocnemius m. (medial portion)
7 Tendon of the gracilis m.
8 Tendon of the semitendinosus m.

6 Once the sartorius, gracilis and semitendinosus muscles have been disinserted, the entire insertion of the popliteus muscle on the medial edge of the tibia, which must be sectioned, is exposed.

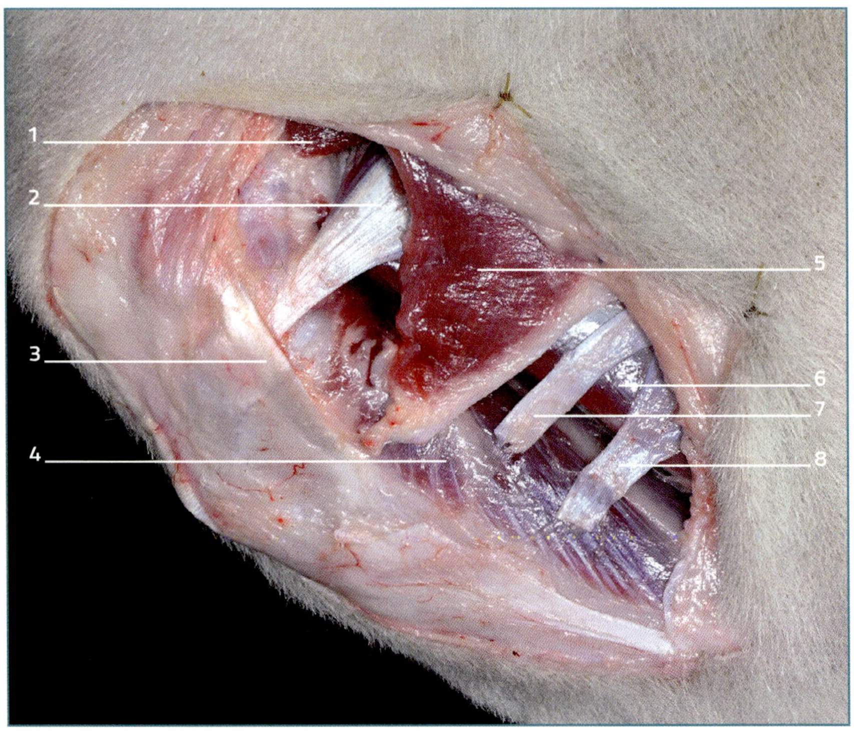

1 Semimembranosus m. (cranial portion)
2 Semimembranosus m. (caudal portion)
3 Medial collateral ligament
4 Popliteus m.
5 Sartorius m. (caudal portion)
6 Gastrocnemius m. (medial portion)
7 Tendon of the gracilis m.
8 Tendon of the semitendinosus m.

7 Disinserting the popliteus muscle exposes the medial edge and the caudal aspect of the tibia at its proximal end. Caution: the path of the popliteal artery and vein must not be disturbed.

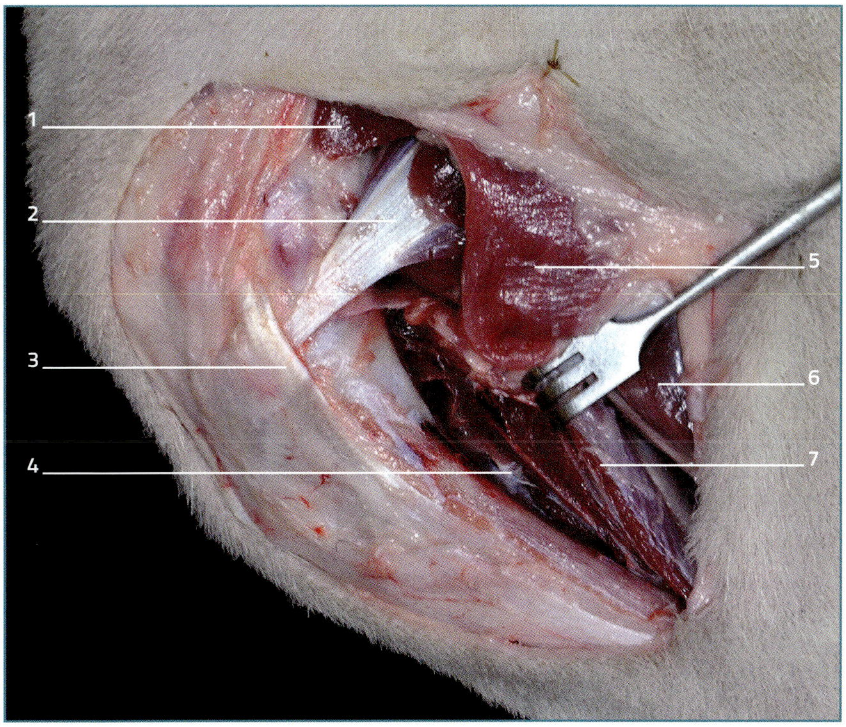

1 Semimembranosus m. (cranial portion)
2 Semimembranosus m. (caudal portion)
3 Medial collateral ligament
4 Popliteal artery and vein
5 Sartorius m. (caudal portion)
6 Gastrocnemius m. (medial portion)
7 Popliteus m.

8 The fascia of the leg, which must be sectioned parallel to the tibial tuberosity, is identified in a cranial view.

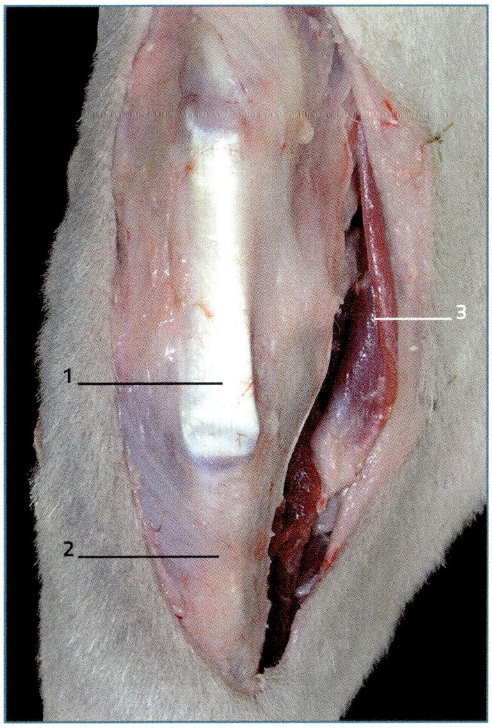

1 Patellar ligament
2 Tibial tuberosity
3 Sartorius m. (caudal portion)

9 Once the fascia has been moved laterally, the attachment of the tibialis cranialis muscle to the tibial tuberosity, which must be sectioned, is identified.

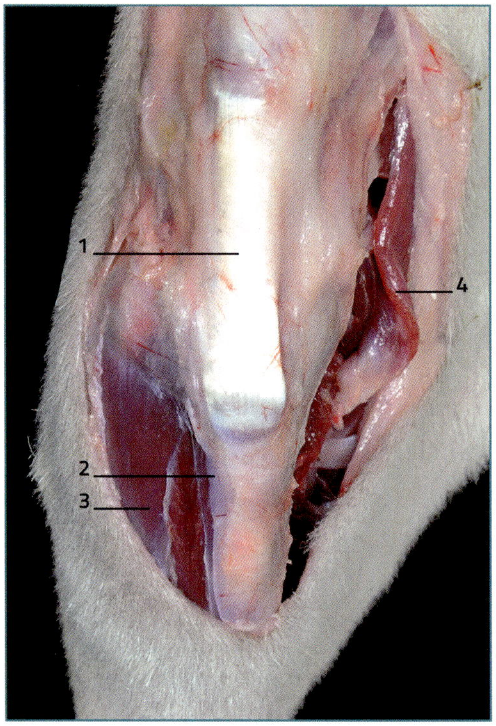

1 Patellar ligament
2 Tibial tuberosity
3 Tibialis cranialis m.
4 Sartorius m. (caudal portion)

10 The lateral muscles of the leg are moved laterally to completely expose the lateral aspect of the tibia. Caution: the path of the tendon of origin of the long digital extensor muscle must not be disturbed.

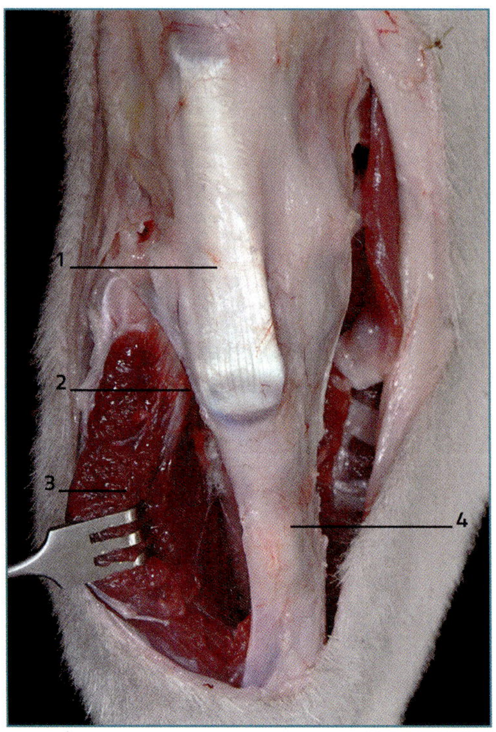

1 Patellar ligament
2 Tendon of origin of the long digital extensor m.
3 Tibialis cranialis m.
4 Tibial tuberosity

BIBLIOGRAPHY

AIKEN, S.W. KASS, P.H., TOOMBS, J.P. Intercondylar notch width in dogs with and without cranial cruciate ligament injuries. *Vet Comp Orthop Traumatol*, 1995; 8:128-132.

ARAGON, C.L., BUDSBERG, S.C. Applications of evidence-based medicine: Cranial cruciate ligament injury repair in the dog. *Vet Surg*, 2005; 34:93-98.

ARNOCZKY, S.P. Surgery of the stifle. The cruciate ligaments (Part I). *Comp Cont Educ*, 1980; 11:106.

ARNOCZKY, S.P., TARVIN, G.B., MARSHALL, J.L., *et al*. Over-the-top procedure. Technique for anterior cruciate ligament substitution in the dog. *J Am Anim Hosp Assoc*, 1979; 15:283-290.

ARON, D.N., SELCER, B.A., SMITH, J.D. Autogenous tensor fascia lata graft replacement of the patellar ligament in a dog. *Vet comp Orthop Traumatol*, 1997; 10:141-145.

BANWELL, M.N., HOSGOOD, G., KERWIN, S.C., *et al*. In vitro evaluation of fluorocarbon leader line for use as a fabella-tibial suture. *Vet Comp Orthop Traumatol*, 2004; 17:35-40.

BAR-AM, Y., KLEMENT, E., FOURMAN, V., *et al*. Mechanical evaluation of two loop-fastening methods for stainless steel wire. *Vet Comp Orthop Traumatol*, 2004; 17:241-246.

BENNETT, D., CAMPBELL, J.R. Unusual soft tissue orthopaedic problems in the dog. *J Small Anim Prat*, 1979; 20:27-39.

BONNEAU, N.H., BRETON, L. Avulsion fracture of the origin of the extensor digitorum longus muscle in two Great Dane dogs. *J Vet Orthop*, 1984; 3:15-20.

BRINKER, W.O., OLMSTEAD, M.L., SUMNER-SMITH, G., PRIEUR, W.D. *Manual of internal fixation in small animals,* second revised edition. Springer-Verlag Berlin Heidelberg, 1998.

BRUNNBERG, L., DÜRR, E., KNOSPE, C. Zu den verletzungen del Patella und Ligamentum patellae bei Hund und Katze I. Patellafraktur. *Kleintierpraxis*, 1991; 36:547-559.

BRUNNBERG, L., DÜRR, E., KNOSPE, C. Zu den verletzungen del Patella und Ligamentum patellae bei Hund und Katze II. Ruptur des Ligamentum patellae. *Kleintierpraxis*, 1992; 37:179-182.

CHAUVET, A.E., JOHNSON, A.L., PIJANOWSKI, G.J., *et al*. Evaluation of fibular head transposition, lateral fabellar suture, and conservative treatment of cranial cruciate ligament rupture in large dogs: a retrospective study. *J Am Anim Hosp Assoc*, 1996; 32:247-255.

CLIMENT, S., *et al. Manual de anatomía y embriología de los animales domésticos*. Conceptos básicos y datos aplicativos. Miembro torácico y miembro pelviano. Sistema circulatorio. Esqueleto de la cabeza. Ed. Acribia, 2004.

CLIMENT, S., LATORRE, R., KÖSTLIN, R., VÉREZ-FRAGUELA, J.L., SÁNCHEZ-MARGALLO, F., SÁNCHEZ, J., CELDRÁN, D. *3D Joint anatomy in dogs. Main joint pathologies and surgical approaches*. Servet editorial - Grupo Asís Biomedia S.L., 2014.

DAMUR, D., TEPIC, S., MONTAVON, P.M. Proximal tibial osteotomy for the repair of cranial cruciate-deficient stifle joints in dogs. *Vet Comp Orthop Traumatol*, 2003; 4:211-216.

DE ROOSTER, H., DE BRUIN, T., VAN BREE, H. Morphologic and functional features of the canine cruciate ligaments. *Vet Surg*, 2006; 35:769-780.

DICKINSON, C.R., NUNAMAKER, D.M. Repair of ruptured anterior cruciate ligamen in the dog: experience of 101 cases, using a modified fascia strip technique. *J Am Vet Med Assoc*, 1977; 170:827-830.

DRAPE, J., GHITALLA, S., AUTEFAGE, A. Lèsions mèniscales et rupture du ligament croisè antèrieur: ètude rètrospective de 400 cas. *Le Point Vétérinaire*, 1990; 22:39-45.

DRAPE, J., GHITALLA, S., AUTEFAGE, A. Rupture du ligament croisè antèrieur (LCA) chez le chien: pathologie traumatique ou dègènèrative. *Le Point Vétérinaire*, 1990; 22:57-64.

DRAPE, J., GHITALLA, S., AUTEFAGE, A. Traitement chirurgical de la rupture du ligament croisè antèrieur (LCA) chez le chien par la mèthode “over the top” modifièe. *Le Point Vétérinaire*, 1990; 22:11-19.

DUVAL, J.M., BUDSBERG, S.C., FLO, G.L., *et al*. Breed, sex, and body weight as risk factors for rupture of the cranial cruciate ligament in young dogs. *J Am Vet Med Assoc*, 1999; 215:811-814.

ENDRES, B. Luxatio patellae congenita des Hundes. *Vet Med Diss*, München, 1977.

ENGELKE, A., MEYER-LINDENBERG, A., NOLTE, I. Die Ultraschalluntersuchung des inneren Kniegelenkes bei Hunden mit Kreuzbandriss. *Dtsch Tierärztl Wschr*, 1997; 104:114-117.

EVANS, H.E. *Miller's Anatomy of the Dog*, 3ª ed. WB Saunders, Philadelphia, 1993.

FRANCH, J., LÓPEZ, C. *Atlas de abordajes quirúrgicos en traumatología de pequeños animales*. Temis Pharma, S.L., 1999.

FRITZ, R.M. Zur Luxatio patellar des Hundes, klinisches und röntgenologisches Spätergebnis nach. Transposition der tuberositas tibiae und/oder vertiefung der Trochlea Ossis Femoris. *Vet Med Diss*, München, 1989.

GEYER, H. Die Behandlung der Kreuzbandrisse beim Hund: Vergleichende Untersuchungen. Vetsuisse Faculty, University of Zurich, Zurich, Switzerland, 1966.

GUERRERO, T., MONTAVON, P.M. Advancement of the tibial tuberosity of cranial cruciate-deficient canine stifle. Video production: University of Zurich, 2003.

HAGEN, B. Untersuchungen zur apophysenfugenlösung und anderen Ossinfikationsstö-rungen im berich der tuberositas tibiae beim wachsenden Bullterrier. *Vet Med Diss*, München, 1991.

HAYASHI, K., MANLEY, P.A., MUIR, P. Cranial cruciate ligament pathophysiology in dogs with cruciate disease: A review. *J Am Anim Hosp Assoc*, 2004; 40:385-390.

HENDERSON, R.A, MILTON, J.L. The tibial compression mechanism: a diagnostic aid in stifle injuries. *J Am Anim Hosp Assoc*, 1978; 14:474-479.

HOFFMANN, D.E., MILLER, J.M., OBER, C.P., *et al*. Tibial tuberosity advancement in 65 canine stifles. *Vet Comp Orthop Traumatol*, 2006; 19:219-227.

http://leibinger-medical.com/en/products/veterinary/tta-rapid/tta-rapid/

https://www.youtube.com/watch?v=xq6JuEiG7HE

https://www.researchgate.net/publication/267103122_TTA_Rapid_Description_of_the_Technique_and_Short_Term_Clinical_Trial_Results_of_the_First_50_Cases_TTA_Rapid_Surgical_Technique_and_Initial_Outcomes

HULSE, D.A., SHIRES, P., ABDELBAKI, Y.Z., HUGH-JONES, M., KEARNEY, M.T. Vascular acess channeling to increase meniscal regeneration in the dog. *Vet Surg*, 1986; 15:414-419.

INTERNATIONAL COMMITTEE ON VETERINARY GROSS ANATOMICAL NOMENCLATURE. *Nomina Anatomica Veterinaria*. Fifth edition (revised version). Authorized by the General Assembly of the World Association of Veterinary Anatomists (WAVA). Published by the Editorial Committee Hannover (Germany), Columbia, MO (USA.), Ghent (Belgium), Sapporo (Japan), 2012.

JAGER, M., WIRTH, C.J. *Praxis der Orthopädie*. Georg Thieme Verlag, Stuttgart-New York, 1986.

JERRAM, R.M., WALKER, A.M., WARMAN, C.G. Proximal tibial intraarticular ostectomy for treatment of canine cranial cruciate ligament injury. *Vet Surg*, 2005; 34:196-205.

KIM, S.E., POZZI, A., KOWALESKI, M.P., *et al*. Tibial osteotomies for cranial cruciate ligament insufficiency in dogs. *Vet Surg*, 2008; 37:111-125.

KOESTLIN, R. Cirugía articular. I Congreso Internacional de la SETOV, Proceeding textbook 90, Cáceres, 2009.

KORVICK, D.L., JOHNSON, A.L., SCHAEFFER, D.J. Surgeons' preferences in treating cranial cruciate ligament ruptures in dogs. *J Am Vet Med Assoc*, 1994; 205:1318.

LAFAVER, S., MILLER, N.A., STUBBS, W.P., *et al*. Tibial tuberosity advancement for stabilization of the canine cranial cruciate ligament-deficient stifle joint: surgical technique, early results, and complications in 101 dogs. *Vet Surg*, 2007; 36:573-586.

LAMPMAN, T.J., LUND, E.M., LIPOWITZ, A.J. Cranial cruciate disease: current status of diagnosis, surgery, and risk for disease. *Vet Comp Orthop Traumatol*, 2003; 16:122-126.

LATORRE, R., GIL, F., CLIMENT, S., LÓPEZ, O., HENRY, R., AYALA, M., RAMÍREZ, G., MARTÍNEZ, F., VÁZQUEZ, J.M. *Color atlas of surgical approaches to the bones and joints of the dog and cat*. Intermedica S.A., 2009.

Matis, U. Zur Drahtzuggurtung distaler epiphysiolysen bzw. suprakondylärer Frakturen des femurs bei Katze und Hund. *Bert Münch Tierärztl Wschr*, 1977; 90:240-243.

Matis, U., Köstlin, R. Zur Kreuzbandruptur bei der Katze. *Prak Teirarzt*, 1978; 59:585.

Moores, A.P., Beck, A.L., Jespers, K.J.M., *et al*. Mechanical evaluation of two crimp clamp systems for extracapsular stabilization of the cranial cruciate ligament-deficient canine stifle. *Vet Surg*, 2006; 35:470-475.

Mullen, H.S., Matthiesen, D.T. Complications of transposition of the fibular head for stabilisation of the cranial cruciate-deficient stifle in dog: 80 cases (1982-1986). *J Am Vet Med Assoc,* 1989; 195:1267-1271.

Newton C.D., Nunamaker, D.M. *Textbook of small animal orthopaedics*. JB Lippincott Company, Philadelphia, 1985.

Patterson, R.H., Smith, G.K., Gregor, T.P., Newton, C.D. Biomechanical stability of four cranial cruciate ligament repair techniques in the dog. *Vet Surg*, 1991; 20:85-90.

Piermattei, D.L., Flo, G.L. *Handbook of small animal orthopedics and fracture treatment*, third edition. WB Saunders Company, Philadelphia, 1997.

Piermattei, D.L., Johnson, K.A. *An atlas of surgical approaches to the bones and joints of the dog and cat*, fourth edion. Elsevier Inc, New York, 2006.

Pond, M.J. Avulsion of the extensor digitorum longus muscle in the dog: A report of four cases. *J Small Anim Pract*, 1973; 14:785-796.

Read, R.A., Robins, G.M. Deformity of the proximal tibia in dogs. *Vet Rec*, 1982; 111:295-298.

Salter, R.B., Harris, W.R. Injuries involving the epiphyseal plate. *Journal of Bone & Joint Surg*, 1963; 45-A:587.

Sandoval, J. *Tratado de anatomía veterinaria*, 3ª ed. Tomo II: Aparato locomotor. Imprenta Sorles, León, 1998.

Schäfer, H.-J. Vergleichende Untersuchung zur chirurgischen Behandlung des vorderen Kreuzbandrissies beim Hund mit der “modifizierten Over-the-Top” und der “Fibulakopfversetzungstechnik”. *Vet Med Diss*, Hannover, 1991.

Schäfer, H.-J., Köstlin, R.G., Nolte, I. Zwei Methoden für die Kreuzban-operation im vergleich: Die Over-the-Top und die fibulakopfversetzungstechnik. *Kleintierpraxis*, 1991; 36:683.

Schaller, O. *Nomenclatura anatómica veterinaria ilustrada*. Ed. Acribia, Zaragoza, 1992.

Schebitz, H., Brass, W. (Hrsg). *Operationen an Hund und Katze*. Verlag Paul Parey, 1985.

Schmökel, H.G., Montavon, P.M. Versetzung der tuberositas tibiae mit einer Kranialisation bei der Patellaluxation beim Hund. *Kleintierpraxis*, 1993; 38:805-808.

Selmi, A.L., Padilha, J.G. Rupture of the cranial cruciate ligament associated with deformity of the proximal tibia in five dogs. *J Small Anim Pract*, 2001; 42(8):390-393.

Singleton, W.B. The surgical correction of the stifle deformities in the dog. *J Small Anim Pract*, 1969; 10:59-69.

Slocum, B., Devine, T. Cranial tibial wedge osteotomy: a technique for eliminating cranial tibial thrust in cranial cruciate ligament repair. *J Am Vet Med Assoc*, 1984; 184:564-569.

Slocum, B., Devine, T. Trochlear recession for correction of luxating patella in the dog. *J Am Vet Med Assoc*, 1985; 186(4):365-369.

Slocum, B., Slocum, D.B., Devine T., Boone, E. Wedge recession for treatment of recurrent luxation of the patella. A preliminary report. *Clin Orthop Relat Res*, 1982; 164:48-53.

Slocum, B., Slocum, T.D. Tibial plateau leveling osteotomy for repair of cranial cruciate ligament rupture in the canine. *Vet Clin North Am Small Anim Pract*, 1993; 23(4):777-795.

Smith, G.K., Torg, J.S. Fibular head transposition for repair of cruciate-deficient stifle in the dog. *J Am Vet Med Assoc*, 1985; 187:375-383.

SOLER, M., MURCIANO, J., LATORRE, R., BELDA, E., RODRÍGUEZ, M.J., AGUT, A. Ultrasonographic, computed tomographic and magnetic resonance imaging anatomy of the normal canine stifle joint. *Vet J*, 2007; 174(2):351-361.

STONE, E.A., BETTS, C.W., RUDY, R.L. Folding of the caudal horn of the medial meniscus secondary to severence of the cranial cruciate ligament. *Vet Surg*, 1980; 9:121-124.

VASSEUR, P.B. Stifle joint. In: Slatter, D. (ed). *Textbook of Small Animal Surgery*, third edition, vol. 2. Philadelphia, Saunders, 2003; pp. 2090-2116.

VASSEUR, P.B., JOHNSON, A.L., BUDSBERG, S.C., *et al*. Randomized, controlled trial of the efficacy of carprofen, a nonsteroidal anti-inflammatory drug, in the treatment of ostearthritis in dogs. *J Am Vet Med Assoc*, 1995; 206(6):807-811.

VÉREZ-FRAGUELA, J.L. Reparación de la rotura del ligamento cruzado anterior mediante osteotomía niveladora de la meseta tibial. *Consulta Difus Vet*, 2001; 83(9):77-90.

VOLLMERHAUS, B., SCHEBITZ, H., ROOS, H. Über die Entwicklung der Insertio ligamenti patellae beim wachsenden Hund. *Berl Münch Tierärztl Wschr*, 1981; 94:255-259.

VOSS, K., DAMUR, D.M., GUERRERO, T., *et al*. Force plate gait analysis to assess limb function after tibial tuberosity advancement in dogs with cranial cruciate ligament disease. *Vet Comp Orthop Traumatol*, 2008; 21:243-249.

WESTHUES, M. Die Operation bei Zerreibug der Ligamenta decussata im Kniegelenk des Hundes und der Katze. In: Berge, E., Westhues, M. (eds.). *Tierärztlichen Operationslehre*. 29 Auflage, S 365, Paul Parey Verlag, 1969.

WHITEHAIR, J.G., VASSEUR, P.B., WILLITS, N.H. Epidemiology of cranial cruciate ligament rupture in dogs. *J Am Vet Med Assoc*, 1993; 203:1016-1019.

ZAERA, J.P. Comparación de la técnica en cuña y la trocleoplastia con y sin ácido hialurónico en el tratamiento de la luxación rotuliana en el perro; estudio experimental. Tesis Doctoral, Universidad Complutense de Madrid, 1993.

ZAHM, H. Die Ligamenta decussata im gesunden und arthrotischen Kniegelenk des Hundes. *Vet Med Diss*, München, 1964.

Published by Servet editorial - Grupo Asís Biomedia S.L.